STRESS AND THE
PERCEPTION OF CONTROL

STRESS AND THE PERCEPTION OF CONTROL

S. Fisher
Department of Psychology
University of Dundee

LAWRENCE ERLBAUM ASSOCIATES, PUBLISHERS
London   Hillsdale, New Jersey

Lawrence Erlbaum Associates, Ltd., Publishers
Chancery House
319 City Road
London EC1V 1LJ

British Library Cataloguing in Publication Data

Fisher, Shirley
    Stress and the perception of control.
    1. Stress (Psychology).   2. Stress
    (Physiology)
    I. Title
    616.8   BF575.S75

ISBN 0–86377–006–1

Printed in Great Britain by A. Wheaton & Co. Ltd., Exeter.

To Reginald William Pittman

Acknowledgments

I would like to acknowledge the hospitality provided by the Faculty of Psychology, Rice University, Houston, Texas, during part of the period when I was writing this book. I was grateful for the provision of facilities and the opportunity for research discussions as well as for the enthusiasm and interest shown.

I would especially like to thank Dr. D. E. Broadbent and Professor J. Reason for reading selective aspects of earlier drafts of this book and for providing many detailed and helpful comments. I would like to thank Dr. E. C. Poulton for encouragement given for some of the experiments reported in this book and for the provision of helpful comments in this respect. Mr. A. Flook and Dr. N. Loveless read and provided comments on very early draft chapters during formative periods in the preparation of the book, and I am grateful for the help they provided, especially in keeping me aware of the contributions of Social Psychology and Psychophysiology, respectively. My thanks are also due to Dr. M. Doward for many helpful discussions and for constant reminders of the importance of psychological factors in illness encountered in general practice.

I owe a debt of gratitude to the typists who tackled the task of converting my written drafts into typed chapters. In particular I would like to thank Mrs. Margaret Greatorex, Mrs. Margaret Grubb, Mrs. Aileen Sandilands, and Mrs. Marilyn Laird.

Diagrams and graphs were prepared by the Medical Illustrations Department, Ninewells Hospital. Photographic work was undertaken by the Photographic Department in the University of Dundee. I would like to thank all those concerned.

Finally, I am grateful to Mrs. Mair Rowan for the help provided with checking the details of the bibliography and particularly for the care taken in this respect. Mrs. Patricia McKillop provided help with the indexing of authors and subjects. An excellent editing service was provided by Communication Crafts, East Grinstead.

Contents

List of Tables

Introduction

STRESS: A PLAYGROUND FOR IDEAS

Within the last thirty years there has been much research on the problem of stress. The research literature is now both diverse and daunting, and adequate accounts of the diversity can really only be provided by means of edited readings. However, there is a very good case for arguing that individuals must, from time to time, attempt to make some sense of it and to provide a theoretical framework. It is inevitable that such attempts will result in selectivity. In order to pursue a theme or argument, some elements of the research literature will be seen as central; others will be seen as less important. It is inevitable, therefore, that books on stress will be controversial; but this can be all to the good in stimulating debate and research.

Stress is interesting not merely because it provides applied problems. Stress is theoretically fascinating. It is a playground for ideas in which some of the important theoretical debates in modern psychology feature strongly. At least one major problem is the level of explanation for changes in behavior in stress. There has been a recent tendency to concentrate on changes in arousal associated with stress; this has dominated the experimental literature, especially in the area of environmental stress. However, of equal importance are the mental processes associated with identifying situations as threatening, deciding on courses of action, evaluating success, and so forth. Despite major contributions by those who take a broader approach and include "life stresses" and symbolic stresses, there has been rather little attempt to draw on this evidence in trying to understand how behavior is affected. Yet, it would be reasonable to assume that being preoccupied with a problem posed by a potentially threatening situation reduces the available capacity for processing other information. Much of the influence imposed by life stresses may require a great deal of cognitive activity and may take place in prospect or in retrospect. One of the main concerns of this book is to develop the notion that stresses are dependent on and impose considerable demand on mental resources.

THE PROBLEM OF DEFINITION

The diversity of the topic of stress is reflected in the difficulty of finding an adequate definition and is evident in the diversity of stressful conditions such as pain, heat, loss of sleep, moving house, getting divorced, isolation, public speaking. In the case of uncomfortable environments, what is stressful could be seen as an extreme level of what is tolerable normally. In this sense stress is just an intense level of everyday experience. Stresses such as noise, heat, pain stimuli could thus be given definition in terms of extreme levels of the independent variable.

By contrast, more complex stresses seem to depend on interpretation and meaning. These stresses depend for existence on "internal directives" such as ambition, intention, perception of personal capability. Not only are stresses such as taking an examination or public speaking best understood in these terms, but even in cases where actual danger is involved there appears to be strong influence of internal directives. Interest in danger sports such as parachuting and hang gliding is testament to the importance of interpretation: One man's stress may be another man's challenge. Moreover, the pleasure obtained may not necessarily be relief from overcoming the danger and responding to a challenge; the apparent enjoyment produced for some people by roller-coaster rides, where skill and challenge is minimum, indicates that the experience itself is capable of different interpretations.

The "independent variable" definition of stress is inadequate in that it fails to provide an effective common denominator of sufficient generality to encompass the wide range of experiences considered stressful.

One solution would be to adopt an operational definition. Thus, stress could be defined as "any condition that causes a stress response." The further difficulty of individual differences in stress response could be overcome on the assumption that stress is "any condition in which the majority of people react by giving a stress response." Thus, pain would on these considerations be considered as stress.

However, the difficulty is to decide on a criterion. One obvious criterion is bodily alarm, associated with high muscle tension and high autonomic arousal: but "happy" mood states may also be associated with high arousal. Although recent research has emphasized specific features in the patterning of arousal in relation to external conditions or mood states, it is still not clear that we can distinguish the nature of the independent variable in terms of the physiological state with which it is asssociated. A theoretical approach developed in Chapter 5 is that the pattern of physiological state may actually reflect decisions about control. We review evidence supporting the idea that adrenaline is likely to be associated with loss of control and noradrenaline with an assessment suggesting that control is possible. Thus, the features of the physiological state may reflect the outcome of specific decisions. This creates difficulties for the use of physiological criteria in defining the existence of stress.

In any case, an operational definition of the existence of stress is made more difficult by fractionation of the relationship between arousal and performance. It is now well established that arousal and performance features are likely to be related in the form of an inverted "U" curve, even if some of the assumptions on which this hypothesis is founded are sometimes challenged. In the early stages of arousal, performance will improve; in later stages, it will deteriorate. This assumption subsumed under the Yerkes–Dodson Law (Yerkes & Dodson, 1908) means that for different levels of arousal the impression given by performance features will be different.

A COGNITIVE APPROACH TO THE PROBLEM OF STRESS AND BEHAVIOR

The problem of definition cannot easily be divorced from problems of approach to the study of behavior in stress. If stress is only partly "out there" and partly determined by directives within the individual, then an approach centered exclusively on stimulus-response concepts would be ignoring fundamental factors. Stress research poses problems for a cognitive science because even attempting to define its existence requires understanding of the acquisition and utilization of knowledge.

The "top-down"/"bottom-up" dichotomy is only of superficial significance in the understanding of the effects of stress. A "top-down" approach could be defined as one in which threat is determined by psychological processes; by restructuring the problem cognitively, the stress is alleviated. A "bottom-up" approach could be defined as one in which the stress is "out there," and action is required to put the situation right and restore equilibrium. The former might suggest concentration on processes such as denial, repression, redefinition. The latter might suggest concentration on forms of behavior or "doing." Effective action depends, however, on a number of processes that depend in turn on knowledge and its utilization: "Doing" is as much "top-down" in orientation as cognitive restructuring and is a legitimate topic for cognitive science.

The approach taken in this book is that stress and its relationship with behavior and with mental disorder must be understood in terms of fundamental aspects of cognition. A central theme is that a person seeks to establish control over his environment, but the occurrence of stressful circumstances generally involves changes in the level of control. Precisely because stressful conditions are undesirable, a person will seek to control them as part of homeostasis, in order to minimize unpleasantries experienced. Both behavior and physiological response form an integral part of the attempt to minimize the duration and intensity of stress. Failure of control maximizes the effects of these conditions and provides knowledge in which failure to cope is represented. Both aspects of control loss may influence subsequent reactions.

A major theme throughout this book is that stresses impose great "mental demand" on a person. As part of the attempt to establish control and minimize the risk of unpleasantries, he must recognize impending situations and organize his resources for effective action. Miller, Galanter, and Pribram (1960) were the first to emphasize the view of performance as being designed with consequence in mind, and organized hierarchically to resolve discrepancies between ambition and reality. A person needs a mental representation of reality and of his ambition, in order to select appropriate action. This formulation contained in the idea of a "plan" as a unit of behavior provides a foundation for the understanding of control.

THE ORGANIZATION OF CONTENTS

Information from both the environmental stress and the life stress literature is brought together in terms of decision making about control. The approach provides a number of links between cognitive and clinical psychology and should be of interest both to academic researchers and to clinicians.

Whereas the book is aimed at researchers and clinicians who already have some knowledge of work on stress, the chapters also provide the advanced-level student with reviews of relevant research. In particular, the central four chapters (Chapter 4–7 inclusive) are concerned with ways in which stresses are likely to influence performance and hence to change the level of control that is possible.

In chronological order, the identifiable themes of the chapters are as follows. In the first chapter, the question of mental demand likely to be associated with stress is considered. The question of interest is why we have been so neglectful of increased mental load as a factor in explaining performance in stress, when there is such a substantial body of work showing that mental load is a factor that accounts for transient inefficiencies in relatively simple laboratory tasks. How much more demanding should it be to recognize and react to the figure of a man lurking in the garden at night than to recognize and react to a letter "A" appearing on the display of a microcomputer. One answer to the question of neglect of mental load in stress is that states of worry or preoccupation are difficult to measure scientifically. Heavy dependence on introspective report inevitably means that rather less confidence can be attached to findings, for there are no objective data. An additional reason may be the fact that much of what has been accumulated about the character of performance in stressful conditions has come from laboratory studies using environmental stresses such as noise and loss of sleep, where perhaps responses such as worry and preoccupation seem less appropriate. Finally, since biological arousal was first shown from early research of Yerkes and Dodson (1908), using animals, to be a variable capable of influencing learning and performance, there has been a tendency to explore the explanation to the full. Research with human beings confirmed that raised tension levels were associated with changes in the quality of performance (e.g., Courts, 1942; Malmo, 1959), and in spite of recent arguments by Näätänen (1973) that the design capitalized on dual task conflicts, the arousal model has continued to provide a dominant source of explanations for performance changes in stress.

Arguments presented in early chapters lead to the view that performance in stress must be seen as being the result of a pattern of independently driven influences with the possibility of interactions at the level of central mechanisms. This provides the basis of a model that is multicausal or composite. Scientists might be more likely to be attracted to single-factor models that generate testable hypotheses. However, the composite model developed in Chapters 5 and 6 of this book is, we believe, more appropriate and more able to unify laboratory and life stresses in explaining behavior in stress. It does have important implications for the interpretation of research findings. It may no longer be sufficient to elaborate and revise the concept of arousal on the basis of an experimentally manipulated change in an independent variable such as noise or heat and a change in performance characteristic.

A central aspect of mental demand is argued to be the assessment of personal control as the determinant of behavior and long-term reaction. The early chapters are concerned with reviewing some of evidence demonstrating the importance of the perception of control in modulating stress effects. The logical requirements are considered of a model that explains how control is assessed. A major requirement is to understand how a person can know that action and consequence are related; how he can be sure that control is being personally caused rather than having a chance relationship with action, and how he knows that he can produce change in the desired direction.

A model of the cognitive basis of control based on the principles of ideomotor theory is proposed; efferent copy signals provide a store of expectancies from which to compare real "action and consequence" information. It is also argued that a "rule-of-thumb" technique might be noting successive changes in the initial discrepancy contained in the original plan. There may be cases where it is sufficient to note successes and infer that this must have been caused by action. The relevance of the perception of control as a factor influencing stressful situations with respect to conditions such as a conflict, interruption, responsibility, and helplessness is emphasized in Chapter 3. If the perception of control is important in stress and if the assessment depends on mental processes, then there is even greater reason to suppose that many stressful situations will be characterized by high mental demand on a person. In addition, biological arousal has been found to reflect the outcome of control decisions. The decision that control is possible is more likely to increase noradrenaline relative to adrenaline, whereas the reverse is the case when perceived loss of control is an outcome. This is incorporated into the composite model by assuming that different arousals coexist in "concurrent state" and interact with incoming arousal influences in determining outcome. The notion of "arousal compatibility" partly dependent on control decisions is developed in Chapter 5.

Chapters 6 and 7 are concerned with exploring how various central influences translate into the detail of performance, and particularly with considering the implications for the perception of control. In Chapter 6, we examine how "plan running" changes under stress. Changes may be due to decision timing or to violation of the rules of plan running. In either case, a person should be equipped to detect his own errors and to discount these trials in assessing control. However, the question of interest is how tolerant he will be of occasional error before he begins to revise his opinion about control. A critical question for future optimism might be whether a person attributes his errors to the presence of stress.

However, if, as indicated in Chapter 8, stresses may operate via changes in processes such as memory and attention to distort the ingredients of plans, a person may relinquish some of the control he would normally expect to have. A number of consequences follow. Firstly, a lack in the availability of essential details on which internal error detection depends means that a person may develop distortions in the perception of control. He may not be aware of the errors he makes unless feedback is provided by consequences. He might, therefore, expect that he is performing well but later discover his inadequacies. In some cases he may never be able to know about these inadequacies; he may relinquish control without realizing it.

In cases where errors are detected, optimism for the future may depend on the attribution made. Original research data suggesting that normal, uninformed people might expect to perform badly under stress is described. The belief might provide the basis for "making allowances" for self-produced performance or the performance of others. A rating experiment confirmed that this might be the case.

The final part of the book is concerned with the origin of clinical states in terms of decision making about control. In Chapter 8, the operation of a number of feedback loops that promote performance deteriorations is described. A person may experience only a transient inefficiency, but if conditions favor the operation of a positive feedback loop, he may lose control progressively to a point of crisis, which is assumed to be total performance incompetence. Research evidence suggests that the average person might resist the implementation of these loops by self-serving techniques or strategies, typically over-representing the amount of contingency, the "illusion of control," which incentive conditions are present. An alternative technique might be to try to find evidence of contingency by predicting the statistical structure of events on a task. Evidence is presented to suggest that the average person might respond in this way. Finally, obtaining control by other means may be useful in preventing a generalization of self-blame or lowered self-esteem. These ideas are discussed again in the final chapter.

In Chapter 9, concern is with the transmission of vulnerability. Research on predisposing and precipitating factors in mental disorder is briefly considered. Early deprivation and trauma are assumed to increase the risk that a precipitant will result in personal crisis. A hierarchical model of decision making in control is developed. It is argued that vulnerability may be represented as a metamemory of decisions: A person who is vulnerable may be more likely to recognise threats and more likely to perceive them as highly probable. Equally, he may be more likely to be unrealistic in control decisions: Inappropriate engagement and struggle when the problem is unsolvable may be as unbalanced a response as helplessness when it is solvable.

It is assumed that these dispositions are risk factors that combine additively or interactively with factors within a stress scenario to determine the risk of crisis. Risk may be represented as criterion positions that determine likelihood ratios for different aspects of decision making in stress.

In Chapter 10, an attempt is made to consider different forms of mental and physical disorder in terms of the pattern of events within a stress scenario. Aspects of illogical thinking in both normal and depressed subjects are described, and the implications for the origins of forms of mental disorder are considered. The role played by causal attributions in preventing or augmenting the development of lowered self-esteem as a response to helplessness is discussed. Finally, forms of both mental and physical illness are related to coping patterns in stress scenarios.

"WORRY" AS A CONCEPT IN STRESS

One aspect of new technology is a greater facility for change in psycho-social environment. Life change as assessed through questionnaire studies has been shown to be an important predictor of changes in mental and physical well-being (e.g., see Rahe, 1968; Holmes, 1978; Kobasa, 1979), likely to be more critical than negative features of experience alone (see Dohrenwend, 1973). So far there is relatively little understanding of the effects of change in terms of the processes required for adjustment. At least one very important aspect may be a change in the content of daily thinking; a person may need to undergo a period in which he frees himself from the old or previous environment or life style and adapts to the new. During this period a person may be preoccupied or "worried," and the content of worry will relate to the demands made by change.

At least one way in which we have begun to study this is in terms of "homesickness" — a response generally understood by most people to be a reaction to a new geographical environment. The results of the study are described in Chapter 1. It is clear from accounts given by subjects who reported strong homesickness effects that there are episodes of thinking accompanied by agitation in which the main theme is mental preoccupation with the "previous" psychosocial environment and life style. One result of this study was to cause a revision of our thinking about the likely ways in which stresses of various kinds may come to influence performance. It was clear from subjects' own accounts that they considered themselves to be working at lowered efficiency levels. At least one plausible explanation was the occurrence of uncontrollable intrusive thoughts about home, which made concentration difficult. Academic records appeared to indicate below-par functioning, but we have yet to establish this by means of laboratory tests and tests of daily efficiency. However, the reports by subjects suggested that we must consider preoccupation with stress problems as a possible factor in understanding performance changes in stress. Strangely, the literature on how stresses might come to produce changes in efficiency has neglected this aspect of explanation. There is a contribution by Hamilton (e.g., 1974) and Sarason (e.g., 1975) that emphasizes the intrusive nature of "task irrelevant" responses in test anxiety, but there is as yet no considered attempt to understand how daily worries might reduce efficiency levels as a function of stresses. This book attempts to redress the balance a little by placing much greater emphasis on the possible role of stress problems as determinants of daily performance on tasks.

One hypothesis developed is that "worry" is functional; it is part of the process of trying to establish control over new situations, and it is a response to the lack of control induced by change in old situations. Part of establishing control may involve retrospective and prospective analysis, in which old contingencies between events and outcomes resulting from action are revised and new contingencies are established. A typical problem-solving approach to a life-event problem may be of the form "If I had taken that course of action, then x could have been prevented," or "If I now try to take this particular action, then x is likely." On some of these occasions, the "environment" involves personal relationships. In these cases, contingency assessment between action and outcome involves the behavior of other people and may therefore be a less certain, more demanding task.

Precisely because we have tried to provide a synthesis of ideas about stressful conditions and their effects on people, it has been necessary to be selective. We apologize to anyone who feels that his research findings have not been given sufficient weighting or to anyone whose research has not been included.

1 Mental Demand as a Factor in Stressful Conditions

THE MENTAL DEMANDS OF STRESS

An intuitively plausible reason why stresses of various kinds influence performance is because of demands made on mental resources. It is a common enough observation that people become worried by stressful encounters and threatening situations, yet the demands made on resources by "worrying" have been to a large extent neglected. Some attention has been paid to the debilitating effects of "task-irrelevant responses" produced in some stressful conditions, such as in tests and examinations (e.g., see Hamilton 1974), but the study of "relevant" demands stresses may make has been relatively neglected.

This chapter is concerned with reviewing "circumstantial," logical, and psychological evidence relevant to the conclusion that stress is likely to be associated with high work load. There are a number of identifiable sources of processing load. Firstly, there may be the processing load imposed by the need to identify whether or not a particular event or situation is threatening or hazardous. This may involve unraveling ambiguous situations. Secondly, there may be processing load associated with the choice of appropriate responses. Thirdly, there may be load resulting from the need to note the consequence of action and to decide how likely success will be. There may be an additional need to take note of the possible costs associated with failure and of likely ways in which failure can be made palatable. Finally, there may be mental activity very like that used in problem solving, when stress is present and ways of attenuating it or avoiding it are maximally uncertain, or when obvious courses of action are prevented by circumstances. Much real-life stress activity may involve anticipatory or reflective thoughts. Of central significance to the understanding of stress is the fact that pressures may build up in advance or after an event and may provide a constant stream of thought content, which intrudes into daily activity. Many life stresses occur while a person is trying to cope with daily tasks; he may thus find himself involved in dual-task activity of a kind that scientists in laboratories have not studied.

Being "mentally busy" or "preoccupied" should result in a reduction of resources available for the rest of daily life. It might be expected that if daily tasks have the status of secondary tasks, there are likely to be failures of various kinds. Thus, the stressed person may not be the best person to be in charge of an aircraft or an operating table.

There has been surprisingly little by way of demonstration that stresses do impose mental processing demands on individuals. Perhaps one reason lies in the methodological difficulties associated with indexing mental load while people go about daily tasks, but also because in conditions of life stress a person may suffer intensive worrying generally only at times when the task he is engaged in is undemanding or of low priority. To some extent, the worried person may have some control over his worries, switching them off and on in accordance with periods of high and low priority in daily life.

If the thesis that stresses do impose considerable mental demands on people is accepted, an important consideration is the degree to which these demands interfere with concurrent activity. Research on the effects of stresses on performance to date has concentrated on high arousal resulting from stress experience. It remains reasonable to assume that being distracted, preoccupied, and generally "mentally saturated" with a stress problem may lead to important changes in performance; a dual task has been created, and dual tasks are normally associated with deterioration of the elements perceived as less important or less salient. This is a notion that is developed further in the central chapters of the book.

This chapter is primarily concerned with considering the possibility that stress conditions impose task-relevant mental demands on people. This leads toward a consideration of what kinds of mental activity may be involved. The theme developed in the next chapter is that a person is likely to be concerned with establishing control, power, or mastery. The evidence suggests that personal control is a very important aspect of stressful circumstances; if control is lost, even an ordinary task may become stressful, whereas in most stressful conditions, being given control reduces the effect of the stress.

Before following up some of these considerations, it is necessary to look at the evidence that leads to the conclusion that people in stress are likely to be mentally busy. For the reasons given above, there is no direct evidence to show that recognizing and responding to threats creates overload on resources; however, comparison with laboratory tasks requiring recognition and response to simple stimuli using tapping tasks and probe tasks to index load lends considerable support to this view. The remainder of the evidence comes from subjective reports and from consideration of the density of decision making likely to be required.

Demands Imposed by "Simple Threats"

A number of states of discomfort produced by adverse environments are generally regarded as stresses. Extremes of temperature, humidity, sound pressure levels, levels of fatigue, degree of loss of sleep, are normally described under the heading of "environmental stresses." On the first consideration, it might be expected that very little information-processing load is imposed: A state of discomfort is produced, and action to relieve the discomfort is taken. In terms of operational definition of demand it could be argued that some of these conditions should impose rather little demand. Experimental studies have established that people are generally fast to respond to intense stimuli. McGill (1963) established that there was a positive relationship between stimulus intensity and reaction time; Broadbent (1958) pointed out that those high-intensity or high-frequency noise signals that were most distracting were also most likely to be responded to quickly when presented as signals in their own right.

Therefore, in operational terms it might be expected that intense signals of any kind would be associated with relatively low mental demand, precisely because recognition is enhanced. However, the opposite would be expected for stresses that involve or cause degraded or weak information.

Any model proposing that stresses are conditions of departure from optimum conditions implicitly assumes that a person's recognition of discomfort is likely to be equal in both directions. In fact, this may not be true; overstimulating environments may impose less mental work in recognition than "weak-signal" environments. However, there are many stresses that involve low or infrequent stimulation; monotony may result from too small a level or too sparse a pattern of information. These stresses, discussed by Cofer and Appley (1964, p.441), do not fit in well with a model that simply proposes only a one-way departure from optimum or tolerance.

Also, a qualification often needed in order to define the existence of threat or stress is that there is an imbalance between the demand made on the individual and his perceived ability to meet that demand. The point made by Lazarus (1966) is that an environmental event or treatment will only be perceived as stressful if the organism anticipates that he will be unable to cope with it. Stress is thus seen as more than just a case of departure from optimum conditions or of intensity of stimulation, or even of imbalance between objectively defined demand and capacity; stress may depend for existence on the *perception* of subjective demand, in turn dependent on the perception of response capability. Immediately, the point that the definition of the existence of stress depends on quite complex cognitive activity is emphasized; a person who perceives his capability to be low may be subject to greater threat but also greater "work load" in subsequent assessment. The question of how threats are identified in very simple situations rapidly changes to one of how it is that the foundation for the perception of "loss of capacity to cope" is provided in knowledge. This is a cognitive problem. This thesis will be developed further later.

Returning to the question of the likely demand made in even very simple situations and forgetting for the moment the issue raised above about coping resources, it is more than clear from laboratory studies involving stimulus recognition and simple reaction that varying degrees of work load are likely to be involved. Studies concerned with presenting two independent streams of information to a subject, requiring a detailed report of the content of one stream and as much as can be remembered from the less important source, have tended to confirm a "pecking order" of interference between tasks, which varies as a function of the specific focus of demand on processing systems. Thus Allport, Antonis, and Reynolds (1972) found that when the less important source contained either visual pictures, visual words, or auditory words, the greatest recall for content was in that order. The research also indicated that combined conditions were associated with attenuated recall on the less important channel as compared with single-task conditions.

The idea of a pecking order of interference has been confirmed by other laboratory studies. Basically, simple identification of a stimulus does appear to require very little capacity; probe response latency studies in which a stimulus or "probe" is made to occur during a task such as a letter-matching task have indicated that encoding the stimulus prior to the match may incur very little penalty as far as a concurrently occurring probe stimulus is concerned (Posner & Boies, 1971). In a review of work in this area, Ells (1973) supports the idea that simple identification of signals may require little by way of processing resources and tends not to interfere with concurrent activity.

The question implied in the above discussions on resource and capacity concerns demands made by the recognition of threatening events. Is there any way in which we could consider that identification of threat is as simple as identifying a letter in a matching task?

Mental Activity in the Recognition of Threat

There are obvious evolutionary advantages to fast recognition of dangerous objects. A question of interest is the extent to which reading of context or preoccupation with likely outcome are important factors.

The early ethologists (see Tinbergen, 1951; Lorenz, 1950) contributed to the understanding of the relationship between environmental stimuli and behavioral repertoires, based on observations in naturalistic settings. Two major issues of interest are contained in their conclusions. The first is whether certain stimuli or stimulus configurations can be reacted to at an instinctive level. If, for example, an animal can identify a key stimulus such as a large shadow as implying threat, then further encoding might be unnecessary. One of the costs might be false positives, but the gain is survival. Although there is evidence that key stimuli such as *big shape*, *moving shape*, or *black shadow* have the capacity to evoke immediate fear (see Russell, 1979), there clearly are configurational qualities present. The efficient organism could reduce encoding demand by developing a configurational template so that certain simple patterns evoked alarm. Equally, he could operate so that one feature, such as darkness or size, had immediate access to alarm. Again the cost is high false alarm rates, but processing load could be reduced.

The second contribution of the work of the ethologists was the notion that internal energy states could raise the tendency to produce a given pattern of behavior to very weak stimuli, or even in the absence of a stimulus. Although this was particularly applied to the analysis of out of context "displacement activity," there may be some useful applications to the understanding of fear responses. Unfortunately there is little by way of specific hypotheses concerning the way in which time and circumstance might combine to lower the threshold of response to stimuli. The "hydraulic" model developed by Lorenz (1950) provided only a very basic description of the interplay between internal energy states and stimulus strength as response determinants.

The ethologists' models were not developed in sufficient detail with respect to fear for clear conclusions about the facilitation of the recognition of threat to be drawn. Tinbergen did favor the view that simple stimulus properties were less effective than "configurational organization" as determinants of fear responses and drew attention to the features of the hawk-like shape used to evoke fear in young birds. "Short-neckedness" was the important quality and could only be deduced from the total configuration presented; the direction the shape was pulled in was important. Tinbergen argued that the innate releasing mechanism could not be operated unless two or more stimuli were present. A similar point was made by Bowlby (1973), who pointed out that fearful behavior is more likely in cases that compound two or more fear stimuli. Some stimuli may provide the context for appraisal — thus the effect of a loud noise may be greater if the individual is in a dark wood.

The reading of a key stimulus may be important in cases of certain fear responses. Instead of identifying the whole configuration, the organism reacts to a factor usually present in threatening situations. An interesting review by Russell (1979) of properties of objects that induce fear suggests that a stimulus frequently associated with predation is movement toward the prey; this is likely to produce protective movements indicative of fear. Movement properties most likely to produce this response are speed, directness, suddenness, and closeness (Bronstein & Hirsch, 1976).

However, there are objects associated with fear responses in which the key stimulus is not clear and the underlying reason for the response is not clear. Fear of snakes is an interesting example. A snake is characterized by a whole number of stimulus properties such as longness and movement properties such as slitheriness, but it is not clear that these sensations alone determine the fear response. Strong avoidance of snakes is shown by some human beings (e.g., Mellstrom, Cicala, & Zuckerman, 1976) and animals (Morris & Morris, 1965)—presumably, the latter are not reacting to symbolic or mythological qualities, as the psychoanalysts might suggest for human beings. Equally, the reaction of chimpanzees to the sight of rubber snakes when there has been no previous encounter (e.g., see Hebb, 1949) suggests that simple stimulus configurations must play a role.

Even when the reading of key stimuli might be responsible for a particular response, a factor of importance may be the context in which the particular stimulus is experienced. Jersild's (1943) early study of fear of the dark drew attention to this point. In a study of young children (aged 2–5), Jersild reported that young children were reluctant to enter a dark tunnel to retrieve a wanted object; however, although 45% of the group would not enter the tunnel, some would if accompanied by an adult. This suggests that fear can be alleviated in circumstances that increase the likelihood of safety.

An important aspect of fear responses in relation to stimuli was developed by Dollard and Miller (1950), who based their ideas on learning theory developed by Hull (1943). They postulated a primary drive to avoid pain: In order to avoid pain, an organism must learn the signals associated with it. The greater the number of unpleasant experiences and the more intense the pain, the greater the learning. However, learning can be extended by the principle of stimulus generalization; different stimuli may be associated with the object causing pain, and hence more and more stimuli may come to evoke the same fear response. Cues may also become "attached" to the primary object of fear, so that objects present at the time the pain occurred may also acquire the capacity to arouse fear. Thus complex stimuli may acquire, by learning and generalization, association with a fundamental stressful event. An implication of this is that rather remote stimuli may come to be associated with fear as a function of previous experience, and the mental work involved may be reduced.

A more recent development has been the proposal that certain stimulus/ response, or stimulus/stimulus associations are prearranged or "prepared" and increase the facility with which learning can occur. The concept of "preparedness" as introduced by Seligman (1971) is operationally defined in terms of ease of learning and relative resistance to unlearning. Evolutionary pressures have been assumed to favor relationships of benefit to "pretechnological man."

One implication of this concerns the ease with which certain stimuli can come to evoke a fear response. Somatic withdrawal responses may be prepared in relation to stimuli usually associated with fear or pain. Some responses, such as relaxation and yawning, may be very difficult to evoke under these conditions. Therefore, the range and uncertainty associated with possible behaviors could be reduced, thus reducing some of the demand made on the organism. An implication is that avoidance responses may be almost reflexlike in availability and speed.

Seligman proposes a continuum in which different weight may be given to learning in stimulus response associations. Thus, at one end responses are instinctive, and at the other learning may be involved. In addition, he proposes a continuum of level of preparedness, from "contraprepared" to high levels of preparedness. An experiment illustrating the prepared/ contraprepared distinction is one by Garcia and Koelling (1966) on the acquisition of learned aversions. Rats were presented with saccharine-tasting water in a "bright, noisy environment." In one condition rats were submitted to X-irradiation while they drank, in another to electric shock. In the former condition, radiation-contingent sickness occurred within an hour, but the rats associated the sickness with the water taste and developed an aversion to water. In the latter shock condition, rats developed an aversion to the bright, noisy environment. Such specific associative links are of evolutionary advantage, since animals who have been poisoned will develop an aversion to the cause of the poison.

The concept of evolutionary advantage is used to explain the apparent nonrandom distribution of fears and phobias across stimulus conditions. De Silva, Rachman, and Seligman (1977) developed a rating scale for estimating the biological relevance of phobias and found evidence for evolutionary significance in 66 out of the 69 phobias studied. However, there is the problem that although these sources of fear may seem rational in the context of man's evolutionary history, there is no evidence to suggest cultural differences that might be expected, since some classes of "threat" are more likely to occur in some parts of the world. Small animals are common sources of phobic fear, and yet there are geographical differences in their distribution.

The demonstration that there may be facilitated acquisition of avoidance responses to some stimuli has been provided by Ohman (1979). Using the technique of presenting pictures of spiders and snakes (fear relevant) and flowers and mushrooms (fear irrelevant) for the conditioned stimulus in a fear conditioning experiment, Ohman reported that in the case of fear-relevant CS content, conditioned fear responses were acquired more rapidly and were more resistant to extinction. Comparable results were obtained when "angry" as opposed to "happy" faces were used as conditioned stimuli.

Prepared associations and stimulus generalization are two possible ways in which there may be facilitation of the recognition and response to threat. If situations imply greater dependence on cognitive processes because of the need to read context and decide on likely courses of action, there may be no benefit from facilitatory effects of learning or preparedness.

The Reading of Context

The noting of context provided by situations or even by instructions in laboratory experiments is an important aspect of stressful appraisals in human beings. Research by Lazarus and his colleagues has shown that threat can be experienced symbolically by human subjects. The technique used involved presentation of harrowing films under conditions in which subjects knew themselves to be personally safe. Provision of an instructional commentary could change the level of stress experienced. "Intellectualization" and "denial" commentaries reduced the level of stress experienced (see Speisman et al., 1964).

The ameliorating effect of "intellectualization" and "denial" instructions may be taken as evidence of the influence cognitive processes may have on the level of the stress response. A similar modifying effect has been reported for pain stimuli. For example, Sternbach (1968) reported a study that demonstrated the effects of instructions on what to expect concerning electric shock. Groups who were led to expect higher-intensity shock reported more pain. A study by Staub and Kellett (1972) varied the information given to subjects prior to their receiving short-duration shocks, which increased in intensity with time. One group was informed about precautions taken to maintain safety in the equipment, whereas the other group was told about physical symptoms likely to be associated with shock. Both these sets of information were provided to a third group. Results showed that those who had both sets of instructions received higher shocks before reporting pain or asking to terminate the trials.

Although in the single condition subjects did not differ significantly, the influence of cognitive factors was demonstrated.

In a different situation, which involved injection of the drug skoline, which produces up to one hundred seconds respiratory paralysis, Campbell, Sanderson, and Laverty (1964) gave advance information to one group, so that the subjects knew what to expect in terms of the effects of the drug. The informed group differed significantly from the uninformed in terms of the magnitude of the stress response to skoline; although both groups showed evidence of being under stress, the effect was ameliorated for the informed group.

There is now a great deal of research pointing to the importance of knowledge and thinking as a factor in the magnitude of the stress response. Lazarus (1966), provides an excellent review of many useful studies in which the moderating effect of beliefs are emphasized. An interesting study by Symington and others (1955) was concerned with the stress of dying; heightened autonomic activity was found to be characteristic in cases where patients remained conscious, suggesting that dying itself is not intrinsically stressful; it is the thoughts and anticipations associated with dying that matter.

It appears that in the absence of instructions or advance knowledge, people attempt to acquire realistic information for themselves. The much-quoted study by Grinker and Spiegel (1945) on flying sorties in the Second World War showed that the actual number of casualties predicted the incidence of nervous breakdown: As casualty rates rose, the number of mental casualties also rose. Moreover, the cause of the casualty, when known, was argued by the authors of the study to provide a focus of concern during flying.

Thoughts of an anticipatory or reflective nature may themselves be responsible for panic or depressive attacks. This has been convincingly demonstrated by Beck (1967, 1970) in the case of clinical patients under treatment. Studies of spontaneous fantasies in patients have shown that they are associated with emotional changes. They may be subject to spontaneous modification in the absence of reality testing. Moreover, the dream content of patients is indicative of clinical factors normally observed.

Even what we have previously described as "simple fears" may have a cognitive basis. In discussing fear responses in chimpanzees, Hebb (1949) remarks that young infant chimpanzees do not show fear of a model of a human or chimpanzee head detached from the body, but older (half-grown) animals do. Hebb draws a parallel with human differences in response to snakes as a function of age; the frequency and strength of fear increases up to the age of seventeen in people who have never been injured by a snake. Hebb points out that these fears depend on a degree of intellectual development.

Anticipatory Responses

Much of human stress behavior is anticipatory or reflective. One of the most interesting aspects of stress is that it is not necessary for the event to be present at the time. One of the most useful of laboratory studies that concentrated on anticipatory shock was conducted by Wherry and Curran (1965). In the study of the effects of anticipated shock, they showed that disruption of current performance reflected a number of important factors such as the proximity of the event, its probability, and the perceived degree of unpleasantness. Anticipatory disruption appears to be realistically based. The characteristic disruption in performance was U-shaped, with some improvement for mildly unpleasant levels and decrement for high amounts.

Anticipatory mental activity preceding a parachute jump has been studied as part of the research programme by Epstein and Fenz (see Fenz, 1964, 1975). The most interesting effect reported was a change in galvanic skin response, described as a monotonic increase, before the jump itself. For experienced jumpers and good jumpers, the response reverts toward base level just prior to the jump; the resulting pattern is thus a V-shaped function. The beneficial effects of experience appear to act in advance of the jump in the case of experienced jumpers. However, the possibility that those who incur a reduction in arousal at the critical moment jump better cannot be entirely discounted.

A study by Epstein and Clarke (1970) was concerned with heart rate and skin conductance levels preceding and following a burst of 107-dB noise. Instructions given influenced the result; one group was led to believe the effect would be worse than it was; one group was led to expect a reduced effect; and one group had an accurate description. Results showed that those who expected the worst had the greatest level of anticipatory arousal preceding the event and showed the greatest reaction to impact.

Although there are clear problems with interpreting anticipatory designs, it is at least reasonable to conclude that informed mental activity occurs in advance of an event. Part of anticipation may not just be thinking about the event to come but may involve manipulation of mental codes that enable a person to take instructions, context, and previous experience into account.

Shannon and Isbell (1963) provided a useful demonstration of the powerful effects of anticipation over a very short time period. There were five experimental treatments of injections in the mouth. On one treatment 2% hydrochloric acid was injected; on another, this was combined with epinephrine; on a third occasion, sodium chloride was used. The remaining two treatments were dummy runs: The first treatment was actual needle insertion and nothing injected, which provides a control for looking at the injection process itself; the second treatment was the instruction that injection would occur under conditions in which the needle is placed in the mouth. Under all five conditions there was a rise in hydrocortisone in the blood, which persisted for up to 15 minutes after the treatment. Since the effect does not distinguish actual drug treatments from dummy treatments, it must be due to the anticipatory effects. In this study the strength of the anticipatory effect is well demonstrated, and the important feature of it is that it is brought about very quickly because little warning was given to the subjects. The powerful controlling influence of mental processes in determining response is demonstrated.

A profile of physiological changes preceding the occurrence of a noxious event was obtained by Birnbaum (1964) in a doctoral dissertation. Using a technique comparable with those used by Lazarus and his colleagues, Birnbaum showed films of various unpleasant industrial accidents. Measures of autonomic activity such as heart rate and skin conductance showed a sharp rise at the appearance of cues that would imply that the accident is likely to happen. At the occurrence of the accident, described as the moment of confrontation, there is a further rise, but this is followed by a drop, although the unpleasant results of the accident are being shown. Again this emphasizes the powerful effects of anticipatory mental activity; the effect is stronger than being confronted with the harrowing scene. The experiments also confirm the capacity to anticipate stresses that are symbolic.

The Demands of Action

So far, it has been assumed that action to combat threat might occur almost at the reflex level and demands very little of the individual in terms of decision making. In fact this may misrepresent the case for many stresses with which a person may be confronted. The notion developed by Cannon (1932, 1936) that the stress response is best understood in terms of homeostasis preparing the organism for a return to equilibrium does not specify the nature of action required for this process. If the physiological response is seen as the controlling variable designed to mobilize resources required for the production of energy, there is no particular need to suppose that the form is variable and situation-specific, although this latter view is in keeping with evidence from modern research. If behavior is seen as the controlling variable that restores equilibrium, it is necessary to assume that it will be situation-specific and may involve complex decisions that could be likened to problem solving in some cases.

The question is what demands the organization and production of effective action are likely to make on a person. It has been hypothesized from early work on refractoriness (Welford, 1952) that time and therefore resources in the nervous system is required for the processing of feedback from responses. Moreover, studies concerned with investigating dual task interference have pointed to the importance of both recall and response organization processes as being most demanding of capacity (see Kerr, 1973). In cases where the organism has to decide on the form of response, it would be expected that demands could be high.

A useful distinction is made by Lazarus (1966) concerning action tendencies in stress. In addition to attack and avoidance, he recognizes actions aimed at strengthening reserves against harm. The individual attempts to influence the actual conditions with which he is confronted, and this involves consideration of the consequences of alternative strategies. At the very least this process would require mobilizing information stored on the basis of experience concerning likely courses of action and likely outcomes. If action is carried out in advance of the anticipated hazard, its impact may be reduced at the time, as with the building of storm shelters to avoid a likely squall. The penalty may be that advanced activities will disrupt efficiency on other tasks at the time. The same argument may be advanced for "mental anticipations": Thinking in advance about an impending problem may produce benefits in the long term but may incur other penalties.

In addition to the varying need to consider alternative courses of action is the need to consider the consequence of a particular action and the cost of action in particular cases. Powers (1973) has argued that the consequence of behavior in terms of the changes on the independent variable is an important neglected aspect of behavior. In stressful conditions a person may be particularly concerned with perceived consequences of different courses of action.

A number of "metaconcepts" may need to be extracted, such as perception of the skills required, perception of the capability of carrying out the skilled action, perception of the likely consequence of desired action. Developing and manipulating these concepts may be part of the process of worry, and failure to perform this work effectively may render the individual vulnerable to an approaching problem and dependent on "here-and-now" decision making. Yet this hypothesis is very conjectural; so far the literature on stress does not contain any significant studies that have attempted to tackle this problem.

An important function of "worry" may be to weigh up the short- or long-term costs of action. A person would need to know that the cost of a particular course of action is not greater than the cost of inaction, which results in the penalty of experiencing the threat. In addition, he may need to weigh the likelihood of desirable cases of action being possible. If "escape routes" are closed, there is a need to evaluate the possibility of direct attack against the penalty of no action. In the case of closed escape routes, a high level of panic is likely (Smelser, 1963). Such perceptions may involve mental checking operations concerned with likely actions, likely outcomes, etc. In a study of the behavior in German concentration camps, Bettelheim (1943, 1960) argued that one of the main ways of controlling escape attempts was to make the penalty attached to failure so great that the action ceased to be a viable alternative in this respect.

The possibility that in disambiguating an imagined scenario in order to decide how threatening it is a person makes use of information about the availability of suitable responses was examined by Fisher (1983g). The study was concerned with obtaining protocols from individuals who were asked to increase the threat potential of a hypothetical situation.

Twenty subjects were asked, individually, to consider the following situation:

> You are a young girl, alone in the house. At about 11 o'clock at night you look out of the window and see a man standing in your garden.

Subjects were asked to generate ten statements that would increase the threat imposed by the imagined situation. Exact protocols from three subjects chosen at random are illustrated in Table 1.1.

Independent judges, who were student volunteers, read the protocol statements and classified each statement according to whether the statement concerned the man (object) or the girl (subject), or whether the statement was concerned with psychosocial environment. In addition, object and subject statements were classified in accordance with whether the concern was with descriptive state (e.g., "looks fierce") or whether action was implied (e.g., "runs toward me").

In general, as illustrated by Table 1.2, about half the statements were concerned with context and about half with subject and object. Clearly, context is an important consideration in contributing to threat appraisal. There was no significant difference in the use of "context statements" between the first and second section of the statements, suggesting that context continues to be important throughout. An important difference was that a greater proportion of early statements concerned the "man" ($p<.01$), and a greater proportion of later statements concerned the "girl" ($p<.01$). In the early statements, "action" and "state" featured about equally; in the latter, action statements predominated for the "girl" ($p<.001$), but there was no significant difference for the "man".

The study suggested that in an imagined situation there is concern with context, and that as far as the content of the "scenario" is concerned, there is a change in the balance of thinking from the "man" to the "girl." Further, action statements concerning the "girl" predominate in the later part of the sequence of thinking.

TABLE 1.1.
Randomly Selected Examples of Threat Recognition Protocols

Scenario: Imagine you are a young girl, alone in the house. At about 11 o'clock at night you look out of the window and see a man standing in your garden!

Instructions: Generate 10 factors which would lead to a positive threat appraisal, or would increase the degree of threat you would sense.

Exact replication of subject protocols to illustrate variety of form.

Subject 1.

1. Man carrying object in his hand
2. Reaction of man to seeing me
3. No one else in the house
4. It's evening or during the night
5. There's no easy way for man to get out of garden
6. The bigger and stronger he looks
7. His face is darkened and not so easily visible
8. How far I am from back door and how easily can I lock it
9. There are no neighbors near the house to shout
10. There is no implement close at hand with which I can defend myself

Subject 2.

1. Is man big with dark hair?
2. When he sees me does he come toward me?
3. Is he smiling or does he look angry?
4. Is he at the end of the garden or is he near me?
5. Is Mummy in so that I am not alone?
6. Is it getting dark or is it broad daylight?
7. Do we live alone or out in the country?
8. Is man carrying anything which he might hit me with?
9. Is he young or old?
10. Has Mummy spoken of a strange man in the neighborhood recently?

Subject 3 (only subject who provided a "problem-solving" account and did not follow instructions).

1. Feel surprise at him being there
2. Notice what, if anything, he is doing
3. If he hasn't seen me, hide and watch him
4. If he wasn't doing anything harmful go up to him and ask him if he knows he is on private property
5. Study him—is he well dressed and shaved. If not then I would feel nervous at approaching him—hands shake, butterflies in tummy
6. In going up to him I would go a way where he couldn't see me until I am near
7. If he is doing some damage, I would feel more frightened and surprised
8. Then I would have to decide what to do and that would be very difficult indeed, especially if there was no one else in the house
9. I would also feel annoyed that he was damaging my property and if this anger grew stronger than my fear I would go straight up to him and demand to know what he was doing
10. To do that I would be very nervous but because I knew I was in the right I would gain strength from that knowledge

TABLE 1.2.
Classification of Statements in Protocols of Imagined Threat Scenario (in Percentages)

	Object (man)		Subject (girl)				
	Action	State	Action	State	Context	Other	Total
1st 5 statements	24.4	18.2	2.1	2.1	50.1	3.10	100%
2nd 5 statements	10.1	13.0	20.4	12.4	42.2	1.90	100%
		102.7			92.3	5.00	200%
$\overline{X}$ Total %		51.35			46.15	2.50	100%

It would appear that when sequential "thought ordering" is imposed, subjects indicate initial concern with properties of the scenario confronting them and gradually increase the proportion of thoughts concerned with possible courses of action. Such a change in the characteristic of threat recognition is in keeping with the analysis provided by Lazarus (e.g., see 1968). In accordance with the Lazarus scheme, primary appraisal is concerned with situational features, whereas secondary appraisal is concerned with consideration of forms of coping available. A later stage of appraisal, termed "re-appraisal," is also identified and is basically concerned with reflective consideration concerning outcome and original appraisals made.

The main difference between responses concerned with disambiguating an imagined scenario and responses in a real situation is that in the former the action is frozen, whereas in real life the scenario is dynamic and not interrupted. One implication of this is reduced time to think; a person is paced by events. Thus, in real life, work load may be high because of increased density of decision making in time.

One way in which the demands of selecting action can be reduced is if a person is pretrained. A pilot trained in procedures for aborting take-off in case of engine fire follows a list of automatic procedures. Alternatively, anticipating likely events, actions, and outcomes in advance could have a similar desirable effect. Janis (1958, 1962, 1974) considers the benefits of psychological preparation for an impending event and uses the term "worry work" to describe the process whereby a person "adjusts to a painful reality situation" (Janis, 1974, p. 375). Janis argues that the person who fails to do the work of worrying adequately does not have plans for meeting contingencies and may feel helpless. He does not correct overoptimistic expectations and fantasies; this increases the chance of disparity. Janis bases his observations on studies of patients faced with impending surgical operations. Those subjects who were told practically nothing about the impending operation were more likely to experience anger on the day of the operation and to develop unfavorable attitudes and greater emotional reaction to the surgeon. The provision of information raised preoperative fear levels and duration both on the day before the operation and on the day of the operation, but it may have provided the necessary internal codes that help to structure the content of "worry work." Janis also found that preoperative anxiety levels had a curvilinear relationship with postoperative adjustment; thus, high levels of preoperative fear could counteract the beneficial effects of worry work.

The Recall of Information on Threats

Mental work in responding to threats of all kinds would be reduced if the information were easily retrieved. One way in which this could be achieved is by an efficient structure in the organization of material in memory. In theory, it would be desirable for a person to be faster to recognize a snake than a raspberry, faster to retrieve the information "snakes bite" than the information "snakes are long" or "snakes are members of the reptile family." Some researchers have begun to give attention to the possibility of a memory structure for fearful objects, but so far the structure has not been probed experimentally.

A possibility raised by Mandler (1975) is that the capacity to threaten may become a property of the object, rather in the way that it has other attributes. Thus a dog has fur and four legs; a history of bad experiences with dogs may lead to the attribution "it bites" rather in the same way. A "dominant node" might develop, in which "bites" becomes a prime attribute.

Work on the structure of semantic memory has suggested that the organization of concepts is hierarchical and related to frequency of usage. Thus, certain items may become highly dominant members of categories; a robin would be an example of a dominant item in the category "bird." Norms established by Battig and Montague (1969) have established dominance levels of category members across a large number of subjects. Little comparable work has yet been carried out with memory for fearful events. A task designed to investigate the dominance of items in memory is the retrieval task in which subjects have to decide whether a particular item is a member of a stated category (e.g., Freedman & Loftus, 1971). Although in general the order of latency of recall supports the organization produced by natural recall, this is not always the case, and in addition the relationship between dominance and frequency is not perfect. Moreover, Gregg (1976) showed that although high-frequency words may be recalled more quickly than their counterparts, the reverse is true for recognition.

It would be of obvious advantage if information about possible threats were organized for maximally efficient retrieval. This should reduce the memory load associated with retrieval. However, there are difficulties with testing the supposition that a hierarchical order might exist for objects associated with fear. The main problem arises because of idiosyncracies in the classification of fear-provoking objects. A study by Collett (1982, unpublished) explored the nature of organization of items in memory for two categories of objects; the first was "disturbing" and described as personal and emotionally charged, the second "enlightening," which could be considered personal but not emotionally charged. Subjects ranked various items for either of these two adjective sets and subsequently responded to those same items on a sentence verification task; they were asked to decide whether an item was a category member. The verification task took place at least one week after the recall task. For fear items Collett used items on the "Augmented Fear Survey Schedule II" (Wolpe & Lang, 1969), standardized by Fischer and Turner (1978).

Collett's results showed that there was a positive correlation between order of recall and response time on the verification task (see Table 1.3); subjects were faster to verify these items, which they themselves had

TABLE 1.3.
Recognition Latencies for Self-generated Items Classified as
"Disturbing" or "Enlightening", Ranked in Order of Production (from
thesis by Collett, 1982)

a. *"Disturbing"*

	Rank position							
	1	*2*	*3*	*4*	*5*	*6*	*7*	*8*
Mean RT	1038	1086	1091	1128	1117	1127	1200	1177
SD	236	290	236	280	217	272	391	387
No. of Ss	13	13	13	13	13	11	9	5

b. *"Enlightening"*

	Rank position							
	1	*2*	*3*	*4*	*5*	*6*	*7*	*8*
Mean RT	1008	1026	1028	1038	1062	1095	1117	1154
SD	162	177	165	178	156	314	206	252
No. of Ss	13	13	13	13	13	13	13	12

recalled early in the sequence initially. A comparable result was obtained for enlightening items. Collett also tested the norms for dominance level in fruit against verification latencies and did not find a positive correlation. However, more experimentation is needed to ensure that order of production was not influencing rather than reflecting the structure of memory.

In spite of idiosyncracies in the way in which different objects are represented in terms of their potential for evoking fear, it does seem that there may be a within-subject structure that is in some ways comparable with the organization of material in semantic memory. One point worth making is that it is likely to be characteristic of feared objects that they are avoided. If events are encountered with low frequency, the dominance structure must be based not on frequency mechanisms but on some other system perhaps relating to priority and danger.

As far as the arguments that have been advanced about mental demand are concerned, operational definitions would imply that since items most feared are retrieved quickly, the memory work would be reduced. In cases where retrieval is slow, memory work is arguably higher. If stressful experiences and objects are given positions in memory that facilitate recall then at least part of the demand will be reduced.

SOURCES OF INTERNAL INFORMATION: "WORRY WORK"

In summary, the evidence is fragmented, but it does seem reasonable to expect that with immediate stresses present in sudden accidents and catastrophes, the individual may incur transient overload of resources because of the need to identify key stimuli, "read" context, organize responses, and process feedback about consequences. The strongest case for proposing that this is likely is that much simpler conditions have been found to produce transient overload in laboratory tasks.

Longer-term stresses may be more likely to provide problem-solving situations where actions and the consequences and costs of actions must be retrieved and evaluated as part of the decision-making process. Life stresses may provide scenarios across a period of time; during this time there may be variable periods when the individual is worried and preoccupied. If he is required to perform other daily tasks, transient fluctuations in efficiency levels may be expected.

Some stresses depend for the greater part of their effects on anticipatory or reflective processes. From the evidence available, it appears that these processes might be effective if relevant information is provided. Anticipatory activity does seem to be realistically based and may be beneficial in the long term. Anticipation may result in disruption on a concurrent task as a function of factors such as the perceived danger or pain, or the imminence and probability of threat. Anticipation depends exclusively on mental activity and may involve elements of rehearsal. Many stresses in life, such as impending illnesses, deaths, disasters, catastrophes, financial losses, tests, examinations, and failures may involve anticipatory elements. During the anticipatory period, a person may be inefficient and "absent-minded." Anticipatory information might be thought of as providing a competing stream, which varies in its capacity to capture attention.

An additional source of information, which may be important to the individual although perhaps seen as task irrelevant in that it is of no benefit to the task, is that concerned with wider implications for the individual. A valuable contribution to an understanding of this aspect of mental demand in stress is provided by research on test anxiety by Sarason (1973, 1975) and on socialization anxiety in children (Hamilton, 1974). Considerations such as the reasons for and the consequences of failure have been shown to be typical responses in test-anxious subjects. Hamilton provides a conceptual formulation in which these task-irrelevant sources compete for limited capacity space and cause loss of resources for the task stimuli. Seen in this way, information-processing demands produced by test environments are likely to be responsible for failure; a positive feedback loop is established.

In general, with the exception of the test anxiety studies, there has been very little attempt to consider the mental demands of stress and the likely implications for understanding performance changes in stress. An attempt is made to rectify this in Chapter 4.

2 The Basis of Personal Control

THE PSYCHOLOGICAL IMPORTANCE OF PERSONAL CONTROL

Inextricably linked to the notion of personal freedom and the principle of free will, the concepts of "personal control," "power," or "mastery" have proved to be of relevance for the understanding of the perception of and the response to stressful conditions. A number of researchers have been concerned to present acceptable definitions of control. For example, Lazarus (1966) introduces the notion of "reversibility": A person has power or control if he can reverse the state of affairs, if he so desires. Mandler (1975), draws attention to similarities between personal control and White's concept of "competence" (White, 1959). Competence is an individual's "felt control" in executing responses that are organized. Rotter and his colleagues (e.g., Rotter, 1966) have emphasized that the tendency to perceive whether control is or is not possible is a personality disposition that varies between individuals. Seen in this way, attitudes to evidence about control may reflect ideological beliefs but also the nature of life history experiences.

The whole question of control is linked to discussions in the previous chapter concerning mental processes under stress. Decision-making load may vary as a function of the uncertainty about whether control is possible. A person who decides that he is never likely to have control may, irrespective of reason, be less loaded in terms of decision making, but more likely to incur the punishment attached to being helpless and to the consequences of failure. The demands made on him may thus be quite

20

different from those on the person who believes he should have control and decides to exercise it when faced with an identical situation. The greater the uncertainty concerning the likelihood of control, the more comparisons will be required mentally. The perception of control will be likely to depend on assessments made in advance of or during the task, and in these circumstances they should add to mental workload. These ideas are developed further in subsequent chapters; personal control is argued to be a problem for cognitive science.

THE PSYCHOLOGICAL BASIS OF CONTROL

Experiments on the Effects of Perceived Control

Many studies concerned with control tend to avoid the problem of definition and also the nature of the correspondence between what is objectively true and what is subjectively true. Thompson (1981) attempts to rectify the former and defines control as "the belief that one has at one's disposal a response that can influence the aversiveness of an event" (p. 89). Averill (1973) concentrates on a typology of control. "Behavioral control" is defined in terms of the availability of a response that can modify objective characteristics, "cognitive control," as the processing of relevant material in order to reduce stress, and "decisional control" as the choice between alternative courses of action. By contrast, Miller (1979) defines four types of behavioral control: "Instrumental control" is the ability to modify the aversive event; "potential control" is belief that control is possible although the necessary action is not used; "self-administration" is a form of control achieved by self-administering the stress; and "actual control" is indistinct but appears to imply an effect on the aversive condition that is separable from increased predictability.

These typologies seem to represent a confusion of methodological issues and stages in the decision making whereby control is assessed and represented. Before discussing concepts of control in detail, it is useful to consider a selection of relevant experimental findings that illustrate the concept itself or difficulties with it.

One of the first studies on self-administration was conducted in 1943 by Haggard. Self-administered shock resulted in smaller skin conductance changes than experimenter-induced shock and was perceived as less unpleasant. In addition, the response was more readily extinguished, and subjects were more aware of contingencies.

However, any self-administered treatment is also subjectively predictable and certain, and it is possible that the effects related to prediction and not to control. Pervin (1963) designed an experiment to resolve this difficulty by introducing three levels of uncertainty and two levels of control and requiring each subject to experience all treatments. A difficulty is presented by the likely existence of order and adaptation effects; however, results suggested that predictability was perhaps the key factor, because the small trend toward amelioration of stress in self-administered conditions was greater in early trials in unsignaled and inconsistently signaled conditions. Subjects were also found to prefer consistently signaled shock.

For arguably similar reasons, most subjects show a preference for immediate rather than delayed treatment of an anxious condition (Maltzman & Wolff, 1970). Also, having been given prior experience of self-administered as compared with externally administered shocks, most subjects will choose self-administered shocks and will give as a reason the preference for uncertainty reduction. In an experiment by Ball and Vogler (1971) 25 out of 39 subjects showed a preference for self-administered shock. It seems that subjects believe predictability to be important, but it may be that they find it difficult to define or express "control" as an aspect.

There have been a number of studies in which choice was available to the subject with regard to the attenuation or termination of unpleasant stimulation. Generally it seems that being given "control facility" is an important factor in ameliorating a stressful effect. A study by Geer and Maisel (1972) involved measurement of GSR during the presentation of unpleasant photographs of victims of violent death and showed that if the subject could terminate the visual exposure by means of a switch, the impact was reduced. Predictability provided by a warning signal was found to be less important in determining the effect.

The conclusions that can be drawn from these studies are not clear with respect to the importance of control. Averill (1973), after providing a detailed account of major experiments on the difference between experimenter-administered and self-administered treatments, concludes that most people prefer to have control over a potentially noxious stimulus, even when that control has no instrumental value in altering the objective nature of the threat (p. 289), but emphasizes that this does not necessarily mean that the preference indicates that the stressful qualities are reduced. Also, Averill remains unconvinced that regulated administration affects anything more than predictability of the nature or timing of threat. However, predictability may provide the basis of the evidence on which a person assesses contingency between his behavior and the world outside; it may be the brick that provides the foundation for the assessment of control.

A series of studies by Glass, Singer, and associates (e.g., Glass, Singer, & Friedman, 1969), investigated the effects of control over loud noise. Subjects could operate a switch to terminate noise. Performance on various tasks was investigated in the presence of loud aversive noise delivered in nine-second bursts. Subjects showed some adaptation to the noise, but later, when two subsequent tasks were presented, there were differences in performance according to the experience of the noise condition. Those subjects who had received a random schedule of exposure to noise made, for example, fewer attempts at problem solving on an unsolvable task. Subjects who received noise at predictable intervals did not differ from controls.

Perhaps the most interesting finding to emerge from the studies was that if subjects were provided with a switch for controlling the source of the noise, there was a marked beneficial effect on performance. For example, on the unsolvable problem task, subjects who had been provided with a switch to control the noise attempted five times the number of puzzles. On a proofreading task it was reported that there were fewer errors (see Glass, Singer, & Friedman, 1969). It seems that merely believing that control is possible can have beneficial effects. None of the subjects reported in this study used the switch. Later, Glass, Rheim, and Singer (1971) reported that this effect remained even when subjects were only able to operate the switch by asking another person to operate it for them.

The first possible explanation of experiments in which an ameliorating effect of the presence of control is demonstrated is that experience of the event is more predictable. However, it has already been argued that predictability may be an element of the perception of control; the existence of regularity may even lead to the false belief that there is control. A more detailed analysis of these experimental situations is, therefore, needed.

Secondly, the presence of control facility may lead a subject to be more tolerant of an unpleasant experience because he can determine the exposure time. In real life, it could be expected that the presence of control facility might be more important in providing the subject with a means of ending an unpleasant experience, as compared with the situation in the laboratory, where the subject is agreeing to cooperate by experiencing an unpleasant situation for a relatively brief period that is known to be finite.

A view advanced by Thompson (1981) is that most of the experimental results that demonstrate a positive effect of control facility are concerned with tolerance; the dependent variable is usually the willingness to endure noxious stimulation. Studies concerned with measuring physiological arousal or performance are less likely to show improvement with control facility.

This is not entirely true for all experiments concerned with either performance or arousal change. For example, in the noise and control experiments by Glass et al. (1969), the cost of exposure to 110 dB loud noise described in terms of "post adaptive" deterioration on a proofreading task was ameliorated by the presence of a control switch (see also Glass & Singer, 1972).

Moreover, an experiment by Gatchel and Proctor (1976) is interesting in illustrating an important need to look carefully at the kind of control operated in the context of the experiment. They report an experiment consisting of two phases, the first of which was a pretreatment of 45 trials of unsignaled loud tones. In one condition, depressing a microswitch four times allowed escape. In another, subjects were yoked to the escape condition receiving the noise that the "escape" subjects received. In a third condition, subjects had to listen passively to the noise. The second phase of the experiment consisted of an anagram test that had to be solved. The important point is that skin conductance levels indicated greater arousal for the group with escape facility.

The most important feature of these experiments, which has not been made explicit, is the operation of control by avoidance. The experiments of Brady (1958), which revealed ulcers in "executive" monkeys who had the control facility for avoiding shock, involves a similar situation without a pretreatment condition. Brady unfortunately did not assign his monkeys randomly to the escape and yoked groups. However, his design is essentially one of control by avoidance, and his results indicate that this is more stressful than being helpless. Weiss first pointed out that control by avoidance may be maximally stressful (Weiss 1971b, 1971c) because of the absence of feedback signals that allow the animal to know whether the response is successful. In addition, the point is worth making that control by avoidance may involve vigilance, expectancy changes, and extra effort, all of which are largely unreported or unmeasured in designs. These issues are developed in greater detail in the next chapter.

The main point to be established is that there may be different ways of establishing control. Control by avoidance may impose new demands on the individual and may be maximally stressful because the individual does not have the information that provides a basis for the perception of control. Thus, he may appear highly stressed in a situation where he exerts control because of the features of the behavior required or because he does not know that he is gaining control. Miller (1979), has developed the "minimax hypothesis." In accordance with this, a person has control in a situation to the extent that he can minimize maximum future danger. In control by avoidance, it may be objectively true that the individual is successfully avoiding shock, but it may continue to be the case that in terms of subjective assessment there is total uncertainty about the chances of minimizing maximum future danger.

The attempt to draw general conclusions about control and its relation to stress are fraught with difficulties, at least partly because of specific details of different paradigms. Also, there may be disparities between what is objectively true and what is perceived to be the case. However, it is argued that there is a sufficiently strong relationship between control and the level of experienced stress, the tolerance of noxious stimuli, and the responses made in the presence of hazard to provide a strong motive for a closer understanding of the mental processes involved in the perception of control.

Contingency as the Basis for Control

If a person indicates that he knows he has power or mastery over the environment, what he is really indicating is that he believes there is a contingent relationship between his action and the outcome. Contingency on successive trials must somehow be represented as a statistic of covariation between action and consequence. On this view, a subject is making the assumption that correlation implies causation; only if he makes this assumption can he deduce that the covariation of action and outcome implies that he has control.

It could be argued that the perception of contingent relationships of all kinds provides the basis of a stable world and thus that beliefs about control have much in common with beliefs about cause-and-effect relationships in general.

It is possible to distinguish "S–S contingency," which is concerned with independent variable events observed by a person in the "world outside," and "S–R contingency," concerned with internal contingencies between stimulus and response. In the case of the perception of control, the relationship of interest is what might be termed "R–S" contingency, or the relatedness of action and consequence. A person perceives control to the extent that action and consequence relate and lack of control to the extent that they do not.

It is also possible to distinguish different aspects of contingent R–S relationships. For example, a person may perceive control because a "no response" has a positive result, or because a "positive response" has a negative result. In the first case, he exerts control by no action, and in the second he is acting to prevent or block events; it is convenient to distinguish this by the label "incompatible contingency." In "compatible contingencies," a positive response results in a positive event or a negative response produces a negative outcome; in "incompatible" cases, the relationship is the reverse.

It is important to make these distinctions, because for any task a number of action/outcome relationships are possible. Which are selected as sources of information on which to base an estimate of control, is important. An example might be if a person were asked to decide whether sunsets at night produce fine weather the next day. He could choose a "sunset" or a "nonsunset" and then note the result: "rain" or "fine weather." Obviously, trials in which a "nonsunset" results in "fine weather" are just as useful in conveying information as cases where "sunset" results in "fine weather." Equally, "nonsunset" followed by "rain" and "sunset" followed by "rain" also provide information.

If we translate this into R–S concepts, then there are, therefore, at least four relationships a person may note in trying to decide whether he has control or not. Some or all of them may occur as a result of chance, and so ideally a person should use a statistical approach in order to make a decision about whether combinations in the stream of event/outcome pairs are greater than chance.

The cognitive task is likely to be difficult; even in relatively straightforward situations a person must notice, store, retrieve, and generalize from two or more types of "data stream" (e.g., "sunset–rain," "not sunset–rain," etc.). The question of interest is how he notices and attends to the different kinds of "event/outcome" pairs when he attempts to assess control overall. Although the research literature is complex, experiments have established that stresses are likely to change features of attention and memory. Therefore, a person trying to assess control level when he is already under some pressure may note aspects of the "contingency data stream" rather differently and may retrieve the representative statistic differently (see Chapters 7 and 8).

Also, people are not good at providing reliable estimates of event frequency. Howell and Burnett (1978) and Marques and Howell (1979) have pointed out the existence of "generator bias" whenever people are required to give overall frequency estimates. This phrase means that what a person believes is true of the system he is assessing will determine the estimates he gives. Put quite simply, if a person believes he is assessing a faulty machine, he will overreport evidence of faults. Could it therefore be the case that if a person believes that he cannot cope with a particular task he will overrepresent the mistakes he makes? This is important, because we have shown in experiments in Dundee that people generally expect to perform badly under adverse conditions. If this is the case, we would expect underrepresentation of control because of enhanced representation of errors and inefficiencies. These considerations are taken up in detail in Chapters 6 and 7.

Despite the complexity and demand presented by estimating and representing control, experiments by Jenkins and Ward (1965) and subsequently by Alloy and Abramson (1979) have shown that people are quite good at assessing the degree of contingency between action and outcome. Fisher and Ledwith (1983) have recently confirmed this. All three studies were concerned with relationships between response and subsequent event when skill was not involved. A subject merely chooses a response and receives the event that was programmed to be either contingent or random; he then estimates the level of contingency as a percentage of the total number of trials. Control assessments are positively correlated with objective contingency in these cases.

An issue of interest in relation to the question raised above concerning whether "generator bias" about poor performance in stressful conditions would lead to underestimation of control is partly addressed in the Alloy and Abramson study. Depressed subjects could be assumed to have a pessimistic "generator bias" because they typically undervalue their own performance (Beck, 1970). However, they continue to remain very logical in their assessments of contingency levels. A possible explanation is that the "generator bias" is very specific in the case of depressed subjects and is confined to cases where self-produced performance is being assessed.

The Alloy and Abramson study has shown that contingency assessment is affected by prevailing motivational conditions; positive features such as produced by the provision of incentive causes normal subjects to overestimate control levels through an "illusion of control." Fisher and Ledwith found that the effect was not true for performance in loud noise. Therefore, not all conditions that are positively arousing are associated with this effect. The issue is discussed in greater detail in Chapter 8.

There are studies that draw attention to the need to include in a model of the cognitive basis of control the idea that "performance relevance," or "success" are features. Both Bowers (1968) and Szpiler and Epstein (1976) have demonstrated the importance of successful task performance in reducing or avoiding the occurrence of a noxious event. An experiment by Coulter (1970) specifically showed that "performance relevance" may be an important feature—if subjects found their performance to be relevant to the reduction of the occurrence of electric shock, then improved performance led to reliable reduction in anxiety levels. Thus, at least one explanation is that control in a "desired direction" had been achieved; the subject had control over shock because he had control over a task that, if successful, would be capable of preventing shock. The number of contingent relationships involved in such assessments must be quite high; the point that control is an assessment that takes into account "intention" or direction of effect of action is emphasized.

In order to establish control, a person must perceive that what he does is instrumental in achieving a change in reality. But more importantly he must perceive that what he does achieves change in the desired direction. There could be a contingent relationship that is not desired, as for example when a person *always* fails examinations. It is possible that exposure to adverse circumstances, by reflecting changes in performance, results in certain regular contingent relationships that are not in the desired direction. A person under time pressure may always fail examinations by producing a certain type of behavior that will not help him to tackle problems. This would be contingency that is a regular and predictable but undesired aspect of this person's behavior.

In order to incorporate this into a model of the cognitive basis of control, it is necessary to include representation of action but also to include codes that will represent the selection of action with respect to the intention. It is useful to begin to develop a model that will provide the logical requirements for assessing control by considering in outline the basis of planned activity.

Figure 2.1, from Miller, Galanter, and Pribram (1960), provides a format for understanding these concepts. They provided the notion of a TOTE unit as the fundamental organizational unit of behavior that enabled a person to behave "with consequence in mind." In other words, behavior is assumed to be purposeful and addressed to a particular desired outcome. Thus, as illustrated by the now famous example of hammering a nail into wood, a person must first note a discrepancy between reality and

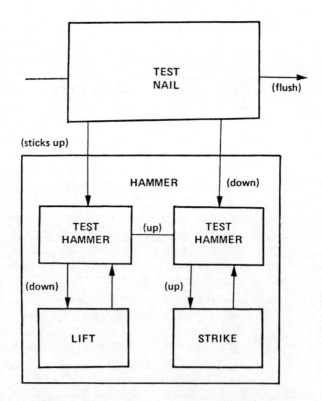

FIG. 2.1. The hierarchical plan for hammering nails. (Redrawn from Miller, Galanter, & Pribram, 1960, with the permission of the authors and Holt, Rhinehart and Winston.)

intention; if the nail is not flush with the wood, action is required. After action selection, the same comparison is made again, and the whole process loops until the nail is seen to be flush with the wood. TOTE thus describes the essential test–operate–test–exist cycle terminated only by a total resolution of the original discrepancy. Since action to strike the nail into the wood necessitates the lifting of a hammer, which in turn involves discrepancy detection and correction, the organization results in an imbedded series of TOTE systems, as illustrated in Fig. 2.1. At any point in the hierarchy of comparisons and decisions, a failure must have significance for the exercise of control and for the perception of control. However, different failures may have specific consequences in this respect; continued failure to hit the nail means that control is reduced, and the perception of control is accordingly modified; failure to detect the original discrepancy produced by the nail not being flush with the wood in the first place may mean that objectively there is loss of control, but subjectively the perception of control is not altered.

A fundamental directive for action is provided by discrepancy between the "state of reality" or the "data base" and the desired state of reality. Comparison between reality and intention provides the code for action selection and is assumed by Miller and colleagues to have energizing qualities.

Modification of the discrepancy produced by the internal code of reality and intention should provide a basis for the assessment of contingency, which includes the degree to which changes are in the *desired direction*. If a person notes that there is contingency between response and outcome but that the discrepancy value is not modified, he will be forced to conclude that he lacks the ability to choose and implement appropriate action. These two elements of information should have a marked effect on decisions about control.

A relevant consideration concerns how actions are selected in the first place. If establishing control requires reducing the discrepancy between reality and intention, it is convenient to have stored representations of appropriate kinds of action. In some cases, knowledge may be obtained by a comparison of previous action/consequence relationships. In other words, contingencies are stored, perhaps in modified form, but in such a way that a consequence may readily be associated with an action. For example, we might come to know that blunt knives squash tomatoes, where serrated-edged knives cut them. Byrne and Morton showed that actions may remain closely associated with stimuli in memory. For example, in generating a list of ingredients required in making an apple pie, ingredients are recalled in the order in which actions are required (see Morton, 1974).

A basis for understanding how action might be chosen with respect to consequence involves the storage and retrieval of action and consequence relationships. A theoretical formulation for understanding this is provided by ideomotor theory as formulated by James (1890) and more recently by Greenwald (1970). A major contribution to the understanding of the cognitive basis of stability in perception is provided by the principle of reafferance (see Von Holst, 1954). Basically, a movement copy (or copy of an efferent signal) is stored against the consequent change in stimulation (reafference). Correlation and comparison processes provide the basis of stability in the visual world. If the environment does not behave in the expected way, then a discrepancy is produced, in that the efferent copy evokes an "expectancy" (or expected reafferent signal) that does not match with the true reafferent signal. If this occurs, the perceptual world is no longer stable; this state may be likened to loss of control in perception. Sensory deprivation effects that involve either total reduction in stimulation or the reduction of pattern in the input to a level of randomness (visual noise) have been interpreted in this way (e.g., see Held, 1961). Basically, stability is ensured only if there is a reliable match between the expected and the obtained reafferent signal; the expected signal is selected by the action chosen.

Turning this formulation on its head, it could be argued that the action selected is chosen because it is likely to result in a reafferent result that is desirable. Thus the store of efferent copies and reafferent contingencies would provide a useful basis for action selection. The efferent signal is specified by the reafferent copy with which it is commonly associated.

Thus, as assumed by ideomotor theory, the efferent signal normally leaves a copy for comparison with the expected reafferent signal (the consequence of movement); the result determines perception and stability. However, this valuable set of reference codes might be used in quite a different way. A discrepancy between reality and intention could be used to specify a desired reafferent result. This, in turn, could then evoke the appropriate contingent efferent copy and thus lead to the selection of action. The storing of internal reference codes about contingency could therefore be very useful.

Cognitive Models of the Assessment of Control

If we now return to considerations concerning how a person may assess and represent control, it is clear that there are at least two possible elements. The first is frequency estimation of action and outcome relationships, and this is generally what experimenters are concerned with when they try to understand the basis of control.

The second element is more appropriate when a person is trying to assess whether he has the capability of changing reality in line with his aims or intentions. Here, it may not be enough to note the frequency of contingent relationships. It may be necessary to note contingency in the desired direction. At least one model we have been considering is a "knock-on" model of progress in resolving the discrepancy between reality and intention.

A reasonable assumption is that the perception of contingent relationships between action and outcome is an intrinsic part of the perception of control. If outcome did not respond to action, then the discrepancy would not be resolved, and there would be no progress. In other words, if action were *not* instrumental in forcing the nail into the wood, then the discrepancy between the position of the nail head and the desired position would not be resolved.

It is at this point that it is perhaps worth reminding the reader that what we are trying to understand is what precisely is involved in making an assessment about whether control or mastery of a situation is possible. There are two cognitive elements: One involves an estimate of the degree to which contingency between response and outcome is present, the other confirmation that progress is in the right direction.

In a pilot study conducted in Houston, using a Radio Shack microprocessor, we attempted to probe the question of what factors influence a person in the assessment of control. There are methodological difficulties with assessment of control mostly because interpretation given to the question may vary. Is it, for example, even meaningful to a subject to give him a hammer and a nail and to ask him to hit the nail on the head to hammer it into some wood and then ask him how much control he thinks he has? He might see fit to answer this from existing knowledge; he might expect 100% control, because hitting a nail on the head is "no problem."

With the help of an engineering student, a pilot study program that represented a long nail as a vertical line on the screen of a microprocessor was designed. A horizontal line at the base of the screen represented the surface of the wood. By depressing a key, a subject could "hit" the nail into the wood, and the vertical nail "sunk" accordingly.

We tried out a number of conditions. In condition A, the subject depressed the switch, and the nail moved by a constant unit each time, so that it took 20 units for it to become flush with the "wood." In condition B, the situation was essentially the same except that the same "hit" produced different movements of the nail, although in the end the same progress had been made after 20 units. In this condition R–S contingency varied from trial to trial, but the nail always moved toward the goal position. Subjects assigned to this condition produced the same 100% control estimates despite the fact that contingency relations varied; the same "hit" was producing different "nail progress"!

In condition C, we used the same design as for condition A, except that on a predetermined 25% proportion of occasions the nail did not respond to a "hit," and so no progress was made. Under these conditions people still continued to estimate that at the end of the task they had almost a 100% control. "Non-hits" were interpreted to be occasions when a person missed the nail.

In condition D, we actually made the nail back up out of the wood on a predetermined 25% of occasions. This meant that subjects "lost ground" in terms of progress toward the end point and could blame this on noncontingency.

Statistical comparisons between the data for seven subjects in each group showed that only in condition D, where the nail was beginning to behave outrageously, did subjects begin to lower their control estimate.

This might tend to suggest that a model such as the "progress model" best describes the basis of the reports. We attempted to clarify this by setting up condition A again and asking subjects what control they had at various points in the task. Only with the first 10 units did subjects give more cautious estimates of control; after that, most estimates approached 100%.

Clearly, however, if "progress information" is used, it is not in a way that suggests that estimates of control increase smoothly with the level of progress indicated by the state of the discrepancy. It is more likely that there is a threshold for decision, and once this is exceeded, estimates favor total control.

Before discussing these matters in greater detail, it is useful to look at the relevance of control as a possible key factor in different "life stress" conditions. It is at least arguable that many traumatic or worrying experiences are identified by changes in perceived control and perceived control loss. We pursue this in the next chapter and then consider possible ways in which control assessment may itself be influenced in conditions of stress.

3

Life-Stress Conditions
and Control

INTRODUCTION

This chapter is specifically addressed to consideration of the possible role played by control in various kinds of experiences people might have to encounter in life. The idea to be pursued is that many life-stress situations involve change in control levels and that response or adjustment depends on the perception of control, which is in turn dependent on cognitive processes. However, the very effect of being under pressure may cause changes in the cognitive processes on which successful adjustment may ultimately depend.

In addition, some stresses may depend for existence on the meaning and interpretation of reality. The assessment of control may be an intrinsic factor in determining the way a person interprets situations.

INTERNALLY DERIVED THREATS AND LOSS OF CONTROL

Discrepancy in Plans

A point made in the previous chapter was that in order to achieve control, a person must reduce the discrepancy between reality, or "the way the world is," and his intention or goal. Contingency assessment may therefore be a necessary but not a sufficient condition for the perception of control; discrepancy reduction across successive trials provides an index of progress. Deducing control level from information concerning discrepancy modification implies noting trial-by-trial information and representing it statistically. There may be critical periods in a person's life where he is faced with life changes or with sudden catastrophe; in these cases the need to assess and establish control may be of paramount importance.

At this point, it is important to emphasize sources of influence on the likelihood of achieving control. The first is that the discrepancy as we have defined it is influenced by two variables: *reality*, or the "way the world is," and *intention*, or what is desired. Both these variables may be independently or jointly influenced to make it easier or more difficult for a person to perform well and establish control.

A person with very high ambition may create a greater disparity by increasing the distance between reality and intention. Equally, the opposite is true for a person of very low ambition. The task of achieving control may be variously influenced by these unknown factors.

In addition, there is the importance of knowledge and capability. A person of poor capability may have, right from the outset, no chance of achieving even moderate levels of control. Therefore the capacity for effective action must be an important variable. In addition, even with adequate capacity, a person rendered less efficient by pressure created by stress will again be reduced in his ability to achieve control.

Although it is outside the scope of this book to consider the ways in which goals and intentions are formulated, there are some important general comments to be made. First of all, many have argued that stresses in modern life arise partly from the pressures for success inherent in Western society. Work by Mills (1973) on suicide rates in young people and also on anorexia nervosa in adolescents has suggested that increases in incidence may reflect these pressures. Mills points out that the rate of breakdown in young people is very high. His figures on anorexia nervosa suggest incidence rates described as about ten times as high as about ten years before. Moreover, he reports that in over 70% of young women between 16 and 23 years of age the time of starting a crash diet corresponded with that of an important examination. Attempted suicide figures are described as reaching 50% of medical admissions for young women in their twenties and 40% for young men. Mills further quotes data to suggest that in one area psychiatrists report that 50% of depression cases involve the age group between 15 and 24 years.

Mills' main argument concerns the pressure of competition, which he sees as a general pervasive influence in society. One obvious way in which these pressures might work is by raising the level of aims and ambition within individuals.

The link between capitalism and protestantism in providing the motive for success was explored by McClelland (1961), who examined the content of childrens' stories. The amount of content that stressed achievement was specifically related to economic development in different countries. In general, studies suggested that the protestant ethic and the capitalist motive encourage work and concern with success. If Mills is right and the pressure for success is increasing, it might be argued that there would be recent evidence of this in the content of childrens' books and games.

A related important point noted by Horney (1937) is that there may be a deep conflict of ideals in society; there is stated concern with ideals of kindness and humility, but society respects and rewards success.

If goals and intentions are variously influenced by pressures, we might expect that there is an increased difficulty for establishing control. A person may feel he cannot possibly achieve the success he desires. On first consideration, this will influence the outcome of encounters in which success in any sense matters. A larger number of situations will come to represent failure and loss of control for a larger number of people.

However, human motive is likely to be more complex and rich than this rather simplistic analysis suggests. Formal experiments by McClelland et al.(1953) and Atkinson (1957) have suggested that the achievement motive is not uniform across individuals. Two kinds of persons can be identified: one more likely to be motivated by fear of failure and one by the need for achievement and success. These two different motives may be reflected quite differently in the tackling of daily tasks. Generally, high achievement is indexed by subjects' performance on the Thematic Apperception Test, whereas fear of failure is indexed by means of a questionnaire designed by Mandler and Sarason (1952) to measure test anxiety.

The achievement- and success-oriented individual is more likely to seek achievement-related activity, whereas fear-of-failure individuals are more likely to protect themselves from it. Therefore, we might expect that the discrepancy generated for the two groups of individuals will differ in that the frequency with which fear-of-failure people encounter difficult situations would be reduced. We might even expect that they would seek to control negative encounters by avoidance. However, the situation is more complex than this. The achievement-oriented individuals are found to prefer and persist with tasks of intermediate difficulty, where success is possible and failure is unlikely, but where there is interest and challenge. By contrast, fear-of-failure individuals will take on very easy tasks or very difficult tasks, because in the first case they cannot fail and in the second they have an excuse for failure because they could be expected to succeed (see Atkinson & Feather, 1966).

There are experimental tests of this distinction. A good example is the ring-toss game, where subjects choose the distance to stand from a target in tossing a ring. High achievers prefer middle distances; fear-of-failure individuals have been shown to select either short or long distances. In a self-selection experiment conducted by Mouton (1965), subjects selected a task from one of three difficulty levels, after having failed or succeeded on a first task. High-achievement individuals chose a high difficulty level if they had succeeded on a first task, but selected the easy task if they had not. Fear-of-failure individuals selected the easy task after success and the difficult task after failure.

Therefore, there are differences that are direct reflections of the anticipated consequences in the discrepancy likely to be generated by individuals. Fear-of-failure individuals may generate an intention, producing a discrepancy with reality that they know they will not be able to reduce. They are protected from the consequence of failure in terms of their own prestige by knowing that no one could be expected to succeed. This, of course, has implications for understanding situations that might be thought to represent loss of control; these situations may also be part of the design and intended by certain sorts of people.

Persistence is equally likely to be affected by the nature of the discrepancy generated. On first consideration, individuals should persist until they achieve total success or establish control. However, persistence is likely to be subject to a number of complex influences.

Persistence and dedication have been argued by Welford (1965) to be important elements in academic success. These might be argued to be indicative of stability and thus to reflect personality an anxiety. However, Furneaux' (1962) classic study of the academic success of University engineering students showed that the relationship between stability and success was far from straightforward. His study showed that the greatest failure rates (61%) were associated with stability and extraversion, whereas the greatest success (21% failure) was associated with instability and introversion. Logically, it is necessary to assume either that persistence is dictated by an instruction that is part of the goal—such as, "keep trying until you eventually get there"—or that the persistence factor is independent and reflects a general personality characteristic.

Feather (1961) presented subjects with an unsolvable mental problem and measured the period of persistence. The success motive was found to have a complex relationship with persistence in that high-achievement individuals, far from persisting for a longer period when they failed to be successful, were found to persist for less time. In other words, the struggle to achieve control was rapidly abandoned when success was not immediately forthcoming.

This might be of some importance in understanding reaction to life events. High achievers who choose to try to succeed with a problem may disengage quickly when the "going is tough." If so, this could be seen as protection against prolonged negative experiences in life and as a manifestation of a rather "optimistic" strategy.

A different formulation is presented by Weiner and associates (e.g., see 1971). They suggest that an appraisal is made of any task at the onset, and this will affect willingness to undertake the task. One important decision concerns whether control is internal because ability is involved, or external because task success does not depend on skill and is a question of luck. Weiner assumes that the causal attributions made by an individual distinguish the high- from the low-achievement-oriented individuals. It is assumed that the attribution determines the form of observable behavior. High-achievement-oriented individuals believe they are in control; low-achievement-oriented individuals believe they are not. Comparisons by Kukla (1972) between subjects differing in achievement motivation showed that when the task consisted of predicting the next number in a series, high-achievement individuals attributed successful predictions to skill and ability; low-achievement individuals correctly attributed success to chance. Moreover, the persistence aspect was also found to be related to causal attribution: High-achievement individuals were found to perceive failure in terms of lack of effort and were more likely to persist, whereas low-achievement individuals were likely to decide that they were not able to control the outcome and were more likely to give up.

These now classic studies raise the point that an unresolved discrepancy may not be stressful per se. It is further interpretation given to this mental representation that is likely to count. Quite clearly, if fear-of-failure individuals will opt for a task so difficult that success is impossible, then failure per se is not critical. It is failure when a person could be expected to succeed that is stressful. Equally, achievement-oriented individuals do not persist when circumstances tell them success is unlikely. Therefore, the struggle for control is not prolonged indefinitely even for those who want to succeed and believe at least initially that control is possible.

It is perhaps important to establish this, because it is otherwise tempting to make some rather simpler deductions. Studies on personality and the perception of control by Rotter and his associates (e.g., see 1954, 1966) have clearly established population differences in control assessments. They are distinguished on the externality/internality dimension. Those who score high on "externality" on the Rotter questionnaire endorse items that indicate that they believe that life is controlled by chance and there is little to be done about it; those who score high on "internality" endorse items that indicate that they believe that the individual has a strong part to play in determining his life. On simplest consideration we might expect "internalizers" to continue to struggle for control, whereas "externalizers" would give up rather easily. Although this view has experimental support, the above considerations must be borne in mind. We will be discussing these and related issues when we develop the notion of a hierarchical model of control decisions later in the book (Chapters 9 and 10).

It is perhaps useful to summarize at this stage the points we have made so far:

1. The size of the discrepancy between reality and intention may be influenced by a number of factors, including chance events in life and pressures that influence ambition and motivation.
2. Failure to resolve the discrepancy and make progress toward achieving control may not always be the important factor in determining the level of stress. There must be a higher-order interpretation.
3. Persistence may not always be an inevitable response to failure to obtain control. High-achievement individuals may disengage when success is not easily forthcoming.

Common Denominators of Stressful Situations

We now consider some of the basic features of situations considered stressful with the aim of looking to see how some of the ideas about the role of control would fit in. Often there are other existing explanations concerned with why particular situations have stressful properties. The "control" explanation may have only the status of an alternative hypothesis. Nevertheless, we believe the idea that change, loss, or breakdown of existing control is a key feature of many unpleasant experiences is worth pursuing.

Conflict

There is a wide and varied literature on conflict. Conflict may be induced experimentally by presenting an individual with two possibilities with strong cost or high positive reward attached to attainment of both, but with the built-in limitation that because of common elements or incompatibilities, both cannot be attempted.

There is a wide and varied literature on conflict. The topic has been an intrinsic part of a number of lines of psychological inquiry. Freud (1943) gave emphasis to conflict within the major systems of the unconscious as a determinant of neurosis in his patients. Pavlov (1928) also gave central position to conflict, produced experimentally by reduction in discriminable difference between critical stimuli, in the causation of neurotic behavior. Many forms of normal behavior have been argued by various authors to be "devices" for reducing or minimizing conflicts. Distortions of thinking and perception, dreams, and imagery have all been argued to represent conflict resolution. Conflict, variously defined, has been cited as a principal cause of strong emotional activity (e.g., Hebb, 1949; Brown & Forbes, 1951) and is measured in terms of automatic activity, disruption of on-going perceptual motor processes, slowing down of response times. Berlyne (1960) makes the point that the degree of conflict should not be identified with the severity of the effects of conflict. The latter aspects are assumed to depend on the kinds of responses that are competing. Both Lewin (1935) and Miller (1944) are quoted by Berlyne as supporting the notion that conflict between approach tendencies may be less evocative and more likely to be resolved than conflict between avoidance tendencies or approach-avoidance conflicts. Berlyne distinguishes the severity of conflict in terms of the nearness in strength of competing factors and the absolute strength of competing response tendencies.

Whereas the "stress-induction" properties of conflict are not in dispute, some authors place very important emphasis on conflict as a primary causal factor in neurotic disorder. For example, Cameron and Margaret (1951) regard conflict as central to behavior pathology and define it as "The natural interference of incompatible systems" (p. 252). This type of formulation assumes that conflict is an inevitable consequence of complex behavior; when many actions are available, then some will be in conflict. An individual richly endowed with "action possibilities" may find not only that he needs more evidence in order to decide what to do but that he is more likely to encounter conflict. The description of conflict situations provided by Cameron and Margaret is based on approach and avoidance factors and results in three major categories of conflict: double approach (positive valence toward two incompatible objects), double avoidance (negative valence toward two objects), and approach-avoidance. The important aspect of conflict is that the individual cannot satisfy both demands, because incompatible or antagonistic response tendencies are invoked. Cameron and Margaret further emphasize that real-life situations involve multiple conflicts.

A contrasting descriptive classification of conflict is presented by Lazarus (1966). Conflicts are described with respect to "source"; external conflicts are engendered by events outside the control of the individual, whereas internal conflicts arise from within the personality system. In the Grinker and Spiegel (1945) study of air crew on active combat missions, each man reported experiencing conflict between fear of danger and the need to appear brave. The source of conflict could be described as "internal," although the distinction is questionable since often an internally produced conflict arises because of acceptance of externally imposed values or acceptance of authority. As mentioned earlier, the psycho-analytic writings of Horney (1937) contain references to deep-rooted conflicts in Western society.

Traditional learning theory emphasizes the notion that the world consists of a universe of punishment and rewards. The principle of hedonism dictates that an organism will seek pleasure and avoid pain. Based on this principle, conflict arises when the organism cannot have one without the other or is forced to decide which of two punishments to take or which of two rewards to accept. Figure 3.1 illustrates the model proposed by Gray and Smith (Gray, 1971), which locates neurophysiological equivalents of the universe of reward and punishment. The key areas are located in the mid-brain (periventricular system). The animal "learns" to avoid activity in the punishment center; a stop system ensures that it terminates all behavior that engenders punishment. Activity in the reward system activates the command "approach" while at the same time having a positive influence on the arousal system. In conflict, both systems are assumed to be activated. Thus the organism is forced to make a decision between the alternatives. During this period there may be vascillation behavior as the animal attempts movements in one direction and then the other. In the case of human beings, the conflict may be more subtle, requiring the weighing-up of consequences based on alternative courses of action.

The possibility that performance decrement in dual-task experiments relates directly to response interference rather than to attentional phenomena has been advanced by Reynolds (1964, 1966). According to this view, competing response tendencies are set up in any situation where more than one response is required. The classic "refractory theory"

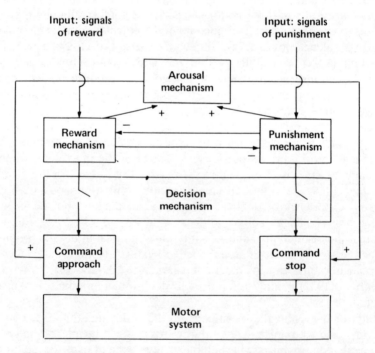

FIG. 3.1.   Part of the Gray and Smith model for conflict and discrimination learning. (Redrawn from Gray, 1971, with the permission of the author and Weidenfeld & Nicholson.)

paradigm developed by Welford (1952), in which two signals requiring two separate responses are made to occur in rapid succession, is argued to involve response tendencies that are in competition. Delay in responding to the second of the two signals is argued to be a function of response competition: The prepotent or dominant response will suffer the smallest delay (see Hermon & Kantowitz, 1970). The response competition model must place emphasis on the production of competing responses; when no response is required, there should be no interference. Both Nickerson (1965) and Kay and Weiss (1961) have reported delays in simple response time when no response is required, although the magnitude of the delay is less than when response production is required. There has never been any suggestion that these situations are stressful.

The existence of response competition alone is not a sufficient condition for stressful experiences. There must be some directive to produce both responses under circumstances when they both cannot be produced. Under these conditions we might imagine that two discrepancies are generated and only one is modified by action-related consequences; the other remains unmodified. In terms of the control model, there will be loss of control regarding one of the conflicting tendencies; conflict maximizes control uncertainty.

In a series of studies on psychological and physiological responses to parachute jumping, Epstein (1967) and Fenz (1964, 1969) have elaborated on the approach-avoidance conflict model as described originally by Lewin (1935) and Miller (1944). Positive valence or approach to the jump is equated with anxiety; avoidance is equated with inhibition. Epstein and Fenz propose that the parachute jump represents a goal with both positive and negative valence. A gradient of anxiety and a gradient of inhibition develops; the latter is assumed to be steeper than the former, and this is assumed to become increasingly evident with repeated successful exposure to the source of the anticipated stress. Epstein and Fenz assume that the interaction between the two gradients reflects a shift in attention para-meters so that the individual has a lowered threshold for environmental cues that are "not relevant to the jump." These may act as warning signals that help the individual to prepare for and adapt to the forthcoming event. This is reflected in the sharp increase in reactivity early in the sequence of events leading up to the jump followed by a decrease, so that arousal at the time of jumping is normal (e.g., see Fenz & Epstein, 1962, 1967). As Figs. 3.2a and 3.2b illustrate, the inverted-V funtion occurs selectively for jumpers; experience and competence seem to be determining factors. For experienced jumpers, the V function is most evident for good performers; poor performers continue at a high level of physiological activity im-mediately prior to the jump, although, as illustrated in Fig. 3.2b there is a slight decrease in arousal after the 1000-ft time marker. In the case of

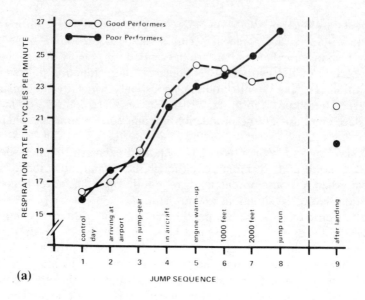

(a)

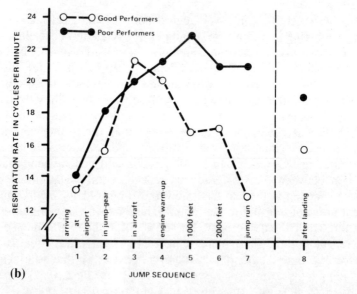

(b)

FIGS. 3.2a and 3.2b.   Respiration rate during a jump sequence of good and poor performers who were novice (top half) and experienced (bottom half) parachutists. (From "Stress and its mastery: Predicting from laboratories to real life," by W. D. Fenz, *Canadian Journal of Behavioural Sciences*, 1973, 5(4), 332–346. Copyright 1973 Canadian Psychological Association. Reprinted by permission.)

novices, both good and poor performers jump at a high base level of arousal, but, as illustrated by Fig. 3.2a, the level of good performers suggests that they have begun to bring anxiety levels down before the jump. The obvious question of interest is whether the group whose arousal levels come down prior to jumping perform better as a result; in other words, whether the reduction in arousal causes the improved jump performance. Alternatively, it may be that—as Fenz argues—the reduction in arousal prior to jumping reflects a change in thinking, which is a prerequisite for good jumping. An important contribution to the "cause-and-effect dilemma" is provided by the data in which experienced and inexperienced jumpers are concerned, because the V is experience-dependent as well as being "good-jump"-related; also, the change occurs in advance of the jump, suggesting that "jump quality" and experience cause changes before the jump occurs.

A study by Fenz, Kluck, and Bankart (1969) showed that the V curve of arousal preceding the jump is lost after a jumping accident. This effect is illustrated in Figure 3.3, which shows the effect of stimuli of different levels of relevance to the jump in terms of the anxiety evoked. After an accident, the anxiety levels to relevant stimuli rise. On the assumption that the level of skill and experience remains the same, such changes must be accounted for in terms of the new "accident information" available to the subject.

These studies have been described in detail, because it is plausible that an aspect of the conflict reported for parachute jumpers that is closely associated with anxiety prior to the jump concerns a mental struggle for control. Experienced jumpers have internal codes on which to base a control assessment and are able to use these to resolve the conflict prior to the moment of the jump. From previous successes experienced, good jumpers are more likely to assess the chances of control optimistically.

Interruption

"Interruption" is a description of a category of conditions believed to be involved in creating tension, and it provides an explanation of common features that are stressful in other situations (e.g., see Mandler, 1975). From the perspective of experimental research, interruption, otherwise described as blocking or thwarting of behavior, has deep roots in psychology. Zeigarnik (1927) studied the impact of interruption on various memory tasks. Performance on those tasks that had been interrupted was enhanced, and this effect was explained in terms of "unresolved tension." Unfortunately, there are now a number of experiments that fail to show the "Zeigarnik effect" (e.g., see Van Bergen, 1968); the evidence must at least be regarded as equivocal.

The idea that completion of a task may have impetus or tension associated with it does emphasize the dynamic aspect of a plan. When

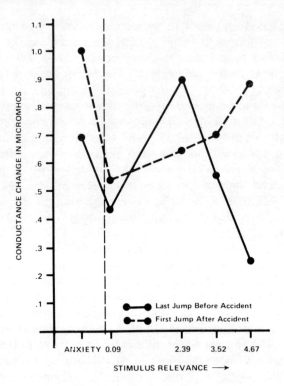

FIG. 3.3.   Galvanic skin response of an experienced parachutist tested on the day of a jump before an accident and again on the day of a jump following an accident. (From "The effect of threat and uncertainty on mastery of stress," by W. D. Fenz, B. L. Kluck and C. P. Bankart, *Journal of Experimental Psychology*, 1969, 79, 473–479. Copyright 1969 by the American Psychological Association. Reprinted by permission of the author.)

Miller, Galanter, and Pribram (1960) introduced the concept of the plan as the fundamental unit of skilled behavior, there was a stated assumption that the plan had energizing properties that created tension toward completion. One possibility is, therefore, that any condition of blocking or thwarting causes sudden release of energy that is experienced as tension and arousal.

Mandler (1975) proposes that interruption of a sequence leaves available the energy engendered by the plan, and that this may have emotional consequences for the individual. The final form of the emotional impact is assumed to be influenced by context. Fry and Ogston (1971) demonstrated that interruption of an "organized cognitive sequence" renders the individual vulnerable to moods induced by a confederate. This is consistent with the experimental findings by Schacter and Singer (1962), which showed that the psychological impact of injected adrenaline depended on the psychosocial context provided for individuals. Mandler further argues that individuals perceive and seek to overcome the consequences of interruption. Mandler and Watson (1966) argue that when "no response is available whereby arousal initiated by interruption can be terminated, the emotion expected would be anxiety, distress or fear" (p. 265). The individual thwarted by circumstances may engage in what Mandler describes as agitated "non-functional behavior." If he cannot open the door of his car, he may shake the door violently or kick the car. Although these behaviors are argued to stem from energy levels that cannot be channelled according to the original plan, the possibility that occasionally some of them may be reinforced by success cannot be discounted.

There is some evidence (Mandler, 1964) that interruption of verbal material produces arousal, and that the more highly organized the material in terms of "tightness and invariance of structure," the greater the probable consequence of interruption (see Mandler, 1975). The evidence is not, however, particularly strong, and there is, as Sher (1971) points out, difficulty due to the confounding of organization with the novelty value of interruption. To make sense of a relationship between the degree of organization and the impact of interruption, Mandler must assume that highly organized plans have greater associated energy and persistence, because the consequences of interruption are direct functions of associated energy levels.

In addition, Mandler argues for the primacy of interruption as a fundamental cause of stress. Data on the effects of nonreward in terms of emotional consequences are readily available (see Amsel, 1962). Mandler argues that the frustrating effects of nonreward may be subsumed within the general hypothesis that interruption has emotional impact. Further, he cites Berkowitz's (1964) studies of aggressive acts, which show that if completion of an organized sequence is prevented, "internal tension is induced" (Mandler, 1975, p. 164).

A general proposition on the effects of interruption as stated by Mandler (1964) is that the interruption of an integrated response sequence produces a state of arousal followed by emotional behavior. In addition, Mandler and Watson (1966) specify (1) persistence toward completion of the interrupted sequence, (2) increased vigor with which the sequence is pursued, and (3) substitution of an alternative element or sequence.

The major consequence of interruption in the absence of relevant ways of continuing or substituting will produce behavior that is characterized by anxiety. This very fundamental effect provides a basis for understanding a number of "scenarios" people and animals find stressful. For example, frustrative nonreward, helplessness, thwarting, blocking, major change, or loss may all fit the basic formula that interruption of an on-going sequence is involved.

There are, however, two embedded explanations, both evoked by Mandler. The first concerns tension release from a blocked plan. The second is that control availability is changed. If there is no alternative for completing the task or problem, a person is left with the perception of loss of control. Mandler and Watson (1966) propose that arousal coupled with unavailability of alternative responses feature when the organism is helpless and are preconditions for anxiety.

There are a number of factors that need more careful explaining. If a greater degree of organization is associated with greater consequences of disruption, this might favor tension release associated with the existing plan as an explanation, rather than problems with establishing control. If a substitute activity is helpful, on the other hand, this would tend to favor the importance of control rather than tension release, because tension should be closely bound to the original sequence of events.

Mandler and Watson (1966) report experiments stemming from a sentence-learning paradigm developed by Mandler (1964), in which a word was presented every 3 sec until learning had occurred, and then the words had to be anticipated. What was described as of importance was not only the degree of organization in the learned sequence, but the relevance of the interrupting event: Relevant interruption produced less behavioral disruption. This could suggest that loss of control is critical, since the more relevant the interrupting event, the greater the chance that it can be absorbed into an existing cognitive framework.

Change

Change is so closely bound up with interruption that, when considering the effect of changes in life, we again face those same theoretical dilemmas. Change involves interruption of previous sequences. It might be "part of the plan" or deliberate, as when a person changes his job; it may be unavoidable, as in enforced redundancy or bereavement.

Stewart and Salt (1981) suggest that control of the change itself might be quite critical. In the case of people in subordinate roles, changes may occur as the result of the decisions of others. In the case of those in dominant roles there is control over others and control over the instigation of change. Females in traditional roles are distinguished from males in traditional roles in this respect. For the same amount of change, males are argued to be likely to become ill, and females to be depressed.

Research has indicated a strong effect of geographical mobility on the probability of ill health. In particular, heart disease and high blood pressure appear to be predisposed by high rates of geographical mobility (e.g., Medalie et al., 1973; Cruze-Coke et al., 1964). In addition, there is some evidence that conditions brought about by antigens also become more likely in those who have moved to work in new unfamiliar environments (e.g., Holmes, 1956; Christenson & Hinkle, 1961). These studies are difficult to interpret because not only is it difficult to infer causation from the occurrence of correlations, but there is evidence to suggest that a geographical move alone is not a sufficient condition for ill health (e.g., Foster, 1927; Tung, 1927; Marks, 1967). It is possible that those who move are self-selected in some way that increases the vulnerability to illness.

Exactly the same argument obtains for mental disorder as a possible reaction. Studies such as that of Leff, Roatch, and Bunney (1970) have indicated the existence of geographical moves as possible factors in depressive disorder. Leff's study indicates that in a sample of 40 consecutive clinical cases, geographical move was the third most frequent in a list of ten precipitants. The occurrence of these precipitants was concentrated in the month preceding the onset of depressive symptoms.

Despite the interpretive difficulties, it does appear that a geographical move may operate as a powerful factor in people's lives. Recent research on the Life Event Scale (Holmes & Rahe, 1967) and the subsequent introduction of the Schedule of Recent Experiences have endorsed the effect of geographical move as a stress factor in people's lives and have underlined the idea that it is the *degree of adjustment* required by change in life history that is important. A life-stress scale of the amount of adjustment required by life events as subjectively assessed (Masuda & Holmes, 1967) was subsequently modified in favor of an index of the number of life-change units (LCUs). The probability of later mental disorder was greater if the number of LCUs was high, irrespective of the nature of the change.

There seems to be agreement that change is a major source of stress in life. It is likely to have a greater effect on the individual than negative experiences, may be associated with cumulative effects increasing the risk of illness and mental disorder, and is likely to have greatest impact on those who are already vulnerable.

Geographical change may provide a major source of other changes associated with housing, employment, education, and life style. It may be associated with preexisting "superordinate" changes resulting in upward or downward mobility. For all these reasons it is difficult to isolate specific factors in the impact of geographical mobility.

It would be fair to say that although the fundamental importance of change as a stress in people's lives has been established, there has been little research into the nature of psychological states following a move and the nature of the adjustment process. There are at least two hypotheses of importance. Firstly, a move may be stressful because it interrupts a highly organized life process that involves detailed plans for daily existence. Alternatively, the important source of the stress may be the encounter with a new environment. A person is faced with high uncertainty about control and may not know what to expect.

A study conducted by the author in 1976 using Edinburgh University medical students and groups of undergraduate students in Dundee was concerned with the phenomenon of homesickness as a reaction to geographical change (Fisher, 1983f). The study was initiated because students reported that their work had been adversely affected by "homesickness" in the first half of the university year. An initial investigation conducted in Dundee simply asked for impressions and experiences in the first half of the university year. Under these conditions, 39% of 25 randomly chosen first-year students used the term "homesick" somewhere in the description given, as compared with 15% of 20 second-year students. All students involved in this initial study met the criterion that there was a substantial geographical distance involved in a move to university and that the previous "home environment" remained in existence. Any move from a geographical location greater than 50 miles from a radius defined by the position of the university was counted as sufficient for a "substantial" move. This might be an important moderator of effect, because geographical distance dictates cost in terms of economic and effort factors, of visits, and of contact with the previous environment.

Table 3.1 summarizes the results of some of the main features of the study. As seen in the table, when given the term "homesickness" to which to respond, more subjects reported the feelings. This was significant statistically for both first- and second-year students sampled.

TABLE 3.1.
Summary of Data from Preliminary Study of Reports of Homesickness
in University Students

	Diary study reports		Homesickness scale	
	1st years	2nd years	1st years	2nd years
'Homesick'	64.1%	13.1%	71.8%	20.2%

Data on homesickness episodes from homesickness diary studies

(4-week reports from 1st year students)

$\overline{X}$ frequency of episodes per day (self-reports)	Range of time occupied by episode	$\overline{X}$ length of episode
2.84	9.3–222.4 min	75.1 min

The main part of the study consisted of providing students in their first, second, or third year of university with a stenciled format that provided descriptions of behavior in terms of whether it was active or passive and whether it was produced in the company of other people or when the subject was alone. Subjects thus attempted to describe their own behavior by hatching in one of four columns against a 15-minute time scale provided down the left-hand side of the page. The four activity descriptions were: active/alone; active/in company; passive/alone; passive/in company. In addition, there was a fifth column, which enabled a subject to record periods of homesickness on the clear instruction that homesickness feelings may overlap with any of these behavior types. All subjects filled in the homesickness column in a way that indicated not a general pervasive state of homesickness but a state in which bouts or episodes occurred during the waking day. In general terms, 64.1% of first-year students gave some indication of periods of homesickness during a two-week period, as indicated by responses per day on these forms. This compared with 13.1% of second- and third-year students. Each reported episode was between 9.3 min and 222.4 min duration. On average, 2.9 episodes per day were reported. The periods reported were not randomly distributed across the 2-hr periods during the day ($0.5 > p < .01$) but occurred with increased frequency during early morning and late evening. A significantly greater proportion of episodes were reported for cases where the subject was alone and passive. There is no way of knowing whether this is a cause or consequence or is merely concurrent with homesickness episodes.

The "homesickness effect," does raise problems for any model that purports to evaluate change in terms of future events only. It is clear that preoccupation was not concerned with the future but with the past. There was a strong longing for the previous "other" environment, which seems counterproductive in terms of getting adjusted to the new one. If it is argued that these preoccupations are functional, then we have to assume that establishing control over a new environment depends on sifting out the old information from the previous environment. Clearly, if this were a prerequisite of adjustment to change, all individuals would report it. The fact that they do not suggests that we might be looking at a population of poor adjusters in whom return to the previous environment where control was possible is preferable to thinking about the future.

The possible advantages of "worry work" in advance have already been mentioned (Chapter 1). Janis (1958) showed that the benefits of anticipating a forthcoming surgical operation may be seen in terms of subsequent emotional reaction and recovery in the postoperative phase. Sarason (1972, 1975) emphasized the debilitating effects of worry that was preoccupied with the self and with thoughts of the consequences of failure in test environments. Neither of these contributions enables us to understand the "homesickness response" to change.

One possibility is that the sifting-through of old plans is, for some individuals, functional as a prerequisite for establishing control of the new environment. Rather as bridge players may benefit from reflecting on possible moves and countermoves after a game, thinking about the "old" life may provide information helpful for the establishing of control in the new environment. Research is needed to find more out about the thinking patterns in those who report homesickness and about their subsequent adjustment to the new environment.

Indications from students who took part in the study suggest that depressed work efficiency results from homesickness. The effect seems manifest in an inability to concentrate on lectures or to cope with written work. Agitation and anxiety and a desire to contact home were described most frequently. Also, students claimed that thoughts were intrusive and that they often felt worried and preoccupied. It would fit well with the theme of the first chapter in this book that a major source of inefficiency in stress may be due to the occurrence of high mental work in stress. Moves may create conditions in which a person is likely to be concerned with thoughts about his home environment. This is "task irrelevant" in the way described by Hamilton for the debilitating effects of test anxiety (see Hamilton, 1974) but may turn out to have beneficial properties in the end. We simply do not have enough evidence formally obtained to enable us to make sense of this at the moment. A study is currently underway concerning homesickness in university students and boarding-school children, and it is hoped to resolve some of the above issues.

Change is also produced by personal loss. Bereavement studies have shown that there is again a reflective component in which intrusive material concerning the person is dominant. Parkes (1978), in his account of both typical and atypical bereavement patterns, describes an anxious searching phase in which there is a tendency to relive events leading up to the death. In atypical grief the period of mourning is more prolonged and is usually accompanied by guilt and self-reproach. A later phase of withdrawal and depression with occasional bursts of panic is common.

There are a number of factors that influence the pattern of bereavement that provide some useful information about the effects of change. Firstly, "anticipatory preparation" afforded by some deaths influences the reaction of the bereaved; secondly, the degree of dependency is a factor; thirdly, being able to talk about the dead person may be a prerequisite for adjustment (Maddison, 1968). Perhaps dominant plans that include the ill or dead person are slowly reviewed and modified. There are possible comparisons with Janis' observations that worry work in advance will modify the adverse effects of surgical operations. It is plausible that there is a balance struck between anticipatory worry work and reflective postevent processes and that both involve roughly the same degree of cognitive reorganization.

Helplessness and Responsibility

The terms "helplessness" and "responsibility" are both closely bound to the concept of control. Helplessness occurs when control is absent. Responsibility has been used to describe conditions in which control has to be exercised over a period of time. Recent research has emphasized that a disposition to react to situations with helplessness can be induced in animals and people as a result of treatments received. Alloy and Seligman (1979) distinguish a perceptual bias toward perceiving noncontingency and an expectational bias toward predicting noncontingency. Both are assumed to occur as a result of treatments. The former leads a person to see noncontingency more readily, the latter to use existing information to predict future noncontingent relationships.

Many animal studies purporting to distinguish responsibility and helplessness have used a yoked design technique so that two animals both receive the same total amount of punishment, but only one of the pair has a means of preventing or terminating the punishment course. Using this technique with rats, Mowrer and Viek (1948) showed greater disruption of learned sequences for the animal who, because of absence of the possibility of control, was deemed helpless. Two groups of rats were fed in a fixed place and then shocked in the place where they had been fed. One group had an instrumental response because jumping to avoid shock was possible; the other group was yoked and received the same punishment. The group with instrumental control showed much less disruption of the previously learned positive response to food.

By contrast, using a similar yoked design, experiments by Brady (1958; Brady et al., 1958) demonstrated that in monkeys the responsible animal who could avoid shock by pressing a lever was the one who developed ulcers. It is possible that helplessness and responsibility are different kinds of stress, with different influences over time. However, one of the problems is that Brady did not allocate monkeys at random to control and executive positions. It remains an open question whether or not there was an interaction with responsibility and "successful avoidance learning," in the "executive monkey" group.

A replication by Weiss (1971) using rats showed that the helpless group were more subject to ulceration than those who were given control (Weiss, 1971). Weiss makes a very important point from the results of his own experiments (see Weiss, 1968, 1970, 1971a, 1971b, 1971c); he noted that the probability of ulceration increases with the number of coping resources but correlates inversely with feedback indicating the success of the response. The most stressful conditions are those in which an animal has to continue to respond but gains little information about the relative success of the responses. As described in previous chapters, Brady's "responsive" animals were achieving control without being provided with information to this effect because successful responses prevented shock. Studies by Mason (1968) have confirmed the high stress levels associated with the exercise of control by avoidance, in terms of high catecholamine and 17-OHCS levels, and have demonstrated the persistence of the stress response across successive episodes. It is important to emphasize that control by avoidance may be operated by responding either passively or actively to avoid events. Some kinds of withdrawal behavior may be a form of passive resistance. The issue is taken up in the latter part of the book.

Seligman (1975) submitted dogs to the stress of uncontrollable electric shock that was both intense and frequent. Each animal was presented with 64 unescapable shocks prior to being placed in an avoidance training procedure with nonshocked (control) dogs. Whereas the control dogs rapidly learned to avoid shock by leaping into a safer part of the cage, two-thirds of the preshocked (experimental) dogs failed to learn. The strength of the acquisition of helplessness is illustrated by the fact that relatively few adaptive responses were made, even when, in the avoidance of condition, escapes were produced by chance, help, or persuasion. The animal could be made to experience the escape response but even in these circumstances appeared to be unable to benefit from it. The experimental dogs were described as passively accepting severe pulsating shock. These experiments were interpreted by Seligman as demonstrating learned helplessness.

A learning theory account of learned helplessness would assume that the animal attempts to learn the probability associated with pain avoidance by producing responses. When the pain stimulation appears independent of any response made, then the animal is learning *not* to produce responses. A difficulty with this, of course, is that the animal passively receiving punishment should also be learning to avoid being passive, or *not* to produce *no* response!

In 1975, Seligman proposed that "helplessness is the state that frequently results when events are uncontrollable" (1975, p. 9). "Uncontrollable" is assumed to mean the independence of voluntary responses and response outcome. Seligman sees "controllability" within the context of learning theory in proposing that in instrumental learning the subject has a voluntary response that exerts control on outcome. In Pavlovian conditioning, the subject does not have a voluntary response available and is helpless. Learning of contingencies is therefore an important element of voluntary learning behavior according to the Seligman model. As far as the Seligman hypothesis is concerned, the important test is whether learned helplessness is a state that arises from intense physical trauma or whether the actual loss of ability to control is the important factor. Using a triadic design with three groups of subjects, Seligman tested the control hypothesis. One group of dogs were given a pretreatment for shock but were given control in that they could terminate the shock by pressing a panel with their noses. A second comparable group were yoked, receiving the same shock as the first but with no control. A third group received no pretreatment. The Seligman hypothesis would predict that the second group, who had no opportunity for control, would be most vulnerable. Significantly, the yoked group were slower to learn the avoidance task, and six of the eight subjects failed to learn any avoidance responses at all. Seligman concludes that it is not shock itself but the inability control shock that is important.

Seligman quotes further support from ane experiment by Maier. Dogs were trained to make passive responses as a form of control in the pretreatment condition. Only by *not* moving their heads could they avert shock. The dogs who had had the passive-control pretreatment first attempted to be passive, but when this did not work they later produced vigorous movements. Therefore, although control is movement-related, passivity or lack of responsiveness can be learned as well as active movement.

The experiments on learned helplessness reported by Seligman and his associates have been replicated with noise avoidance in human beings by Hiroto (1974). Using a design involving a finger shuttle box where a given avoidance response could terminate exposure to noise, Hiroto found that although task instructions indicated to subjects that they were able to terminate the noise, uncontrollable pretreatment subjects were slowest in learning escape procedures. Hiroto and Seligman (1975) further demonstrated that the presence of trauma is not a precondition for helplessness in human subjects; unsolvable discrimination learning tasks were shown to produce subsequent impairment on an anagram task.

These experiments support the notion of the transmission of helplessness, so that it can be produced inappropriately in normal subjects. Thus, as Seligman asserts, "Uncontrollability distorts the perception of control" (Seligman, 1975, p. 37). Together with Miller, Seligman demonstrated a "negative cognitive set" to provide a likely explanation. In a card-sorting task, subjects who had been given a pretreatment of uncontrollable loud noise were subsequently unable to locate possible responses that could aid success or failure.

Taken collectively, the experiments favor "expectancies in cognition" rather than changes in specific information content or in the learning of specific associations. The important point about learned helplessness in the context of the Seligman experiments is that it is a nonveridical perception.

Distortion of reality has been produced by a previous treatment in which the animal's perceptions and reactions are veridical. Experiences with poor chances of positive outcome may thus prime a person to react pessimistically.

CONTROL AS A FACTOR IN LIFE STRESSES

Life stresses are likely to involve instances or combinations of the conditions we have been describing. It is at least plausible that the perception of these conditions as stressful depends on perceptions about control. Some cases may involve loss of control, as in bereavement, loss, and in conflict where only one choice is possible. Other cases may involve reduction of control or uncertainty about control, as when a person is in a new and changed situation.

It is argued that in most life stress cases, some demand may be made on a person to assess and predict his chances of achieving acceptable levels of control. This may involve conceiving plans, working out the likely outcome of action, and testing this against an internal code representing a perceived discrepancy value. A person may work out in advance that he cannot cope and is helpless. A wide range of life stresses could be providing a person with situations demanding "implicit" plan formulation and control appraisal.

The outcome of decisions about control has the same consequences for the individual, irrespective of whether there are distortions or not. The perception that control is possible has been shown by Houston (1972; Holmes & Houston, 1974) to reduce reported anxiety and also physiological arousal in advance. Coulter (1970) has shown that if performance is shown to be relevant in reducing the frequency of electric shock received, improved performance is associated with reduced anxiety.

One of the interesting issues to arise directly from the research by Seligman is that expectancies about personal control can be transmitted across successive experiences. Seligman pointed to what for human beings may be a critical question when he asked "Why are we not all helpless?" Generality and stability of decision making about control are issues considered at greater length in Chapters 9 and 10.

The Cognitive Basis of Control

Two requirements for the perception that personal control is possible are, firstly, that a person stores the occurrence of R–S contingencies and, secondly, that he notes that the contingencies are in the appropriate direction. One possibility is that the change in the original discrepancy

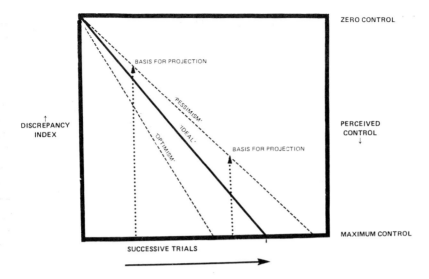

FIG. 3.4. Ideal representation of perceived control as a function of modification of the discrepancy index across successive trials.

between intention and reality provides a progress report. However, without noting actual contingency data, a person could be fooled into thinking he was personally responsible for changes that are due to circumstances.

Figure 3.4 provides an illustration of the use of a value of "discrepancy modification" as a basis for prediction either in advance or at the time of a life-stress event. At any moment in successive trials, a person could use this information to predict likely control and should make a prediction based on progress so far. However, from pilot studies of the "nail test" reported previously, it seems likely that subjects will not behave like this but will collect evidence up to some criterion point and then generalize. If this is true, "optimism" and "pessimism" may reflect in the number of trials required to decide, as much as in the actual decision made.

Part of estimating control must be not merely noting that reality and intention are related, but noting that the effect is being personally achieved. Until this point it has been assumed that a person summarizes R–S contingency data in some form and deduces that the effect is in the right direction by a progress check involving the discrepancy index. A more efficient method could be operated by means of manipulation of internal codes that describe expectancies.

Figure 3.5 illustrates the possible way in which the outcome of internal contingency assessment has implications for perceiving stress. Based on the ideas of ideomotor theory, it is proposed that a mismatch between what is

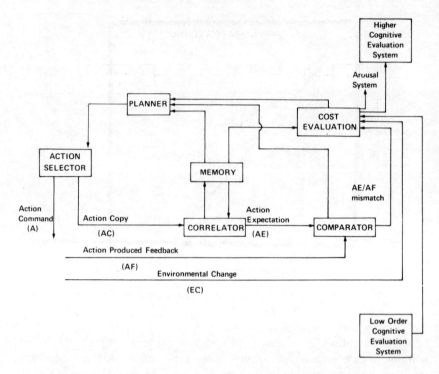

FIG. 3.5. Representation of processes in the perception of control as a function of personal influence (based on ideomotor theory).

expected and what is actually obtained as a result of action will provide a possible basis for the perception of control. The requirement is for a correlator, which keeps a store of action and consequence relationships, and a comparator, which compares what was expected and what actually occurred.

This model will have the advantage of informing the subject not only that he has made progress, but whether he has been *personally responsible* for progress. If the discrepancy is modified in the desired direction but internal evidence suggests that what was expected on the basis of selected action did not occur, a person then knows that some other factor must have coincidentally caused the changes. This may provide a basis for understanding the origin of pessimistic or depressive tendencies; a person may note even a positive outcome under conditions that inform him that he is not responsible.

There has been little research on ways in which loss of control might or might not be stressful. There are many cases in real life where failure occurs and does not result in the perception of threat. Therefore, the meaning and context surrounding loss of control must be considered.

MODEL DEMONSTRATING FACTORS WHICH DETERMINE
FINAL STRESS EXPERIENCE

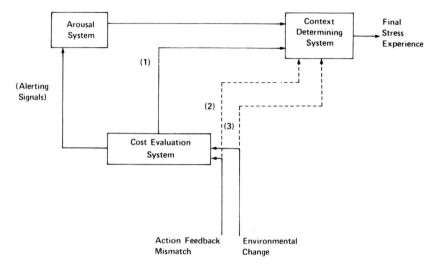

FIG. 3.6.   Representation of factors that determine final stress experience:
1. cost evalutation
2. control loss
3. environmental change

The input to an arousal system cannot be made solely from the perception that the discrepancy is not being modified across trials or from the perception that there is low correlation between action and outcome. There must be some cost weighting attached to the information. According to the minimax hypothesis proposed by Miller (1979), the presence of control may minimize the maximum effect of stress, and the cost of likely consequence would be given a weighting in determining outcome in loss of control. A person may fail to play a game of darts very successfully without necessarily incurring a stressful penalty unless he plays under conditions in which his life is at stake or his personal prestige is threatened. Therefore, the cost of loss of control and the probability of the unpleasantries actually occurring must be weighting factors that influence the stress response.

Figure 3.6 illustrates further that the outcome of the mismatch and cost weighting decision may provide a basis for the context in which the emotional response to threat is determined. This is in line with the empirically supported arguments by Schacter and Singer (1962) that the emotional features associated with injected adrenaline are determined by contextual cues.

Control Assessment in Stress

One possibility that has not been thoroughly explored is that the processes on which control assessment depends may themselves be modified by the effects of the presence of stressful conditions. In the next four chapters there is an examination of the effects of various stressful conditions on the detail of performance. There are grounds for hypothesizing that stresses can produce a shift in the locus of control because of ineffectual performances and that the perception of control may be differentially influenced.

4

A Composite Model
of the Effects of Stress

INTRODUCTION

This chapter is concerned with examining the effects on performance of stressful conditions. The previous chapters have been concerned with exploring the effects of control on the response to potentially stressful conditions. Central to the concept of "control" is the question of performance efficiency. In most conditions in real life, a person is required to make decisions that will enable him to operate control facilities effectively. However, if stressful conditions influence operating efficiency in either a positive or a negative direction, the ability to exercise available control facilities changes.

In this chapter, ways in which stressful circumstances may influence performance are examined. A particular need is to understand how the effects of stress on mental activity might come to influence performance. The foundation for the hypothesis that mental demand is an important but neglected aspect of the effects of stress is provided in Chapter 1. This has implications for a theory of performance changes in stress. There are also other likely sources of influence of performance changes, some of which are specific to certain stress conditions and others that are general in character. These considerations have led to the proposal of a more flexible model in which demand on mental resources and arousal are independently driven sources of influence.

The phrase "composite model" is convenient to describe a model that allows a number of independently driven effects to influence performance. The term "composite" was first used by Poulton in developing his model of noise effects, in which masking and arousal are separable kinds of influence (e.g., see Poulton, 1979). The model developed in this chapter has fundamentally different origins and differs from Poulton's model in having no constraints on the direction of performance change as a function of each influence, but its fundamental formulation is similar.

In real-life situations, a person may encounter multiple stresses simultaneously—a man stranded in the mountains in winter may simultaneously experience cold, pain, loneliness, hunger, sleep deprivation, and fatigue. This is not in itself a case for a different kind of model. Each of these various influences could interact via a common mechanism such as arousal.

A composite model is required because there are no good grounds for ignoring a number of discernible influences. A situation that produces pain may not only provide arousal increase, but may result in, for example, a person reading the context in which the pain occurs and working out alternative courses of action to cope. The case for requiring a composite model rests on the hypothesis that a single stressful condition has a number of identifiable influences.

In terms of the dependent variable, there is evidence that in historical perspective, researchers change their minds about how to explain the effects of stress. The case with noise is clear: Twenty-five years ago Broadbent (1958) reported three common denominators of situations in which deterioration of performance in noise was likely. He linked them with a model that suggested that noise had its main effects on performance because of its distracting properties, which resulted in the occurrence of failure in attention. Subsequently, there was a change in emphasis to take account of the arousing features of noise (Broadbent, 1971); noise effects were seen to be better understood in terms of the influence of arousal on decision making resulting from changes in arousal. A further development has been the hypothesis that decremental noise effects are best explained in terms of the masking of cues and of inner speech (Poulton, 1976b).

A natural conclusion, looking back over 40 years of noise research and theory, is that once noise was seen as a distracting stimulus capturing attention, then as an arousing stimulus increasing the likelihood of attention change, whereas all the time masking effects were being neglected.

There has been a tendency to try to explain all existing dependent variable changes in terms of the new model. Thus arousal increase is assumed to produce a change in the criterion for reporting signals (Broadbent, 1965), a shift in the whole signal and signal plus noise distribution (Welford, 1973), a restriction of cue utilization (Easterbrook, 1959), a tendency for nondominant responses to dictate behavior (Broen & Storms, 1963), a vector change in operating state (Hamilton Hockey, & Rejman, 1977).

The approach taken by Poulton in explaining noise effects has been innovative not just in introducing the idea that noise might act as a masking stimulus producing performance changes because of feedback deprivation or inner speech suppression, but in developing a composite model to explain changes in performance in noise. Noise is assumed both to arouse and simultaneously to mask cues. Performance is the result of the two simultaneous effects. Poulton, however, proposes that arousal change is responsible for positive effects of noise; masking is responsible for negative effects (Poulton, 1979). There are therefore constraints on the direction of influence produced by arousal and masking, respectively.

In this chapter, the idea that any one stressful condition may simultaneously influence performance via a number of routes is developed. One of the reasons it is felt that a flexible new model is required is that at the moment a great deal of potential influence is ignored. Those who have been concerned with meaning in relation to the existence of threat have emphasized varied cognitive activity. Yet in explaining changes in performance we have ignored this evidence. Also, data masking and distortion may be significant influences of stress that are sometimes ignored. There seem to be no good grounds for ignoring the range of potential influences that could act concurrently to determine performance features.

Before developing the argument any further, it is useful first to consider some of the modes of influence on biological and psychological states likely to be associated with different stressful conditions.

THE MODES OF INFLUENCE OF STRESSFUL CONDITIONS

Pain and Arousal

A stress, or aspect of other stresses, associated with fear, avoidance, and high levels of arousal is pain. Many conditions that normally might produce discomfort can at more intense levels produce pain; pain is produced by intense stimulation. Thus, all environmental conditions such as noise, heat, glare, electrical stimulation will at sufficient intensity produce pain.

A number of stimulation studies have located brain centres for pain reception (see Olds & Olds, 1965). In particular, periventricular centers, when stimulated, will produce avoidance behavior in animals and reports of pain in human beings. Whereas the role of the hippocampus in the mediation of pain is not clear, the presence of a 4- to 9-cps rhythm associated with pain has been reported, together with desynchronized cortical activity normally associated with increased cortical arousal (see Gray, 1971). Mere registration of the existence of pain signals in the hippocampus may not provide a basis for the selection of action; further discriminative activity may be required for the selection of approach or avoidance action. Since Kluver and Bucy (1939) showed that lesions in the amygdala abolished the ability to distinguish between punishment and reward, the role of the amygdaloid body has been established as the center for further discriminative activity. Thus it appears that information provided by pain signals is an important prerequisite for action selection.

There are at least two kinds of influence associated with pain. The first is the arousal component; both autonomic and cortical arousal changes are characteristic. The second is information processing demand. One source of demand may arise from a need for elaborate avoidance in cases where reflex avoidance is impossible. A second concerns context, shown to have an important moderating effect on the tolerance of and reaction to pain. A demonstration of the effects of context in moderating pain experience concerns the giving of prior information. Relevant studies were reviewed in Chapter 1. It is possible to mislead subjects concerning the sensations they feel. Nisbett and Schacter (1966) found that the administration of pills with specified effects that were alleged to be similar to—or, in another case, not similar to—those produced by shock could "fool" subjects into misattributing the symptoms of shock, and at least for a low shock condition into tolerating *more* shock in conditions where the symptoms were attributed to the drug. Therefore, there must be some labeling of bodily reactions that affects the tolerance for shock-induced pain.

It is not clear from these studies whether what is being affected is sensitivity per se or the criterion for reporting pain. A study by Clark (1969) using a signal detection theory analysis suggested that if a placebo "pain reliever" is given to subjects, they will tolerate higher levels of pain, but the tolerance is a criterion effect; sensitivity remains unchanged.

An attempt to make sense of the possible role of cognitive factors in the detection of pain was made by Melzack and his asssociates (e.g., Melzack & Wall, 1965; Melzack & Casey, 1968). They suggest that there are two systems of pain input: a fast system with immediate access to the nervous system and a slower system capable of moderation by inputs from higher centers. Thus pain input may be attenuated by information provided because of the activities of higher centers.

The evidence suggests that pain is accompanied by arousal increase, by emotional reactivity, and by information processing demand. The difficulties of requiring people in pain to complete laboratory tasks is evident, so there is no way of obtaining accurate assessments of the effects of pain on performance of tasks. A study by Wherry and Curran (1965) has provided a convincing demonstration of the strength of anticipations about pain as disrupters of performance. Any reliable model of the effects of stress on performance should take this into account.

Problem-Solving Demand

A particular aspect of stress that occurs spontaneously in daily life is that problem solving is required. If simple avoidance is impossible, more elaborate plans are required to reduce, attenuate, or terminate the unpleasant circumstances, often while maintaining efficiency on a current task.

Problem-solving demand may thus create a dual task environment. Priority may be assigned to one or other of the tasks, and attention may not be deployed across all aspects. Performance on the main task may reflect decisions taken about priority, which may, in turn, reflect the importance of the problem. A person who has to tackle landing an aircraft in the presence of loud noise coming from a faulty radio receiver may be expected to give rather more of his resources to the task of landing than a person who is faced with the same task when there is a fire in the cabin.

In other situations, a person may "see" his performance on the task as a possible way of solving the problem. A pilot may fly his aircraft in such a way as to put out an engine fire. A driver on the motorway may drive faster in order to leave the motorway before the fog worsens. These compensatory aspects of behavior cannot be easily studied in laboratory conditions but may be operative in real-life conditions where a person perceives that the way he performs the task "controls" the source of the stress he finds unpleasant.

A possible reason for relative neglect of this aspect of stressful conditions may be that most detailed information about performance in stresses is provided by means of laboratory tasks. The advantage of the laboratory task is obvious; greater control of factors is afforded. The disadvantage is that only selective aspects of the likely effects of stresses may be investigated. Equally, a person may be more prepared to tolerate unpleasant circumstances in a laboratory as part of the pact implicitly made with the experimenter, and may even relish the challenge.

Laboratory tasks do provide some evidence to suggest that subjects may make assessments of the likely effect of stress and then try to make compensatory adjustments. Fisher (1983b) showed that on a memory and search task, performance in noise was superior than in quiet in that the task was completed more quickly. However, closer examination of the data showed that subjects worked harder to achieve this result, because more items were inspected more quickly in order to locate targets. At least one viable explanation is that subjects expected to be less efficient and as a result worked harder to compensate.

Equally, in an experiment involving the production and self-rating of choice responses (Fisher 1983a), subjects in noise reported increased slowness on a rating scale whereas in fact their performance was faster. On a hypothesis that performance reflects some degree of compensation for perceived or expected inadequacy, a person in stressful condition may need constantly to check and adjust his performance to maximize any gains and minimize the losses. This kind of response is difficult to establish objectively. If true, then problem solving demand even during a task may be quite high. This issue is discussed again in Chapter 7.

Stimulation Levels and Arousal

Stressful conditions and complex tasks may both be associated with raised stimulation levels. The relationship between high levels of stimulation and states of arousal has never been made explicit. It is generally assumed that arousal is related to external stimulation levels. One possibility might be that arousal represents "captured energy" from external stimulation. An alternative is that intense levels of stimulation are alarming and cause changes consistent with the mobilization of resources for attack or avoidance.

Complex tasks might also be thought of as increasing stimulation, because as long as a person undertakes a commitment to a complex task, he is likely to be engaged in a task with high requirement for attentional deployment across sources or memory work. The density of stimulation might be high in cases of uncertainty. However, a task may not stimulate merely because it is complex. Wilkinson (1964) showed that merely making a dull task more difficult did not help to ward off the effects of loss of sleep; it was incentive that appeared to be critical.

Arousal and Performance

The notion that stimulation, arousal, and change in performance were related was first introduced by Yerkes and Dodson (1908), who demonstrated that when levels of electric shock were raised, there was a curvilinear relationship with trials required to learn to criterion in animals, as shown in Fig. 4.1. There are two important elements of this work. Firstly, as shown in Fig. 4.2, arousal is assumed to relate to performance in the form of an inverted U curve. Performance first improves and then deteriorates as arousal level increases. A number of "base positions" on the dimension are possible and whether performance improves or deteriorates is a function of two variables: base position and direction of movement. Thus, an individual with low arousal improves with increased arousal, whereas an individual with high arousal shows deterioration of performance. Secondly, task complexity levels are associated with different positions of optimum performance. As illustrated in idealized form in

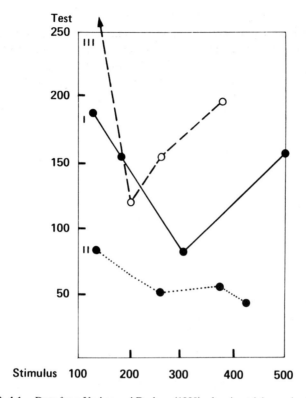

FIG. 4.1.   Data from Yerkes and Dodson (1908), showing trials required to learn to criteria against intensity of electric shock.

I = moderate difficulty task

II = easy task

III = difficult task

Fig. 4.3, difficult tasks were likely to be associated with lower arousal optima than simple tasks.

Whereas the Yerkes and Dodson research anchored performance changes to states of the independent variable, later research in the 1940s and 1950s tended to relate performance changes to central states, supposedly states of activation, usually indexed by the measure of a single variable.

As illustrated by Fig. 4.4, dynamometer tension has been shown to relate to performance in the form of an inverted U curve (Courts, 1942), and to the level of anxiety as indexed by different scores on an anxiety scale (Matarazzo, Ulett, & Saslow, 1955). In the latter case, the authors point out the methodological difficulties inherent in the use of F and t tests on

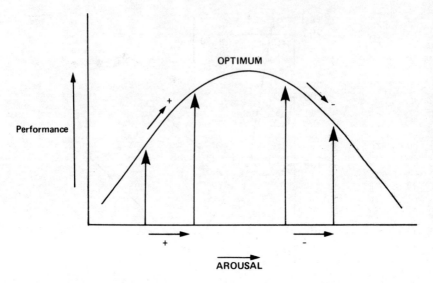

FIG. 4.2. Idealized representation of inverted U curve of arousal and performance.

group data that are ordered with respect to an experimental variable. Additionally, the strength of the relationship is not tested (pp. 85–89). On the results of regression analysis, the authors conclude that a moderate but significant relationship of anxiety and time to learn exists. However, results by Matarazzo and Matarazzo (1956) on a pursuit rotor task showed no relationship with anxiety as measured by the Taylor scale. Thus internal states and performance may not always afford reliable U relationships.

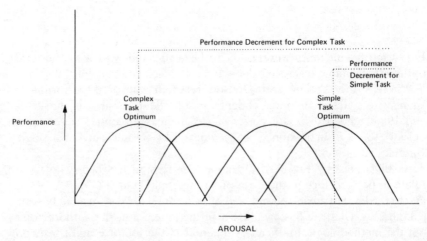

FIG. 4.3. Idealized representation of the Yerkes–Dodson Law.

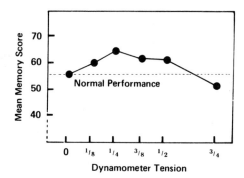

FIG. 4.4. An inverted U relationship between muscle tension and memory score. (Redrawn from Courts, 1942.)

Use of the arousal model in explaining performance changes in stress involves a number of difficulties. Firstly, there is a danger that the model could be used to explain away any data. There are two unknowns: The first is base arousal level, which would be expected to be different for different individuals and to vary with factors such as time of day; we cannot assume that at any one time individual base positions are distributed around optimum. The second unknown is the direction of the effect of a particular arousal agent. In a priori terms, noise could be argued to increase stimulation or to mask existing stimulation.

The second problem has been partly solved by the work on stress interactions. If pairs of stresses or drugs and stresses show interactions, then the same mechanism must be involved; the likely direction of effect of the agents that interact can be "pegged" by comparing results from a series of pairs of such interactions.

There are a number of useful accounts of stress interactions available (see Broadbent, 1963a, 1971; Poulton, 1970). A reported interaction between the effects of tranquilizers and incentives (e.g., see Steinberg, 1959) establishes great weight for the idea of incentives as activators. A reported interaction between the effects of sleep loss and incentives supports the suggestion that sleep loss is a deactivating agent (Wilkinson, 1961). Equally, the interaction between sleep loss and noise (Corcoran, 1962) establishes noise as an activating agent.

These interactions indicate that a common mechanism mediates the effects of stresses such as noise and sleep loss as well as incentives and tranquilizing drugs. However, there are still problems. Some stresses, such as heat, for example, do not interact in this way; either arousal change will not explain the effects of heat, or a different kind of arousal is involved (see Pepler, 1958; Broadbent, 1963, 1971).

Näätänen (1973) has argued that the basic paradigm on which the U function was derived involved a possible artifact. The design commonly used involved asking a subject to create increased tension by his own

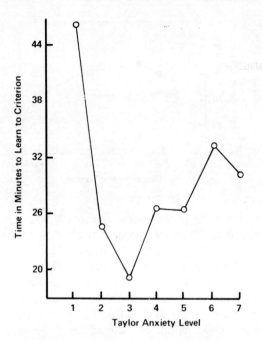

FIG. 4.5. An inverted U relationship between different anxiety levels and time to learn to criterion. (Redrawn from Matarazzo, Ulett, & Saslow, 1955, by permission of the author.)

efforts. An example quoted by Näätänen is that of increasing the pressure on a dynamometer to increase muscle tension. Performance is generally found to be related in a curvilinear fashion to induced muscle tension, but tension is increased by the subject's own efforts. Näätänen points out that the design is a secondary task design; as the subject increases his muscle tension further, greater pressure is required, and greater attention might be expected to be devoted to the task. Using a bicycle ergometer to produce levels of "prior arousal," Näätänen provided data in which there was no obvious U-shaped relationship between arousal and some aspects of performance. Prior arousal level was set by requiring exercise on a bicycle ergometer set at different power levels. Level of activation was indexed by heart rate. Experimental tasks included arm movement and reaction time. Results are illustrated in Fig. 4.6. In both cases there was no relationship between heart rate and the performance measure. However, if heart rate and reaction time were measured during cycling rather than after it, the expected relationship obtained. Therefore Näätänen's suggestion that the performance deterioration observed in cases of induced muscle tension may be a function of the dual task design is supported by his data. It is possible to argue that the prior arousal technique used involves other difficulties, the most important of which, as acknowledged by Näätänen, is that arousal is not stable over the time period of the test.

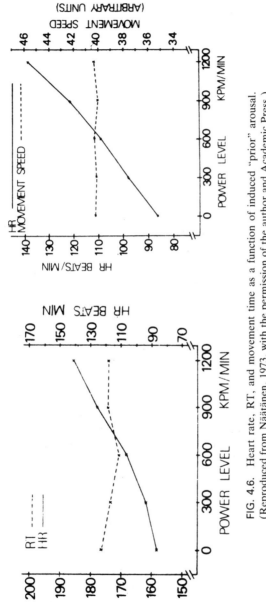

FIG. 4.6. Heart rate, RT, and movement time as a function of induced "prior" arousal. (Reproduced from Näätänen, 1973, with the permission of the author and Academic Press.)

There is also a problem of the sensitivity of certain tasks to the effects of stress. Broadbent (1971) proposed a 2-mechanism model and suggested that different classes of task might be differentially sensitive. Abnormally high or low arousal influences the lower mechanism but may not influence performance unless the upper mechanism is impaired. The upper mechanism is "cholinergic" and based on recent learning; the lower mechanism is "adrenergic" and based on more "remote" learning. Unfortunately, relatively little has been made of this distinction, which is anchored to experiments on animal learning and the effects of acetylcholine and blocking agents (see Carlton, 1963), as well as differences between the locus of action of barbiturates as compared with tranquilizers and amphetamine. Although relatively little attempt has been made to work the details out, it might be expected that classes of tasks such as simple reaction time would not be sensitive. However, in Näätänen's experiment it was the case that reaction time was sensitive during work on the ergometer.

Control and Catecholamine Balance

The arousal model, although with it origins in animal learning, has generally come to be thought of as physiologically committed. However, recent physiological evidence has provided a serious challenge to the assumptions of the model. It is now clear that far from being a bland central state of featureless high energy, arousal is actually likely to be richly patterned and there will be a varied interplay of hormones.

One aspect of arousal pattern may be determined by situations. Early research suggested that situations associated with fear have different physiological patterns from those associated with anger (Ax, 1953). The degree to which situational determinants operate may be limited; Levi (1965) found that watching a tragic war film as compared with a comic film could be distinguished behaviorally, but not in terms of physiological pattern.

A second aspect of arousal pattern variability may be response-determined. Funkenstein, King, and Drolette (1957) demonstrated that anger-in and anger-out were modes of response to perceived failure with different associated arousal patterns. The former response was accompanied by changes symptomatic of raised epinephrine, the latter by changes symptomatic of raised norepinephrine.

In fact, the difference between situation-specific and response-specific elements may be confused in real-life conditions, where individuals may seek out some events rather than others. Carruthers (1974) considers noradrenaline to be the "kick-hormone" that some individuals seek. He describes studies of noradrenaline changes accompanying racing driving. Noradrenaline levels were doubled immediately before a race and quadrupled by the end. The effect of noradrenaline increase is described as "getting a glow" by racing drivers. Carruthers implies that the effect is sought. Irrespective of whether arousal patterns are sought or spontaneously determined, the important point is that they may only create an apparent unitary dimension. Lacey (1967) considers that gross systems of behavioral, cortical, and autonomic arousal only exist in "temporal parallelism," which may be dissociated by the influence of drugs, surgical ablations, and naturally occurring feedback loops.

The point developed in the next chapter is that *compatibility* between arousal influence and concurrent state of arousal may be an important determinant of final outcome. The point of importance for this chapter is that a number of different arousal influences may be simultaneously operative in a stressful condition.

Frankenhaeuser (1971) has drawn attention to a number of factors that influence adrenaline/noradrenaline balance and draws attention to the importance of the relation with personal control: "...adrenaline secretion has been shown to decrease successively as the degree of situational control exerted by the subject is systematically varied from a state of helplessness to ability to master the disturbing environmental influences" (p. 257).

Mason, Brady and Tolliver (1961), using monkeys, confirmed that novelty or uncertainty was associated with raised adrenaline, whereas stereotyped and unpleasant situations were associated with noradrenaline. Mandler (1967) suggested that response availability might be a critical factor; if there is no control available, adrenaline secretion increases, whereas if there is, noradrenaline level is raised. Experiments by Frankenhaeuser and Rissler (1970) showed that increasing situational control was accompanied by higher levels of noradrenaline and a corresponding decrease in adrenaline. Weiss (1970) confirmed that noradrenaline level in rat brains was elevated in rats able to avoid shock, but not in controls who were yoked. These findings are of importance because it is possible that the pattern of arousal changes during exposure to task and stress, as a function either of the degree of objective control or of perceived control. In either case, the change in arousal pattern might alter the detail of performance directly. Changes within or between tasks may be accounted for in this way.

Distraction and the Attentional Demands of Data

Changes in congruity between past and present events have been found to have alerting properties (Hunt, 1965). Interruption of a regular series of events or responses has also been found to be alerting (Mandler, 1975). Sudden bursts of stimulation may have orienting properties at moderate levels, but at high levels may provoke a startle response (Landis & Hunt,

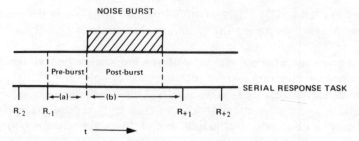

FIG. 4.7. Schematic illustration of occurrence of noise burst during serial task performance. (Redrawn from Fisher, 1972, with permission of *Perception*.)

1939) or defence reaction characterized by negative attributes such as withdrawal, aversion, and protective behavior (Sokolov, 1960, 1963).

There are, therefore, good grounds for supposing that there will be a relationship between the intensity, suddenness, and interrupting characteristics of stressful stimuli and behavioral orientation or alertness. However, the likely effect of stress in creating moments of distraction has been relatively neglected in recent explanations of performance change.

An experiment on the distraction effects of short burst of noise on a serial choice task by Fisher (1972) showed that there was a small localized effect on the serial response currently being produced at the time of occurrence of the noise bursts. Even at fairly low levels of noise (80 dB), a small effect was obtained. As illustrated by Fig. 4.9, the effect was confined entirely to the response currently underway. By analyzing the components of that response into preburst and postburst components as illustrated in Fig. 4.7, it is possible to test the hypothesis that the delay occurs because of a brief distraction rather than because of any "knock-out" or paralysis effect. As shown in Fig. 4.8, distraction theory would predict a constant added delay to reaction time: the preburst (a) and postburst (b) components should remain positively correlated. On the supposition that a noise burst produced a knockout effect (paralysis theory), the onset of a burst should "jam" all processing, and therefore the postburst component should be equal to or greater than one reaction time. As illustrated by Fig. 4.10, distraction seems better supported by the form of the data.

This fits with the view advanced by Broadbent (1958), suggesting that noise produces moments of lapse due to distraction and interruption of the flow of task information. This view is well supported by data that suggest that very intense signals are both good distractors and, when presented as signals for response, are associated with fast reaction times (e.g., see McGill, 1963).

Whereas the effects reported by Fisher were small and contained entirely within one response latency, an effect reported by Woodhead

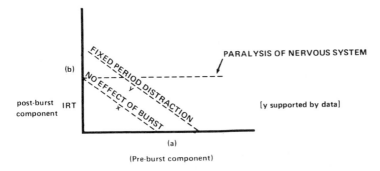

FIG. 4.8. Schematic illustration of the preburst and postburst relationships for "distraction" and "paralysis" hypotheses. (Redrawn from Fisher, 1972, with the permission of *Perception*.)

(1959) involved a localized effect of much greater duration. Woodhead used a task involving the continuous matching of a stationary card with 10 moving cards. One-second bursts of 110-dB rocket firing noise were presented during the task. Overall results in terms of the percentage of correct and incorrect decisions showed no effect of noise, but more detailed analysis suggested a pattern of intermittent gaps in response over the next few demands of the task. Woodhead's data is more consistent therefore with the idea of longer-term changes perhaps mediated by arousal.

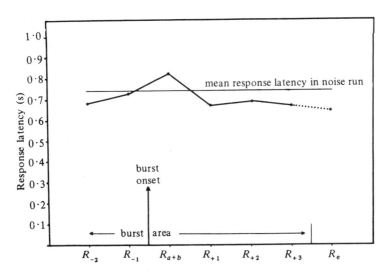

FIG. 4.9. The localized effect of the onset of a noise burst. (Redrawn from Fisher, 1972, with the permission of *Perception*.)

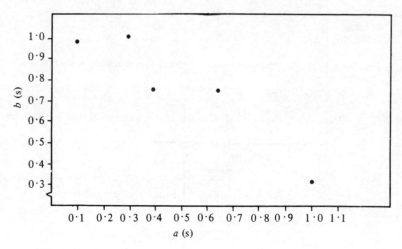

FIG. 4.10. Data showing form of preburst and postburst component of delayed serial response. (Redrawn from Fisher, 1972, with the permission of *Perception*.)

Distracting stimuli are normally considered as being external sources of information that impose on the organism. By definition, they are task irrelevant and intrude into task performance. However, the source may vary. Many distracting stimuli may be thought of as internally generated. There are also many sources of internal distraction that intuitively seem to affect thinking and performance and about which little is known. Pain and illness are two obvious sources of distracting stimuli that may have short- or long-term effects on the performance of tasks. Since individuals are aware of states of discomfort, it is logical to suppose that information is available at some level in the nervous system. Equally, bouts of preoccupation may accompany the continued attempt to solve a problem. In each case, it is possible to think of streams of stored "worry" material coexisting with task data and constituting a possible source of highly intrusive distracting material.

Information Processing Demands

Information Processing Constraints and Capacity

A number of sets of experiments carried out in the 1950s—stimulated by Shannon and Weaver's publication on Information Theory (Shannon & Weaver, 1948)—provided a notion of basic constraints on information processing capacity. As illustrated in Fig.4.11, a person was shown to be limited in the rate at which he could respond to successive stimuli (Welford, 1952). He was slowed in his response to a stimulus by uncertainty

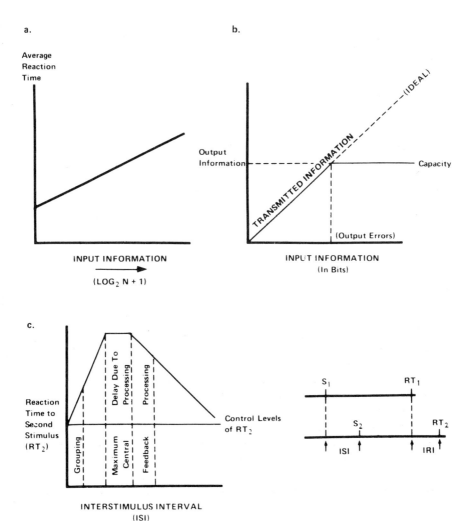

FIG. 4.11.   Idealized representation of three constraints on the processing of information.

a. *Hick's Law:* increased slowness as a function of increased information;

b. *Capacity for absolute judgments:* Increased errors when input information exceeds capacity;

c. *Psychological refractoriness:* Increased slowness of second response as a function of processing time for the first.

about the likelihood of its occurrence (Hick, 1952; Hyman, 1953). He was limited in the number of accurate judgments he could make, and when his capacity was exceeded, he would begin to make errors (Garner, 1962). Despite qualifications introduced as a result of subsequent research, the main features are not disputed.

Studies of the effects of practice on a skilled task have shown that some tasks or task components may become organized at a lower level in the nervous system, thus freeing the central decision systems for additional input. Bahrick and Shelley (1958) showed that time sharing between tasks reflected the degree to which one of the tasks was automated. Interference is reduced as a function of automation. Equally, research on dual task environments has established evidence of a pecking order of degree of interference determined by features of the tasks involved. Some components of a task such as simple encoding may proceed in parallel with elements of another task (Allport, Antonis, & Reynolds, 1972; Kerr, 1973, Trumbo & Milone, 1971).

These considerations are important because, if as argued previously, stressful conditions may spontaneously create dual task environments, the degree of interference will be a factor in performance. If the interference can be reduced because one task is overlearned and automated, or because its demands in terms of processing resources are low, the benefits will be evident in performance. On this formulation, the precise nature of the task will be a very important determinant of the effect of the stress. This is discussed in Chapter 5.

Mental Load and the Concept of Capacity

Many preceding arguments have led toward the suggestion that stresses may create changes in performance because they capture resources required for the task. The situation may involve a concurrent psychomotor task that has to be maintained although unexpected stressful conditions have arisen. Alternatively, the time scale may be longer. A person may have to maintain a level of efficiency in his daily life while coping with a problem such as the break-up of his marriage.

The problem with measuring mental load or work load is that as long as a person is operating within the confines of his own limitations, he will produce error-free performance, and the degree to which he is reaching his own limitations remains unknown. Introduction of a secondary task provided a method of indexing spare capacity. This technique has been used by two researchers to show that even stresses such as loud noise may demand capacity.

Figures 4.12 and 4.13 illustrate two related methods of investigating the mental demands made by a task. If a task is perfectly performed, there is no way of knowing how much capacity is required. An approach developed

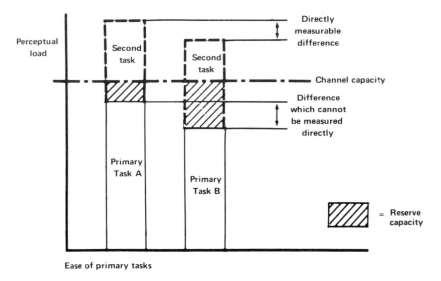

FIG. 4.12.   Illustration of the use of the secondary task technique to index level of mental load. (Redrawn from Brown, 1964. By permission of the author and AIMO Transactions, The Royal College of Surgeons.)

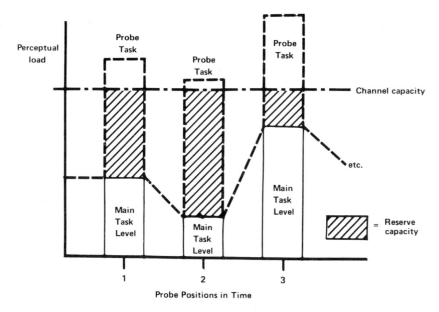

FIG. 4.13.   Illustration of the use of probe reaction time as an index of reserve capacity fluctuations on the same task.

by Brown (1964), illustrated in Fig. 4.12, shows that use of a secondary task can provide an index of the difference in resource requirements between two levels of difficulty of a main task. An illustration of the use of the technique is provided by Poulton (1958), who compared a 2-dial watching task with a 6-dial watching task and indexed the difference by means of a secondary task.

Figure 4.13 illustrates how the same principles are involved when a secondary "probe" signal is presented at various points during the performance of a task. Probe response studies have shown that load levels fluctuate during a letter-match task; identifying the signal is shown to require less capacity than the matching operation (Posner & Boies, 1971).

In both cases, a difficulty is the assumption that capacity is fixed, whereas it may be expanded to meet increased requirements in cases of overload or stress.

Figure 4.14 illustrates attempts by Boggs and Simon (1968), and independently by Finkleman and Glass (1970), to use subsidiary task decrement as an index of noise effects. Boggs and Simon (1968) varied the level of main task load by the introduction of incompatibility into the display/control relationship on a 4-choice reaction time task. The noise characteristics were not varied, but the effect of introducing the noise was to cause deterioration in subsidiary task performance in the condition where it was paired with an incompatible task. The authors of the study conclude: "The introduction of the noise used up some of S's reserve capacity, that is, S had to draw from his reserve so that primary task performance would not suffer as a consequence of noise" (p. 152).

By comparison, Finkleman and Glass (1970) varied the noise characteristics, keeping primary and secondary task features constant. Predictable noise was assumed to be "low demand," unpredictable noise was assumed to be "high demand." Performance on a main compensatory tracking task did not distinguish the two conditions, but performance on a secondary task involving delayed recall of digits showed impairment for unpredictable noise. The results suggest that noise reduced capacity as a function of its demand characteristics.

Slightly weaker evidence for the idea that noise absorbs capacity is provided by Weinstein (1974). He examined the detection of errors on a proofreading task and found that in high noise subjects maintained comprehension but failed to show accurate detection of errors that depended on context, as compared with errors that did not. One explanation considered was that different cognitive apparatus may be required for different types of error detection. In addition, the possibility of an artifact was considered since contextual errors appeared subjectively to be less frequent. In general, Weinstein considers that arousal theory with its emphasis on change in an undifferentiated bodily state is incapable of

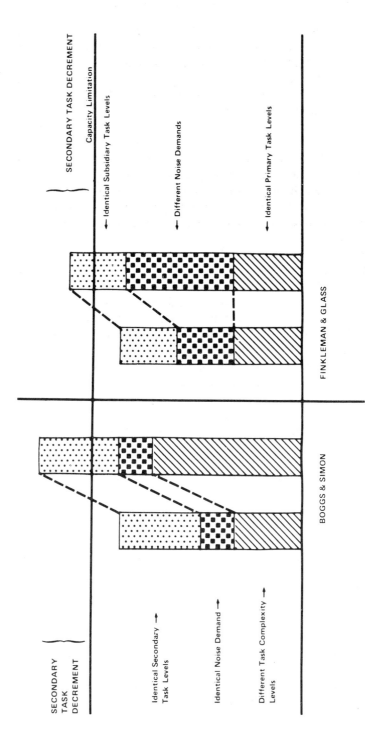

FIG. 4.14.   Illustration of the way in which noise is assumed to require capacity. (From designs reported by Boggs & Simon (1968) and Finkleman & Glass (1970)

dealing with "the relatively complicated pattern of heterogeneous effects observed in this experiment" (p. 552). The possibility that detection of context errors requires more processing space and that noise uses up available reserves is not considered specifically, although Weinstein does point out that difficulty level alone cannot be the crucial variable since "for both types of errors the effect of noise was no greater on difficult lines than on easy lines" (p. 552).

Evidence that indicated the possibility that noise absorbs capacity was also provided by Millar (1980). The dependent variable was reaction latency to a probe that occurred at a number of points during a letter-matching task (Sternberg, 1969, 1975), in which a decision was required as to whether or not a letter was present in a previously learned target set. Normally, the constancy of search times suggests that each additional member of the target set prolongs the search by 35–40 msec. Probe signals were positioned 50 msec, 150 msec, and 250 msec after the occurrence of the test stimulus.

Results suggested that when memory load and display load variables were high for the main letter-match task, the probe latencies were lengthened in noise, which supports the Boggs–Simon suposition that noise acts to deplete reserve capacity. In addition, probes occurring 50 msec after the occurrence of the display stimulus showed greatest lengthening, which implies that points in the main task where demanding operations are required may be particularly vulnerable.

Overload may be a feature of many situations that are considered stressful. The idea that an effect of overload is demonstrated by "overspill" inefficiencies needs qualification. Miller (1962) identified a number of strategies that might be brought in as adjustment to overload. Miller argues that these adjustments imply an active organizational process. Examples include not processing certain stimuli (omission), processing some signals incorrectly (error), delaying responses during heavy work periods (queuing), selectivity in information processing (filtering), giving approximate responses (approximation), making use of alternative channels where possible (multiple channels), and escape (leaving the situation or taking steps to terminate input). Therefore, in many cases it might be quite wrong to think of overload producing a passive "overspill" change in behavior; there may also be adaptive changes to consider.

An issue of interest is precisely how much control a subject has over the organization of input features in situations of overload. He may be too overloaded to be able to produce an orderly adaptation to input features. A study by Fisher (1977) on the effects of overload in a dual task design suggested that the ordering of the attention process involves an independent mechanism, since increased load did not introduce disorganization into the elements of performance but introduced selectivity in time sharing.

However, there is also the possibility that certain operations on which successful performance depends are impaired or changed by overload. There is evidence, for example, to suggest that thinking may reveal pathological features in overload. Flavell et al. (1958) used a word-association test and showed that normal individuals under time pressure produce phenomena such as "perseveration" in associative thinking, which were comparable with associations produced by schizophrenics. Usdansky and Chapman (1960) showed that under time pressure, normal subjects show inability to ignore distracting associations in a word test in a way exactly comparable with schizophrenic responses. They suggest that the effect of overload is to "drive" responses in advance of normal processes being completed, with the result that processing is more superficial; responses recently completed are more readily available, and the memory check that would result in inhibition of repeated response is curtailed.

Although there has been some demonstration that noise overloads resources, it is not clear how an unpleasant condition might require processing space. It could be argued that there is nothing to process. In cases of test anxiety, interfering thoughts about the self and consequences of failure are argued to occur. Sarason (1975) describes self-preoccupation characterized by self-doubt and self-awareness. Wine (1971) emphasizes the attentional demands of "task-irrelevant" responses characterized by thoughts of failure. Hamilton (1974) develops a logical formula for describing how task-irrelevant information might compete for resources and detract from capacity required for the task. It is simply not clear what the content of this intrusive information would be for classes of stress such as sleep deprivation, fatigue, noise. A person might conceivably be preoccupied with the discomfort feelings he has; he might have imagery associated with sleeping if sleep deprived, or cool conditions if he is hot. This may seem intuitively plausible, but it has not been formally demonstrated. As argued earlier, a possible source of information for classes of environmental stress might be provided by concern with success or failure; a person may monitor performance more closely, perhaps compensating for error. Again, there has been no formal demonstration of this.

In addition, there is the possibility of strong situational and individual difference factors in determining the degree to which interference responses are generated. Wine (1971) suggests that attentional training before the task might reduce negative effects on performance. Sarason's studies have shown that reassuring instructions before a test improve the performance of the high-test-anxiety group but may not facilitate performance for a low-test-anxiety group. Additionally, research on cognitive modeling has shown that the high-anxiety group is particularly helped by demonstrations of how problems might be tackled (Sarason, 1973). The nature of the internally generated interfering responses has been investigated (Doris & Sarason, 1955), and from introspective evidence it appeared that high-test-anxiety subjects had interference centered on self-blaming responses; low-test-anxiety subjects were more likely to blame the situation—"it was a bad exam." Sarason further quotes work by Read (1974) concerned with the Uruguayan rugby players whose aircraft crashed in the Andes. Whereas one group of survivors were "task-oriented," a second group of "self-occupied" individuals were described as worrying about themselves and their comforts and being more likely to anticipate disasters.

A further point of importance concerns the nature of capacity. The idea of a fixed capacity limitation has increasingly been replaced by the idea of a finite but expandable system in which decisions can be made about how to allocate resources. Therefore, stresses may not just be sources of extra demand for a limited resource, but might better be seen as situations that require a change in priority about how these systems are used. This, in turn, may provide an important source of mental work.

Loss and Distortion of Data

Some stressful conditions are likely to have effects on the data a person receives when working on the task. In this case it could be argued that performance is influenced not because of stressful qualities per se but because critical information is lacking.

Data Masking

Internal masking may be said to occur when one stimulus interferes with another. Walley and Weiden (1973) propose that centrally based recurrent lateral inhibition between cortical cells may be increased in conditions of arousal. Because of enhanced recurrent inhibition, complex cognitive tasks may be associated with degraded performance in stress. In effect this implies that incoming data may be attenuated or distorted centrally. Walsh and Cordeau (1965) suggest that facilitation of recurrent inhibition may increase as a function of the duration of arousal. Therefore, the tendency for increasing suppression of internal evidence may be a feature of prolonged stress exposure.

Interference between two different kinds of input must be a function of properties they have in common or of conditions attributable to one input stream which directly changes the character of the other input stream. An example of this is the interference produced by noise on a task with auditory components, or the effect of vibration on visual information.

One of the most interesting theoretical debates concerning the effects of noise on performance is the issue of whether noise achieves changes because of the masking of task information, or whether effects are better explained in terms of arousal or distraction. The debate is important and relevant to the theoretical position taken in this chapter. However, there are a great many finely argued points ranging across a number of experiments of different types, and we do not have the space to represent all the detailed arguments that have been developed. With apology to those involved in the debate, we will present only a selection of the experimental findings that support the arguments and counterarguments. The interested reader is invited to read the original development of the debate, which involves a sequence of articles (Poulton, 1976a, 1976b, 1977a, 1977b, 1978a, 1978b, 1979, 1981a and b; Broadbent, 1976, 1977, 1978; Hartley, 1981a).

From some early observations on work and comments by Stevens (see Kryter, 1950; Stevens, 1972), Poulton (1977) noted that Stevens failed to find an effect of noise that is distinct from its effect in masking sounds. This provides a basis for the strongest statement of the masking hypothesis as advanced by Poulton, namely, that all negative effects of noise on performance are explained in terms of the masking of acoustic cues and feedback, or by the interference with inner speech and rehearsal.

Poulton reexamined a number of experiments in which negative effects were reported and provided alternative explanations in terms of masking. In the case of deterioration in noise on the 20-dials test (Broadbent, 1954), Poulton suggested that because of display-control incompatability, there would be increased dependence on the sounds made by a cancelation, and this would be attenuated in noise. A finding reported by Broadbent and Gregory (1965) of a shift toward use of extreme confidence levels in noise was reinterpreted by Poulton in terms of the consequences of internal masking (Poulton, 1978b). The reported finding of increased attentional selectivity toward biased central sources on a secondary detection task (Hockey, 1970a and 1970b) was explained as an effect of the masking of cancelation feedback, which was particularly effective for weak and uncertain peripheral responses (Poulton, 1976b).

In replying to Poulton's criticisms, Broadbent (1978) points to three criteria that can be used to demonstrate that acoustic masking is not responsible for a reported effect: if the same response gives no deterioration in noise when some nonacoustic condition is changed, if different response mechanisms give the same harmful effects in noise, and if acoustic manipulations leave the effects unchanged. Broadbent then shows that he applied one or more of these checks to his own and other criticized experiments. Poulton (1978b) criticizes the criteria in relation to experimental detail and claims they are not water-tight (p. 1074).

The strong statement of the masking hypothesis incorporated in Poulton's composite model assumes that negative changes in noise are attributable to masking, and positive changes are due to arousal. Poulton (1979) also claims that continuous noise does not increase arousal, apart from a transient increase when noise is switched on. It is implicit that any arousal change is moderate; Poulton does not attribute negative changes to hyperarousal.

Strongest support for the notion that masking is a factor that causes performance change because of attenuated task information comes from the demonstration that a change in acoustic properties of noise produces a change in the effect on performance. Poulton and Edwards (1974) showed that reducing the frequency of high-intensity noise prevented adverse effects on the 5-choice serial reaction task.

On exactly the same task, experiments by Hartley (1973b) and Hartley and Carpenter (1974) raise rather a different question, namely, whether masking can be inferred from the detail of performance when the task is performed under different noise conditions that vary the masking factor. These experiments were conducted on the 5-choice serial response apparatus, which in traditional form involves tapping one of 5 appropriate brass contact discs set into a paxolin board with a metal-tipped stylus. Response delays greater than 1.5 sec are scored as "gaps"; the numbers of errors and of correct responses are also scored. The task is serial, pseudorandom, and self-paced. Hartley (1981a) claims that there is no evidence that noise impairs performance by masking acoustic cues on this task and dismisses the composite model in its strongest form.

When the detail of the experiments is examined, it is clear that there are changes in the nature of impairment as a function of the noise characteristics and the method of delivery. The Hartley–Carpenter result shows that headphone noise has a larger effect on gaps (response delays greater than 1.5 sec), whereas free field noise is associated with errors. The results at first imply that headphones plus noise cause attenuation, which translates into gaps. The authors favor a two-factor explanation in which free field noise is associated with greater perceived loudness (Kryter, 1970). Headphone noise is assumed to mask ambient sound and thus increase gaps because of dearousal from increased monotony. The authors evoke a special version of the masking hypothesis.

The results of Hartley (1973b) produced two main findings. The comparison this time involved continuous and intermittent noise and the wearing of ear protectors. Both continuous and intermittent noise resulted in increased errors, but there was a reduction in gaps in intermittent noise. There was a significant three-way interaction of ear protection, noise, and time on task; the proportion of gaps was reduced in the first 20 min. Hartley claimed two sequential effects, one due to arousal increase (decreasing the proportion of gaps) and one to masking, because of increased task monotony, caused reduced arousal, and thus produced a relative increase in the proportion of gaps. Poulton (1977) argues that the gaps are due to the masking of feedback concerning off-target responses or bounces, and that at the early stages of the task a person compensates by tapping more loudly (citing as support Chase et al., 1961).

The position adopted by those involved in the masking controversy is extreme; Broadbent does not consider the possibility that negative effects might be due to masking; Poulton does not accept that negative effects are due to arousal. Hartley allows for negative effects on performance due to masking because of increase in task monotony, but does not accept that suppression might also affect vital task information. Equally, Poulton makes use of the arousal model, but does not allow for arousal to have negative influences as would be expected because of the inverted U relationship between arousal and performance.

A plausible and less extreme alternative is that arousal and masking are independently driven influences associated with noise. Task characteristics determine which influences operate. A task with minimal dependence on auditory cues will be less influenced by masking. Arousal increase is more likely to produce deteriorations in performance if the task is complex. A composite model, in which constraints on the operation of independently driven influences are situationally determined, could provide a plausible account of performance in noise and could reconcile the positions of Broadbent and Poulton in this respect.

Information Deprivation

Stressful conditions may create or derive from lowered stimulation or low density of information. At work, high machine noise may prevent communication, thus enhancing the boredom associated with a monotonous task and increasing the risk of depression in workers (see Broadbent 1982). Equally, poverty may create isolation, restriction of mobility, and lack of opportunity for change: Brown and Harris (1978) argued that these variables were causal factors in depression in working class women at home.

Early laboratory studies of sensory deprivation (Kubzansky & Leiderman, 1958) or exposure to a bland environment with visual noise (Bexton, Heron, & Scott, 1954) provided evidence to suggest profound effects such as perceptual distortions, illusions, or hallucinations resulted. The human need for information was demonstrated.

However, later experiments have shown that even in severe deprivation cases only a small proportion of subjects is affected. For example, Ruff, Levy, and Thaler (1961) showed that only 2 of more than 60 subjects exposed to a wide variety of deprivation conditions reported changes. They identified 8 categories of variables likely to influence the outcome; these included expectancies, instructions received before treatment, and attitudes taken by subjects.

As with pain, sensory deprivation effects may depend on existing knowledge. Although adrenal activity has been shown to increase during deprivation (Mendelson et al., 1960), corticoid responses may not be increased (Murphy et al., 1955). The degree to which deprivation per se is stressful may depend rather more on situational factors than was initially thought.

Task Monotony

Work on human monitoring tasks has shown that when signal rates are low, a subject's ability to detect signals deteriorates. The classical experiments by Mackworth (1950), requiring the detection of a double jump of the hands of the clock, showed that there was a 30% deterioration in performance within the first half hour of the task.

Again situational factors may operate; the characteristics of the decline function show differences. Studies by Ditchburn (quoted by Mackworth, 1950) reported an increase in detection time within a few minutes. Equally, Jerison (1958) and Singleton (1953) reported almost immediate signs of decline. Nearly all studies describe an initial steep decline followed by a plateau. Jerison argues that the plateau is likely to be constant for different experimental conditions within a task (see Jerison & Wallis, 1957).

An influential view of vigilance decline has been that there is a drop in arousal. This is supported by findings that suggest that stimulating conditions ward off the vigilance effect and that in addition to signal rate being an important factor, the total variability of stimulation is important.

The "expectancy" view is given support by the finding that the regularity and size of the intersignal interval is important. Observations by Mowrer (1940) showed that if signals were spaced at predictable 10-sec intervals and a 21st signal was made to occur at a variable time interval from the 20th, reaction time to that signal increased with temporal distance from "10 sec" in both positive and negative directions. The fact that a greater percentage of signals is detected and that detection times are faster for high signal rates (e.g., see Deese & Ormond, 1953; Jenkins, 1953) can be explained on the assumption that high signal rate gives a person more information on which to base his hypothesis about likely times of occurrence. In fact, expectancy theory can cope better with the "two-state" form of decline in watchkeeping; deterioration is usually greater early in the vigil. The expectancy hypothesis assumes that there is maximum difficulty resulting from uncertainty about event behavior during the early period. Expectancy theory can also cope with the improvements brought about by high event rates on the assumption that small intervals are easier to assess than long ones (e.g., see Woodrow, 1951). The effect of signal intensity, magnitude, and duration can be explained on the assumption that the evidence on which expectancies depend is better provided (e.g., see Baker, 1963).

An important contribution was made by Colquhoun (1961), who showed that the number of signals present is less important in determining efficiency levels than the ratio of wanted/unwanted signals. If there is a high proportion of defective (unwanted) signals, vigilance deterioration increases. One of the critical findings in Colquhoun's experiment was that the rate of false reports changes in relation to the number of correct detections during the vigil. This suggests that a change in the criterion for reporting signals is an important factor in vigilance (see Broadbent, 1963b).

Irrespective of the reason for the decline, the experimental evidence indicates that the vigilance effect has great generality. Performance on watch-keeping tasks is likely to be inefficient. In addition, however, monotony as well as total restriction of stimulation is likely to be stressful. One of the important situational determinants of whether monotony is stressful or not is whether a person has control over it. In working life, a person may need to cope with a boring job for every day of his life. In the laboratory, he merely elects to take part for a short specified period. The two situations are different with respect to perceived control.

There is now evidence from hormone studies for different occupations to suggest that repetitive tasks are stressful. Jenner, Reynolds, and Harrison (1980) conducted routine studies in the village of Otmoor in which levels of adrenaline and noradrenaline were measured. Manual repetitive workers were shown to have unexpectedly high levels of adrenaline and noradrenaline. A comparable finding was reported by Frankenhauser and Gardell (1976) in a study of saw-mill workers. Repetitiveness at work resulted in high adrenaline levels and low self-rated levels on "well-being."

However, against the suggestion that boredom always results in increased arousal, the Otmoor study also provided evidence that showed that in comparison with white collar workers, those blue collar workers with manual jobs are more likely to be bored, to be physically tired, and to have low adrenaline levels (Reynolds, Jenner, Palmer, & Harrison 1981). Boredom may thus be a complex stress that varies in influence as a result of situational factors.

Monotony may be a by-product of the masking of varied input, either because of an environmental mask such as noise or vibration, or because of isolating conditions. The effects of monotony may depend on whether experience is long- or short-term, how it is produced, and whether there is control over its occurrence. Repetitive tasks at work are likely to have low control and to be associated with increased anxiety. Other manual tasks may be monotonous but self-paced, and thus the subject maintains a slow level of output and feels bored. When conditions favor enforced exposure to monotony, the effects of increased arousal associated with irritation may obscure any tendency to show lowered arousal due to boredom.

FEATURES OF THE COMPOSITE MODEL

The arguments developed so far suggest that we need a model that will allow for a number of independently driven effects and a number of interaction or control points that permit current influences to combine additively or interactively. The notion of a single dimension of arousal seems better replaced by a number of different kinds of arousal. Interactions will occur only if arousals are compatible. This will be discussed in the next chapter.

Equally, we have developed the idea that stress situations are likely to place high demand on mental activity, for a variety of reasons. We argue that a person's "operating state" at any one time may be a function of a number of independently driven influences on mental and biological resources. Not all influences associated with particular stresses will operate all the time and in all conditions; therefore, the *pattern* of independently driven effects is a variable.

One obvious implication is that the pattern of responses to a particular condition will be a complex function of the specific modes that operate. There may be some "rules" that will provide a prediction about the level of impairment likely in a given population.

1. The greater the *number* of modes that operate, the greater the *probability of general impairment of performance.*
2. The greater the *intensity or magnitude* with which a mode operates, the *greater the probability of general impairment.*
3. The greater the *duration* of the operation of a particular mode or mode combination, the greater the probability general impairment of performance.

The implication for the understanding of the effects of stress in daily life is that it is necessary to itemize all possible kinds of influence and where possible to design experiments that vary these factors one at a time.

The implication for research in the laboratory is to be more concerned with alternative explanations of reported changes. Eventually, computer simulation of a system under stress may help to test and check the rules of performance.

5

Situational Determinants
of the Effects of Stress

INTRODUCTION

This chapter is concerned with analysis of the situational determinants that appear to modulate, summate with, or interact with the effects of stress on performance.

One of the most important sources of influence concerns the task, including the paradigm that describes the stress and task condition. It is important to distinguish cases where the stress *is* the task, or the task itself becomes a source of stress, from more complex designs where the task has to be performed in the presence of stressful circumstances. Although the latter paradigm characterizes most laboratory studies, it is also characteristic of many life stress situations where a problem arises and a person needs to solve the problem and maintain daily efficiency. This approximates a dual task design, and we now know that difficulty levels and instructions are likely to influence the priority structure that obtains.

Secondly, there is the "concurrent state," by which is meant the biological and psychological state at the time of onset of stressful circumstances. Part of the latter state is the "disposition to perceive control." There is now a great deal of evidence that distinguishes "internalizers" who consistently believe that situations can be personally controlled from externalizers who believe that what happens is a matter of luck and chance. The tendency to "internalize" or "externalize" appears to be an enduring disposition, which will have important consequences for the treatment of evidence presented by task or stress environments. Both biological and psychological states provide memories for the effects of previous stressful and nonstressful encounters as well as providing short-term memory of prevailing conditions.

Thirdly, there are factors due to the person and the constraints imposed by total working conditions. Thus there is duration of exposure to task and stress, pacing conditions, and factors such as work posture and flexibility in taking rests.

In this chapter some of the evidence indicating that these factors are important determiners of the nature of performance change in stress and should be included in the "composite model" is considered.

SITUATIONAL DETERMINANTS OF PERFORMANCE IN STRESS

Task Factors

Task factors may contribute to existing modes of influence of stress, for example by increasing stimulation. Equally, the nature of the task to some extent determines the criterion for assessing performance. Sensitivity of the measure afforded determines whether a particular effect of stress is recorded. Finally, the task may be relevant or not relevant to a particular stress influence; a task with no dependence on auditory information should be unaffected by the masking effects of noise.

Task Complexity as a Determinant of Impact

Complex tasks may create conditions of information overload or may create conditions of incentive, because generally increased complexity raises task interest. Additionally, complex tasks are characterized by high involvement of cognitive activity, and there may be specific vulnerability of these processes in stress.

The assumption that conditions of high uncertainty increase processing load or that the addition of many elements in a task increases mental demand, considered in relation to the notion of man as a limited-capacity system, provides a basic hypothesis that task complexity should have a monotonic relationship with performance efficiency. If stressful conditions are assumed to demand capacity because of "worry work," a secondary task should indicate gradual deterioration, even when perfect performance on the main task is preserved. Moreover at a later stage, main task performance will be increasingly represented by "overspill" errors as capacity is exceeded. The stress, because of its priority, may effectively become the main task, performance on which remains constant, whereas efficiency on everyday tasks begins to break down.

The "overload" model does not predict an improvement in performance as a function of increased task complexity and will not easily provide a basis for understanding improvements that may occur when complex tasks are performed in dearousing conditions. Also, as argued in the previous chapter, the idea of a fixed capacity system is better replaced by the concept of a flexible but finite capacity system in which allocation of resources is made in accordance with different demands.

The Yerkes–Dodson Law makes provision for understanding the motivational properties of complex tasks. Thus, complex tasks are less tolerant than simple tasks of arousal increase produced by external conditions. An alternative way of expressing this is that simple tasks are more likely to benefit from increased arousal than complex tasks. The idea of a curvilinear relationship between arousal and performance is retained, but there are different levels of tolerance of arousal increase or decrease as a function of task complexity.

However, the reason why task complexity affects the location of optimum arousal for performance is unclear. One possibility is that complexity adds stimulation, which will combine additively or interactively with existing stimulation levels. A different explanation is that subjects might try harder with complex tasks because of the intrinsic interest or incentive provided. However, the possibility that all complex tasks are intrinsically interesting and provide incentive is not supported by experimental findings. Wilkinson showed that sleep-deprived subjects can sustain performance for up to 80 hours into the vigil without showing impairment if the task is complex. His data provides a pecking order of the likelihood of performance impairment, with simple monotonous tasks being the most vulnerable (Wilkinson 1964, 1965). However, he also showed that it was not difficulty level itself that was important. Merely increasing the number of decisions by introducing uncertainty into a response task—by increasing levels from 4- to 10-choice—did not lead to a significant improvement.

Battleship games and chess games are both complex and interesting. Wilkinson favors the view that the incentive provided by the task is what is important. The incentive value must somehow help a subject to maintain arousal, although this will be at some biological cost. Both Wilkinson (1965) and Broadbent (1971) favor the view that it is possible for arousal to be sustained by compensatory effort. Seen in this way, a complex task simply helps a subject to ward off the effect of dearousal that results from sleepiness. Further support for this is provided by the finding that the magnitude of the effects of incentives is greater for sleep-deprived than for non-sleep-deprived individuals (Wilkinson, 1961).

A problem is how a person can make use of interest and stimulation in the effort to sustain arousal. Studies by Murray et al. (1959) have shown that given the chance to do so, subjects undergoing a sleep deprivation vigil will change tasks. The relationship is in the form of an inverted U, since this activity first increases and then, after 40 hours, decreases.

Task involvement may be a factor; in quite a different context Harrison et al. (1981) showed that women at work did not appear to show the differences in hormone levels as a function of the work characteristics in the way that men did. However, when the women were classified according to the occupation of their husbands, it was found that Social Class I and II women have higher adrenaline outputs, both on work and rest days. This suggests that even being given a certain kind of task on a daily basis will not necessarily produce daily change in arousal level in some populations, although it will in others. Task *involvement* would appear to be a factor in deciding the incentive value of job characteristics.

In vigilance tasks, traditionally regarded as "stress vulnerable" (see Mackworth, 1950), the complexity factor is again important. In experiments by Jerison (1956, 1957), subjects were required to keep track of flashing lights and to count the number of flashes to criterion. A three-source version of the monitoring task was different from a one-source version in that although performance was at a lower level, there was no evidence of the expected decline in performance with time, and the task was more vulnerable to noise. Equally, Broadbent (1951) showed that there was a significant drop in efficiency in noise on a complex 20-dial monitoring task; additionally, the relationship between display and control had some degree of incompatibility.

At least some of these changes may occur because of the vulnerability of component processes such as memory and attention (Chapter 7). Complex tasks place greater reliance on higher mental processes. It is conceivable that a strategy of lowering the level of performance reflects perceived high demand. This might account for the result reported by Weinstein (1974), in which the presence of high noise caused subjects to be more superficial in the detection of errors on a proofreading task; detection of simple errors, such as letter transpositions, was unchanged, whereas more complex errors that depended on the reading of context were less easily detected.

Task Appropriateness

If the task has features that are *relevant* to the likely influences of the stress, we would expect impairment because of data distortion. Thus glare may mask visual events; loud noise may mask auditory information and reduce the cues available from responses; vibration may impair performance on a skilled precision task (e.g., see Poulton 1970, 1977a). The task may operate like a gating device, which determines which of a number of potential influences will be operative. For example, if auditory cues are irrelevant, then the masking influence of noise on acoustic cues will not be influential.

Task Requirements

Other qualities of the task contain implicit directives that influence performance. For example, task events may be externally paced; the rate of occurrence of the external events then defines the rate at which accurate performance must be sustained in order to avoid "blank" trials, which will be recorded as errors of omission. The subject cannot always adjust his timing to match the demands of the stress.

The task may dictate the attitude to performance in that a standard of performance may be implicit. In a series of skilled task experiments conducted in the 1930s, Mace (1935) argued that performance depended to a high degree on standards of performance adopted by the worker. Research on knowledge of results (KOR) as a performance aid usually emphasizes that benefits obtaining from being given such feedback result from the effect of information in relation to standards. Mace showed, however, that urging subjects to do their best could have beneficial effects. Therefore the subject must have some idea of what "best" is. This information can only come from the task definition or from explicit instructions that indicate the criterion whereby performance is judged.

Ambiguous instructions stressing both speed and accuracy are common in experimental designs. There is evidence that shows that settings for speed as compared with accuracy have different implications for the speed/accuracy trade-off (see Chapter 6); thus, how a subject interprets ambiguous instructions may have important implications for the character of performance. We do not yet understand how global instructions are held and executed. An instructional "set" that changed the microstructure of performance was reported by Fisher (1975a). On a dual task design, attention was ordered between the stimuli in such a way that the pattern of events that occurred when instructions favored one task was quite different from the pattern of events when instructions favored the other. Increasing the "load" of the main task also changed the structure of the distribution of attention (Fisher 1977).

Instructions also indicate to a subject what the important features of performance are. In the detection and reporting of signals, a subject may be told how critical signal detection is. Changes in criterion for report may also be affected by stresses. Colquhoun and Goldman (1968) showed that raised body temperature increased the proportion of correct detections and false reports. Equally, the use of a confidence scale may change in loud noise in that subjects give more "extreme" estimates and are more definite about decisions (see Broadbent & Gregory, 1965; Fisher, 1983b).

Finally, as early as 1958, Broadbent emphasized the importance of sensitivity of task measurement (Broadbent, 1958). In keeping with the view that stresses such as noise and sleep loss produced failures in attention, it is important that such failures are recorded. Continuous tasks or tasks in which the stimulus occurs on a random time basis, as in vigilance tasks, provide a method of sampling behavior randomly and are likely to be sensitive.

Concurrent State

An additional factor that is likely to influence performance character is the biological and psychological state of the individual *at the time of occurrence* of a particular stress. We consider just a few of the aspects of concurrent state likely to be important.

Biological States

A biological state may be thought of in terms both of energy and of information. The energy state is both arousal level and associated mobilization of resources on which it depends. The informative element is represented by the relative levels of resources and by the particular pattern of change associated with energy release. Biological memory may also be described in terms of long-term factors such as genetic dispositions and may be tuned gradually as a function of experience.

Biological states of arousal are influenced by the fact that although organs may be capable of prolonged activity, the resources on which they depend are finite. Thus in persistent stress, sugar and fat reserves may be depleted. A long-term biological memory is therefore based on rate of resource depletion. A short-term memory exists because responses are dependent on chemical changes likely to have pervasive but short-term influence.

Energy State and Homeostasis.   The proposal formulated by Cannon (1936), that energy mobilization has a purpose and functions to aid homeostasis, provides a useful basis for considering the relationship of physiology to performance. Mobilization of resources is needed in order that performance should be successful. Fight or flight needs the production of energy. This instrumental view of physiological change emphasizes that the success of performance is maximized. Given that physiological state resulting from stress was seen by Cannon as bland and unidimensional, there is no possible way in which the directional aspect of performance can be influenced.

In some cases, arousal is raised to levels that in operational terms are not beneficial. An obvious question is why natural selection does not favor the operation of a "stop rule" that maintains the level of physiological activity at optimum for performance. Although there are built-in negative feedback loops, their operation may not always be to advantage. Lacey (1967) describes research on the existence of a negative feedback loop, whereby high pressure in the carotid sinus will trigger the activity of barroreceptors and will damp down cortical arousal. Thus, raised autonomic activity might have a counterproductive effect in terms of the programming of performance.

It is possible that a balance between efficiency and physiological cost may be controlled by decision. Frankenhaeuser's research has shown that the response to increased task demand is either to maintain performance at some physiological expense, or to maintain the same effort levels and allow performance to deteriorate. When subjects were required to complete an arithmetic task in the presence of loud noise or were required to complete a color-naming task in which extra conflict was introduced by means of a different dimension, they appeared to meet these extra demands by increased effort; this change is described by Lundberg (1979) in terms of the subject's attempt to "pull himself together." Equally, Selye (1974) suggests that the increased task demand may be met by "raising the body's thermostat of defence," so that performance remains at stable levels.

However, when instructions give less emphasis to sustaining performance, subjects may then allow performance to deteriorate. Increased noise intensity following early experience of low noise level may thus merely be accompanied by deterioration in performance and no change in effort (Frankenhaeuser & Lundberg, 1977).

Stimulus and Response Specificity.   The idea that arousal is best represented by a single physiological dimension that varies only in intensity has been superseded by a model that allows for different kinds of arousal to coexist. The particular mix of hormones and effects produced in a given situation could determine the nature of performance. On the hypothesis that base arousal at the time of incoming influences is an important determinant of performance effects, the existence of different arousal states raises the question of *compatibility* of concurrent states with incoming influences.

Catecholamine balance.   In the previous chapter we began to consider the possibility that the two hormones, adrenaline and noradrenaline, which differ in details such as locus of action, and temporal features, may reflect different emotional and cognitive response styles. Perhaps more importantly, they may distinguish different external conditions in terms of the facility available for control. Although in males and females adrenaline levels rise daily and become particularly pronounced under conditions of mild stress, levels are greater in males than in females. This could be an occupational effect. Population field studies by Jenner, Reynolds, and Harrison (1980) have shown that overall, white-collar workers incur higher daily adrenaline levels than blue-collar workers, but that repetitive manual tasks are associated with very high levels. The implication for understanding the possible effects of accidental events as well as for coping with problems in daily life are great. If a person is already at a high level of adrenaline production, the effect of a stressful event should be to produce hyperarousal and performance deterioration.

As described in the previous chapter, specific conditions may dictate catecholamine balance. A useful illustration in the context of stress at work is provided by Frankenhaeuser and Gardell (1976), from studies of jobs operated in a saw mill. As shown by Figs. 5.1, 5.2 and 5.3, conditions such as restricted work posture are associated with feelings of irritation and with high noradrenaline. Repetition and duration of work cycle affect feelings of well-being and relate to increased adrenaline output. Moreover, as illustrated in Figure 5.4, control of work pace is an important factor; people are more irritated, with high noradrenaline levels, when the work pace is controlled by machine.

Repetition and external control may often go together; available evidence suggests that a person doing fast repetitive work may be both anxious and irritated. These work-related factors may provide a state that continues after work, which determines reaction to events at home and the response to daily problems. Equally, a person coping with a problem at home may be in a state that renders him irritable or anxious at work.

Raised adrenaline levels were found by Mason, Brady, and Tolliver (1968) to accompany avoidance learning in monkeys. During trials, when by responding to a warning animals could avert shocks, urinary adrenaline levels were high. Therefore, having control is associated with high-stress response in circumstances where an animal operates control by avoidance and has to remain alert. This supports the view advocated by Weiss as outlined in Chapter 3. However, Mason's results also showed that across successive monthly spaced sessions, the magnitude of the adrenaline response diminishes although the effect remains present. Thus it is possible that "meta-learning" occurs and leads to a gradual change in state as a function of experience.

In an early laboratory study of "situational specificity," Ax (1953) studied anger- and fear-producing situations in terms of 7 out of 14 autonomic measures; anger was accompanied by a rise in diastolic pressure and an increase in muscle tension and skin response, together with a drop in heart rate. By contrast, fear increased respiration rate, skin conductance, and the number of muscle tension peaks. Ax believed that the anger profile could be linked to the effect of adrenaline and noradrenaline together, whereas the fear profile is similar to the effect of injected adrenaline alone. Similarly, by use of film material, Averill (1969) distinguishes sadness and mirth in terms of underlying correlates; although both appeared to involve increased activation, cardiovascular changes appeared

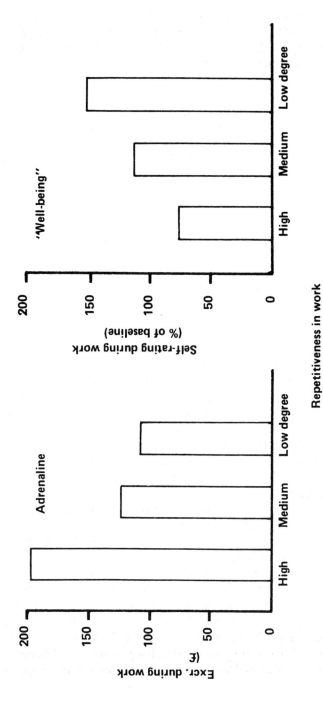

FIG. 5.1.   Adrenaline levels and "well being" assessments as a function of different degrees of task repetitiveness. (Redrawn from Frankenhaueser and Gardell, 1976, with the permission of the authors and *Journal of Human Stress*.)

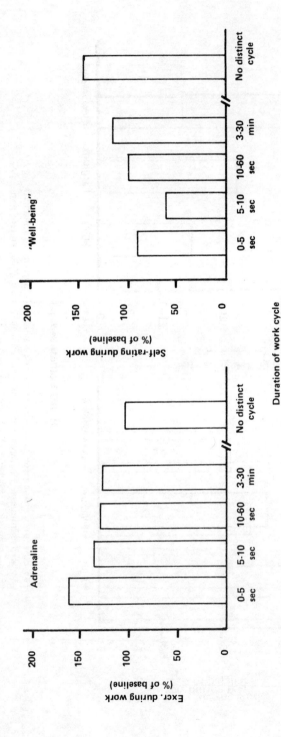

FIG. 5.2. Adrenaline levels and "well-being" assessments as a function of work cycle and duration. (Redrawn from Frankenhaeuser & Gardell, 1976; with the permission of the authors and *Journal of Human Stress*.)

98

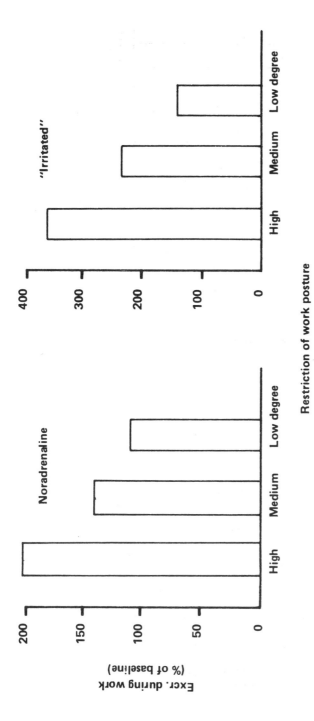

FIG. 5.3. Noradrenaline levels and irritation as a function of work posture. (Redrawn from Frankenhaeuser & Gardell, 1976, with permission of the authors and *Journal of Human Stress*.)

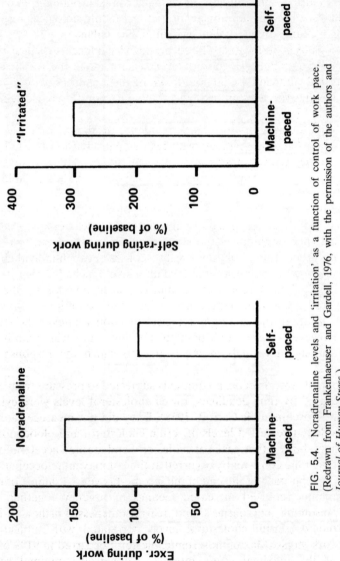

FIG. 5.4. Noradrenaline levels and 'irritation' as a function of control of work pace. (Redrawn from Frankenhaeuser and Gardell, 1976, with the permission of the authors and *Journal of Human Stress*.)

to characterize sadness, and respiratory change appeared to distinguish mirth.

It is also possible that different individuals show differing patterns of reaction to the same situation. Funkenstein, King, and Drolette (1957) identified anger-out (other-blaming) as the cognitive response style to perceived failure in some individuals and anger-in (self-blaming) in others. They found a different accompanying pattern of physiological response suggesting a change in adrenaline–noradrenaline balance.

Frankenhaeuser and Patkai (1965) produced evidence to suggest that adrenaline predominance is more likely to characterize the responses of "well-adjusted" individuals and noradrenaline the responses of "inhibited" personalities. Depressives are likely to be characterized by low catecholamine levels.

Malmo and Shagass (1949) reported evidence of idiosyncratic response modes to pain. Neurotic patients with high somatic tension reacted with increased muscle tension, whereas cardiac patients reacted with increased heart rate responses. This supports the idea of a prevailing biological response disposition.

Finally, in a more careful test of the response specificity hypothesis, Lacey et al. (1953) used exposure to four different types of stress—mental arithmetic, hyperventilation, letter association, and cold pressor test—and reported differentiation of physiological responses between individuals. In terms of autonomic tension scores (maximum level reached during stress), and autonomic lability scores (maximum displacement scores), the evidence favored a constant pattern across all stress conditions. "Maximal activation occurs in the same physiological function whatever the stress" (p. 19). However, the authors pointed out that there was quantitative variation among individuals in the degree to which the response was stereotyped.

In a group of American tax accountants subjected to pressure from work demand caused by time deadlines, raised cholesterol levels were evident (Friedman, Rosenman, & Carroll, 1958). They did not measure catecholamine levels but recorded levels of serum cholesterol and blood clotting time. Results showed that peaks of cholesterol and marked acceleration of blood clotting time consistently occurred at time of maximum occupational stress. At the approach of the end of the income-tax year, a sample of male tax accountants reported increased feelings of urgency together with irritation, insomnia, nervousness, and quarrelsomeness. Further, in individuals studied, serum cholesterol levels correlated with subjectively assessed work stress. Maximum serum cholesterol occurred in 91% of the subjects at the maximal stress interval. Conversely, minimal serum cholesterol occurred in 76% of the subjects at a time of minimal stress.

If we are to understand the impact of concurrent state envisaged as a state of existing activation or arousal, it is clear that the existence of stimulus and response specificity effects is important. Until now we have thought about arousal as a nonspecific state; implicit in the arousal model is that performance is a function of base level *and* the direction of effect of a variable. If we now consider the possibility that base level is in fact a *pattern* of activity, we have to consider the possibility that some patterns "mesh" with new effects and some may not.

For example, imagine a hypothetical situation in which an individual is engaged in a dull repetitive task. In the old formulation we might have imagined this to be dearousing. In fact, we might have to consider the possibility not only that it causes high adrenaline levels, but that A might respond with high heart rate, whereas B might respond with increased muscle tension. The occurrence of a new event falls on a state of heightened cardiac activity for A, and this could mean lowered cortical arousal. For B the state is one of high muscle tension, and there is no reason for assuming lowered cortical arousal. Therefore, it becomes inappropriate to use the simple formulation of (baseline arousal + stress), to describe the likely change in performance. We need to consider the pattern of activity and its likely change in stress. Imagine a case where the concurrent state is one of increased cardiac activity in most subjects, and the incoming event is more likely to affect skin conductance; we would expect the combination to produce different results from a case in which the new event is also likely to influence heart rate. It would be necessary to think about specific physiological preparation for specific events.

One of the important characteristics of autonomic activity is high dependence on hormonal activity. The influence is gross and persistent. For this reason we would expect knock-on effects—one influence preparing for the impact of another. Thus, we may think of an individual as irritable or anxious from one experience; this renders him likely to overreact to another. There is no research that has looked at the likely effects of a stress as a function of its position in a sequence of events.

It may also be the case that some arousal patterns may prepare for poor performance more readily than others. For example high heart-rate responding may increase pressure in the carotid sinus, which has been shown to lower cortical arousal (Bonvallet & Allen, 1963). As a result, performance may be impaired. Thus, if high heart rate characterizes an individual's response to stress, we may predict an increased probability of impaired performance. If a previous task "prepares" for this by producing increased heart rate as a typical response, we might argue that a knock-on effect is increased probability of poor performance to the new task.

What has been described are forms of short-term biological memory. However, it is also possible to think about a much longer-term biological memory: Early experiences may tune and refine the autonomic nervous system in such a way that it has special properties or structures.

A number of studies have demonstrated the possibility that individuals may be prepared in terms of autonomic tuning. For example, as a result of experiments involving the early stressing of rats, Levine (1966) argues that one effect might be to speed up the maturation of the pituitary adrenocortical system, because there are observable physical differences in these animals, including the early appearance of body hair, body weight changes, and increased brain weight due to a speeded-up rate of myelination. There is direct evidence from the adrenocortical response to cold pressor stress: A decrease in ascorbic acid, which indexes the adrenal response, can be observed within 12 days for prestressed rats and not until 16 days in controls.

In addition to the notion that prestressing speeds up the development of mechanisms that mediate stress responses, Levine's original idea was that some emotional immunization takes place in the prestressed animal so that the system would respond less intensely to subsequent stress. Haltmeyer, Denenberg, and Zarrow (1967) showed that prestressed rats produced greater autonomic response to shock in adulthood, but when shock was terminated, the return to the resting state was faster. This provides evidence of greater control over the slow release of hormone. However, if instead of shock the animals are later submitted to the "open field test," the level of autonomic response is greater in controls (see Levine et al., 1967). Autonomic tuning may therefore be situation-specific. Levine and Mullins (1966) propose that early stress experience may mean a more varied adrenocortical response later in life. There are obvious parallels here with the development of skilled responses; the greater the number of experiences, the greater becomes the possibility for the organization of effective responses. The range and competence of response patterns may be tuned by early experience.

Base state of autonomic arousal involving selective disposition to respond may be features of autonomic patterning, tuned by the effect of experience on a genetically determined template. It may be that there are evolutionary pressures; an animal who mobilizes his energy resources effectively produces the "right state" for efficient responses. Further, fast return to rest state will mean that his energy resources are not wasted unnecessarily. Efficient control of the energy responses may therefore have survival value.

It could be argued that cases where trauma is beneficial in formative years is against the learned helplessness model (Seligman, 1975) in that an animal is exposed to unpleasant conditions when he is too young to cope effectively. However, specific conditions of the experience may be critical determinants.

There is evidence to suggest that early trauma reduces the probability of "freezing" in an "open field" test, speeds up resumption of drinking after shock interruption, reduces susceptibility to conflict-produced ulcers, and increases the speed and efficiency of avoidance learning (e.g., see Denenberg 1964; Gray, 1971). These positive effects would favor the notion that there is an advantageous aspect of unpleasant negative experiences; the animal may be learning that such experiences are self-limiting, or can be controlled.

However, there is evidence to suggest that early trauma does not always favor adaptive responses. The type of trauma most likely to engender maladaptive responses is exposure to high or very restricted levels of stimulation. Gray shows that response to shock is a function of the intensity of shock to which the young animal was previously exposed (Gray, 1971, p. 98). Also, effects of early trauma may interact with genetic strain. The role of genetic factors is demonstrated clearly by Hall (1951) and by Broadhurst (1960). The basic demonstration that selective breeding produces vulnerable strains of animals as indexed by defecation scores leaves open the question of prenatal and postnatal influences. By cross-fostering (interchange of reactive and nonreactive litters) and reciprocal crossing (reactive mated with nonreactive partners), it is possible to isolate genetic from "pre"- and "post"natal factors. By these techniques, the genetic influence has been demonstrated unequivocally.

There is the possibility that deprivation and restriction of early environments merely serve to enhance the *novelty value* of subsequent situations. Restricted environments may lead to impoverished structure, so that in cases of normal stimulation the contrast is overwhelming. Thus Hall's open field test, involving exposure of the animal to an arena of bright lights and loud noises, produces an environment that is ideal for testing the effect of restricted environments.

The corticoid response. In addition to changes in catecholamine secretion, changes in the production of ACTH and the consequent secretion of corticoid hormones are mediators of the stress response. In a detailed review of 17-OHCS production in animals and humans, Mason (1968) concludes that the hormone level reflects psychological influence sensitively. Activity appears to be increased in any condition where there is an undifferentiated state of "arousal, alerting or involvement—perhaps in anticipation of activity or coping" (p. 592). He cites evidence of changes from a resting state level of about 12% to stress levels of about 20%. The situations most closely associated with 17-OHCS production are novelty, unpredictability, suspense, anticipation, and—in psychiatric conditions— intense disorganizing emotional reactions. In the latter cases, levels of

30–40% may be observed. There are in addition a number of nonpsychological determinants of 17-OHCS; these include sex, age, and body weight. The avoidance training procedure involved depressing a lever to avoid the occurrence of shock. Results showed a three-fold increase in 17-OHCS excretion level during the avoidance periods. As with the adrenaline response, when there were a number of sessions across monthly intervals, the magnitude of the response diminished but the effect was still large. The authors established by means of free shocks that this was not due to depletion of resources and suggest that dampening mechanisms come into play before resources are exhausted.

Highly significant correlations were reported between 17-OHCS response and lever pressing; the higher 17-OHCS, the lower the avoidance lever pressing rate and the higher the "preavoidance" pressing rate. This might be taken to suggest that in the former case the task has become predictable and control is established, but in the latter case control is not established so that lever pressing is more randomly dispersed. Therefore, although control by avoidance is, as Weiss argues, maximally stressful, the correct use of the response facilities may have ameliorating properties.

These effects might be better understood if we allow one kind of arousal to be associated with the absence of control and one with the operation of vigilance required for avoidance. These considerations suggest that the concurrent state of the organism may provide quite a complex format for incoming material.

With regard to the health of the organism, ACTH production may increase the risk of physical illness by lowering the biological antibody defence system (Amkraut & Solomon, 1975). The result will then depend on the availability of antigens and the relative capacity of the antigen to establish itself before it is countered by an antibody. A "waiting time effect" might operate: Frequent production of ACTH would increase the probability of infection, because an antigen would be more likely to occur during a period of depressed antibody production (Feller, 1966; Fisher, 1973).

Biological Time: Resource and phasic changes. As described so far, biological state is described as if it remains constant in time. However, all available evidence indicates that there is likely to be a time course of events. Firstly, resources are limited and likely to become depleted. Secondly, there will be short-term changes in arousals resulting from the influence of rate of change and production of hormones in circulation. Finally, there will be long-term influences of circadian rhythms. Both mood states and performance features will be subject to these influences as well as to unknown drift factors.

One foundation for these ideas is the work of Selye (1956) on the

General Adaptation Syndrome (GAS)—a triphasic response of the adrenal glands to continued stress. The most important aspect of Selye's work in terms of the arguments to be developed here is that he showed that the concurrent stage of GAS is an important determiner of the degree of resistance to an additional stress. Selye argued that the adrenal cortex was mediator of three phases of stress. In the presence of constant stress such as low temperature, the adrenal cortex first discharges all its fat granules with the cortical hormone (alarm stage), then becomes laden with extra fat and hormone supplies (resistance phase), and finally loses fat and reserves of hormones (exhaustion phase).

The three phases definable in terms of hormone and fat levels produce a triphasic time course of stages. Selye showed that with rats kept in cold temperatures, during the "resistance" phase there was ability to withstand even colder temperatures than in the "alarm" phase, whereas in the later "exhaustion" phase this resistance was lowered and the animal could not withstand temperatures presented in the alarm phase. The middle phase therefore appears to be the phase of enhanced resistance. The animal may be maintaining resistance at the expense of his reserves and energy resources. Selye proposed that the resistance phase is largely mediated by the glucocorticoids that are able to mobilize additional sugars by transforming nonsugars into sugars. These hormones have antiinflammatory properties that make them useful mediators of prolonged stress responses when actual physical assault is involved.

Studies purporting to demonstrate phasic change in affective response to a stimulus have been reviewed by Solomon and Corbit (1974). The observed time course of events is that onset of stimulus, whether positive or negative, produces a rapid peak followed by a steady period of diminished response. Termination of the stimulus then produces a peak rebound effect. An example is provided by an experiment by Solomon and Wynne (1953), in which a dog is given uncontrollable shocks and then suddenly released from the restraining harness, and the shocks are terminated. The peaking and flattening of negative effect during the shock is followed by excitement and tail-wagging on its withdrawal. Solomon and Corbit explain these results in terms of an *opponent process model*, in accordance with which there is a slave effect: The first change is a prerequisite for the second change. The later change is assumed to be an automatic adjustment which brings the organism back into equilibrium. A similar effect is described by Berlyne (1960) in terms of the "arousal jag." Individuals may enjoy a dangerous or unpleasant experience because of the pleasure they obtain when they stop. Practice is an important determinant of the form the temporal characteristics take, presumably because learning that an unpleasant event only lasts for a short period reduces its effect. Since rebound effects are also found when drugs are withdrawn and in cases when stages of sleep are selectively deprived, there is some support for the hypothesis that the effect is biologically based.

Time-based changes in concurrent state may be likened to a short-term or "working" memory. Characteristics based on chemical processes thought to mediate arousal change may be thought of as having some persistence and pervasiveness, which means that the organism may remain in some phase of the stress response long after the source of the problem has been removed. In cases where experience with stress has been prolonged so that resources required for the response have actually been depleted, the state may be thought of as "vulnerable." The response to an event is then a slave to an earlier process. In the short term, this could mean that a person responds less effectively to an event and as a result has to cope with more problems. In the long term there may be risk of both psychological and physical health disorder.

Biological rhythms. Discussions so far have assumed that there is some constant biological state of the organism and that impending events occasionally "push" this state to a temporary extreme position. This ignores totally the fact that a number of quite complex biological and psychological rhythms exist that are likely to provide a fluctuating base for incoming influences. Although detailed review of the work in this area is beyond the space allowed within the confines of this chapter, it is important not to forget long-term rhythms as elements of concurrent state. Therefore, some consideration of the findings in this area is useful. (For detailed discussions and reviews see Blake, 1971; Colquhoun, 1971; Luce, 1973; Folkard, 1979, 1980).

Since the observations made by Gates (1916), implying the existence of a sleep/wakefulness rhythm, and the observations of Kleitman (1939, 1963), suggesting that there was a rhythm for performance efficiency and for body temperature, there has been increasing evidence that might be taken to indicate the relationship of time of day with physiological and psychological changes.

Examination of data on daily body temperature fluctuations (Colquhoun, 1971) showed a steep rate of temperature increase between 07.00 and 10.00 hrs, which is roughly five times the normal rate of increase in succeeding hours, followed by a flattening-off of rate of increase, but a continuing gradual rise toward an early-evening peak. After the peak there is a rapid decline to a low spot of 97.16°F at 05.00 hrs. This data, based on the oral temperature of 70 young men recorded for three minutes at hourly intervals, suggested not only the correspondence of body temperature readings with the active and sleep phase of each 24-hour period but suggested that biological activity may be distinguished within those phases. Kleitman observed that capacity for efficient performance appears to parallel the curve observed for temperature (Kleitman 1963), a conclusion based on observation of a number of tasks such as card dealing, card sorting, hand steadiness, body sway, and tasks such as multiplication and translation. This has been replicated in many subsequent experiments.

Kleitman favored the view that the temperature and performance curves coexisted in parallel and did not attempt to explore the possibility of causal changes. The extensive review by Colquhoun (1971), which considers the detail of both laboratory and shift work studies and the associated methodological difficulties, indicates that whereas there are systematic shifts in efficiency levels during the 24-hour period, the periodicity is not fully understood. Complexity and mental demands of the task may be an important variable, not just as a determinant of the relationship with temperature, but they may influence fluctuation in efficiency throughout the working period.

Colquhoun (1971) rejects the notion of a causal relationship and retains the parallelism notion advocated by Kleitman. Support for this position comes from work by Rutenfranz, Aschoff, and Mann (1972), which failed to find a relationship between temperature and performance when scores were summed across different times of day. Also, the postlunch dip observed by Blake (1971) appears to be an efficiency drop that does not relate to temperature change. The view taken by Rutenfranz and his associates, that temperature and performance are "in phase" with one another, appears to be the only conclusion tenable given the evidence.

Efficiency changes are explained by Colquhoun in terms of arousal change. There is support for this form work by Fiorca et al. (1968) and Alluisi and Chiles (1967), because sleep loss exacerbates the daily change in efficiency levels. The obvious explanation is that a lowered base arousal level allows for performance improvement as the daily increase produces a shift toward optimum. The post-lunch dip is explained as a sudden drop in arousal in normal conditions. Further evidence from comparisons, suggesting that noise, knowledge of results, and extraversion influence performance rhythms (e.g., see Blake, 1971), indicates the involvement of a central mechanism such as arousal. However, a point made in discussions in the previous sections is that arousal is unlikely to be single and unitary. The rather simple formulation of a daily rhythm operating in terms of the shift of a single variable may have to be revised.

Recent work has indicated important changes in higher mental activity during the day (see Folkard 1979, 1980). Early work by Ebbinghaus (1885) showed that learning was over 20% faster at 11.00 hrs than at 10.00 hrs, but slowed down by over 30% at 18.00 hrs. However, there was no evidence from Ebbinghaus that the time at which a list was learned influenced its retention. Folkard (1979) confirms the general finding of diurnal variation in ability on memory tasks and suggests that the changes are best seen in terms of "qualitative changes in the way subjects process information" (Folkard, 1980, p. 38). His results show that whereas time of day effects appear more pronounced for more "realistic" tasks, immediate recall seems to be favored by learning in the morning, and delayed recall by afternoon presentation. Interpretation in terms of arousal theory is difficult. If the differential effect on memory characteristic is described as increase in semantic processing during the day, then it follows that arousal is assumed to increase semantic processing. In fact, Weinstein (1974) reports processing to be more superficial in loud noise. Eysenck (1974, 1975) suggests that retrieval of dominant items in memory is more likely to be favored by increased arousal, whereas nondominant items are attenuated. This could be taken to imply a reduction in the amount of semantic processing under high arousal. Folkard argues that results point to the notion that different circadian factors are responsible for memory and nonmemory aspects of performance. The important point is that these are long-term changes likely to provide shifting base efficiency levels across a variety of tasks as a function of time of day. The custom in stress experiments is either to forget these long-term rhythms or to assume that subject testing times are eventually distributed across all possible times during the working day. Few studies investigate interactions with time of day. The fact that time of day has a complex relationship with different kinds of tasks under normal circumstances suggests a need to consider the effect in relation to the impact of different kinds of stresses. Of particular interest is the change in memory characteristic, because, generalizing from the Folkard studies, afternoon activity favors "elaborative" rather than "maintenance" processing, with greater possibility for long-term rather than short-term recall.

Psychological States

There are two aspects to psychological state with respect to the influence on decisions made about incoming material. The first is the existence of interpretive schemas or structures that select and categorize incoming information. Related to this is the content of the existing memories. The second aspect is transient "load" resulting from levels of data being processed at the time. This may be an important determinant of immediate responses to stress; for example, a person preoccupied with a difficult task may fail to detect incoming information at a critical moment and incur the penalty of an accident.

Interpretive Schemata.   Following Observations of Henry Head, Bartlett (1932) proposed that memory is not merely a reduplicative or reproductive process but is "an affair of construction" (p. 205) based on schemata. Any reaction that "has more than momentary significance" is assumed to be determined by schemata. Bartlett suggested that there were a few basic schemata that provided the basis of consistency, but that as behavior developed, there was an increase in the number and variety of reaction. The role of such structures in determining the impact of incoming stimuli was made implicit. "A new incoming impulse must become not merely a cue setting up a series of reactions all carried out in a fixed temporal order, but a stimulus which enables us to go direct to that portion of the organised setting of past responses which is most relevant to the needs of the moment" (p. 206). Bartlett presented a series of demonstrations in which the content of what was remembered or perceived from presented material showed the influence of beliefs and attitudes, some of which were of social origin. Moreover, in the case of serial reproduction of material from one person to another, Bartlett found evidence of omissions, rationalization, and transformation of minor details. Such selectivities varied from group to group, in accordance with varying group interests or conventions, and produced an effect that was so great that the final version could not be easily connected with the original version without knowledge of the intermediate stages.

The recall of life experiences may be the factor of importance in determining the extent to which a person is influenced by stressful conditions. There may be a "metamemory" for control, based on previously experienced conditions and outcomes. This topic is developed in later chapters, but it is useful to note some of the main features about selectivity in recall for normal subjects, at this stage.

Rapaport (1961) has provided a useful review of the effects of the "hedonic character" of information, including life experiences in determining the properties of recall. One of the problems with some of the early work was that the actual proportions of pleasant as compared with unpleasant experiences were not controlled for. This was true of a study reported by Kowalevski (1908), in which school children were asked to recall vacation experiences. Data showed that 62% on first test recalled more pleasant than unpleasant experiences, suggesting that people might be "memory optimists" in normal conditions. Rapaport concludes, after considering the results of a number of experiments in which main methodological difficulties were absent, that there was only a minority of experiments in which there was better retention of pleasant rather than unpleasant experiences; intense experiences, whether pleasant or unpleasant, tended to have better recall. However, there was some evidence to suggest a time decay factor in which unpleasant rather than pleasant experiences were actively changed (Stagner, 1931).

Recent work by Bower, Gilligan, and Monteiro (1981) involving the reading of text has suggested that induced happy or sad moods at the time of reading are influential in determining the nature of recall. Incidents compatible with induced moods were better recalled. One possibility is that the salience of emotional stimuli are enhanced selectively by a prevailing mood. Induced mood during recall rather than reading had no such effect. These findings are important because the tendency to depression or optimism might lead to selectivity in what is noticed in the environment: A person who is depressed might note mainly negative features of his progress on a task. One result could be a tendency for moods to be self-perpetuating; a person who is depressed may see previous outcomes negatively and lower his assessments about the possibility of control. Hedonic set may have important properties. Certain key events could subsequently form the basis of impressions.

Decision Criteria.   Psychological state could also be thought of as a state of bias in decision making. The concept of a decision criterion evolved in the context of Signal Detection Theory (Tanner & Swets, 1954) and described behavior where a person must choose whether or not to report a signal. As an inspection vigil increases, there is an increased tendency to miss signals and an accompanying decrease in false reports.

Whenever there are two alternatives that have properties in common, the likelihood of one choice rather than the other is described by criterion position. A person walking in snake-infested territory where snakes are known to be dangerous may be expected to over-report seeing a possible snake (false reports) but will not miss the real object if he encounters it.

Criterion position may describe a person's behavior in a number of threatening situations as well as in benign ones. In Chapters 8, 9, and 10, the possibility is considered that a profile of criterion positions may provide a basis for understanding how decisions about control are made. Life events may be thought of as selectively priming criterion positions for decisions between alternatives.

A point of importance is that stress and arousal may cause a shift in criterion position. Evidence for this has been reported by Broadbent and Gregory (1965) and Fisher (1983b) from examination of features of performance in loud noise. The general finding is that subjects appear to make more definite decisions based on weaker evidence. If this finding is robust across a number of stressful conditions, it may be necessary to identify transient representations of psychological state in terms of criterion position.

The Memory for Control.   An interesting question discussed again in Chapters 8, 9, and 10 concerns the memory for control. If helplessness can be transmitted across successive experiences, there must be representations in memory. An important issue is how the conditions and outcome of an experience can be represented and made available as information that determines reaction in a subsequent experience. In Chapter 3 it was suggested that a person can assess control by detecting and representing action and outcome across successive trials. In order to know whether control is in the desired direction, a check is required on the degree to which the original discrepancy between reality and ambition is reduced.

A model proposed by Link (1978) in a different context provides some insight into how specific instances may come to produce a reference code that can have generality and stability. Link proposes that on successive trials each new stimulus presented is compared with a standard by means of a subtraction. The subtraction results in a discrepancy value; if an accumulated discrepancy is smaller than the threshold, one kind of response occurs; if it is greater, then a different response occurs.

This comparison and modification process could provide a basis for establishing the "gist" of whether control is possible or not in specific situation. A similar process could provide the basis for generality if a person then compares data from a different experience at a sufficiently abstract level.

Thus, memory for control may be an aspect of concurrent psychological state that has general, stable qualities. This means that decisions about likely outcomes of near stressful situations that arise can be predicted in advance. Memory for control could be an essential factor determining anticipatory as well as interactive responses to stress. In fact, the available evidence suggests that there are very strong dispositions to anticipate level of control. Level of control is often given the status of ideology and regarded as a personality trait. There are a number of scales designed to estimate whether a person expects to have control over events (internality), or expects that outcomes are determined by chance (externality). Of all the scales, the one developed by Rotter (1966) is perhaps best known, but there a number of others (e.g., Nowicki & Strickland, 1973; Reid & Ware, 1974).

Locus of control appears to be stable and to determine a number of relevant cognitive activities including attention to detail, the level of information actively sought, the level of deferred gratification accepted, and the level of attainment achieved. Level of anticipated control may be hypothesized as an important determinant of stress influence. An initial decision that there is no possibility for control may mean that a person does not "engage the problem" but that he has to suffer the punishment because he cannot avoid any negative consequences. The best analogy is shown by the Seligman dogs (Seligman, 1975). An initial decision that control is always possible leads to a different kind of stress influence. A person engages in the struggle for control, and outcome will depend on his success or failure. The balance of hormones may reflect either initial or subsequent decisions about perceived control. Control ideology might, therefore, be the critical determinant of the kinds of stress influences that come into operation.

"Control ideology" decisions could determine the kind of stress experience of a person in a specified situation. Many aspects of information may be different; internalizers seek information. One of the earliest studies that looked at this was by Seeman and Evans (1962) on tubercular patients. Internalizers were found to have more knowledge about the disease than externalizers. Subsequently, Seeman (1963) went on to show that reformatory inmates who were internalizers showed enhanced recall of parole information when it was relevant but not when it was incidental. A comparable result was reported by Phares (1968): All subjects learned 10 pieces of information about 4 men and were later asked to select appropriate female partners. Internalizers were able to give 50% more reasons for their decisions. When only correct reasons were counted, the difference between internalizers and externalizers increased further. A study by Rotter and Mulry (1965) indicated that when skill is involved, internalizers take longer to make decisions on a matching task and less time when they believe chance is involved. Equally, Julian and Katz (1968) reported that decision time for internalizers reflects task difficulty levels. Finally, attention also seems to distinguish the two groups. Lefcourt and Wine (1969) observed behavior toward an assistant who behaved oddly as compared with one who behaved normally. Not only did internalisers later make more observations about the odd assistant, but they looked at his face more often.

The origins of control ideology are not clear. If control ideology is represented as a metamemory from successive life experiences, then adverse experiences with failed outcomes might lead a person to expect that he has little hope of changing events. Therefore, he might come to be external in his thinking as a logical response to the way outcomes have turned out. This being the case, the poor, the underprivileged, and minority groups would be expected to have higher externality scores. Griffin (1962) attempted to explain the way in which Negroes score higher on externality in this way (see Lefcourt & Ludwig, 1965).

If control dispositions originate in the form of a metamemory from experiences, it is necessary to work out how the move from "particular" to "general" occurs. There must come a time when a person no longer thinks "I cannot control X, Y, Z," but begins instead to think "I cannot control anything ..." If we imagine both that the standard concurrently available reflects previous experiences (see previous discussions on Link's choice reaction time model), it is difficult to explain the inductive process. However, if we imagine that there is a criterion operating so that successive modifications (or lack of modifications) of the discrepancy index result in an outcome (to continue or not continue) and a threshold operates to determine whether the modifications are acceptable or not, we can explain the development of an ideology in terms of criterion setting.

The question of interest is whether stressful experiences are more likely than nonstressful experiences to cause a change toward externality. On the one hand underprivileged groups can be expected to have more basic stresses and less power to change them. We might therefore imagine that a discrepancy index standard might differ. On the other hand, as already described, the criterion for interpreting the discrepancy index may change in stress. We do not know to what extent this effect has generality, but if criterion changes do occur, we would expect a more definite decision on relatively weaker evidence of change in the discrepancy index: more optimism or pessimism.

Transient Processing States.   Implicit in the concept of "mental load" is the notion that overload of resources impairs available capacity. Normally this assumption is applied to dual task conditions overall; decrement on the task considered of secondary importance reflects loss of capacity (see Brown, 1964). The state of relative overload will be an aspect of concurrent state and may provide a sensitive prediction of response to an incoming event, including an alarming event or hazard.

This was found to be the case in the response changes on a main 5-choice serial response task when a secondary digit-addition task occurred concurrently (Fisher 1975a). The structure of each dual task interval was found to be a useful dependent variable; on some occasions the serial task would be interrupted until the digit response had been given; on other occasions there would be one or more serial responses after the occurrence of the digit stimulus and before the answer had been given. A powerful predictor of the time sharing structure was found by Fisher to be the precise time of occurrence of the digit in relation to the last response produced on the serial task; if the digit was close to the last response made, interruption was more likely than if it was distant in time.

There are two possible explanations of why this might be the case. Firstly, it is possible that in the early stage of the production of a serial response decision load is high and an incoming auditory event will block further processing. Rather than start again, a person, interrupted already, deals with the digit. An alternative explanation could be termed "might as well finish"; some internal time-based criterion is set up so that if a response is almost ready to be produced, production continues, whereas early on in the process production is aborted. In either case the concurrent state of the individual is a determinant not just of overspill errors on the secondary task, but on this occasion of the total patterning and hence the attentional organization of the time-sharing interval. The possibility that this effect occurred because there was an internal criterion that led the subject to choose to complete or interrupt was given support by a second experiment, in which the instructions favored the digit task. On 79.1% of occasions the subject interrupted the response, as compared with 22.3% when the serial task was the main task. Such a change occurring as a result of instructions illustrates the power situational determinants may have for changing performance detail.

One way of envisaging the impact of concurrent state is, as illustrated by Fig. 5.5, in terms of a "random walk model." In accordance with the model, motor readiness or attention may be described in terms of a time-varying parameter subject to random drift. Biases may also operate, so that there is a drift toward one alternative rather than another.

As illustrated by Fig. 5.5, a drift or step function orientation toward a particular source of information translates immediately into level of

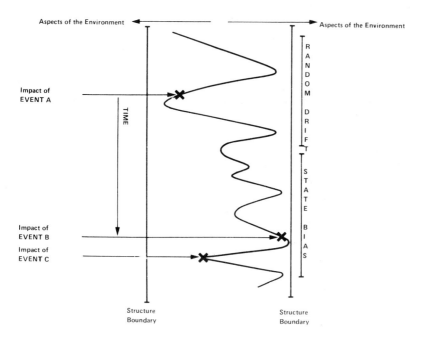

FIG. 5.5. Schematic representation of random walk model applied to descriptions of concurrent states of the nervous system. (Impact is computed from drift or bias position.)

performance efficiency; the individual is ready or not ready, or makes one kind of response rather than another. The question of interest is how much control there is over drifts. On the assumption that at least part of concurrent state is determined by criterion for decisions based on perceived priorities, there is control. To the extent that criterion position is determined by ideology based on previous experience, there may be nonveridical and noncontrollable elements in the drift process.

Duration and Performance

The length of the work period is a complex factor in determining stress effects. We discussed the "vigilance effect," where maximum deterioration appears at the beginning of the work period, that is, within the first half hour of a vigil. The last half of a 30-minute work session has been established as the vulnerable period for noise (Broadbent, 1953; Corcoran, 1962; Wilkinson, 1963). In a vigilance task used by Jerison (1957), it was the last part of a 1½-hour test that was vulnerable in terms of the proportion of missed signals. Sleep deprivation interacts with time on test, so that performance deteriorates gradually (see Warren & Clarke, 1937). Although Mackworth (1950) and Caplan and Lindsay (1946) observed a deterioration toward the end of the task with increased temperature, heat is generally thought to exert maximum effect early on and is a complex stress.

The difficulty with duration effects is to know whether they are underlying changes anyway and the stress just happens to tap a proportion of these inefficiencies, or whether there are changes in resistance or sensitivity to an unpleasant condition. The model proposed by Broadbent (1971) assumes that there are changes in internal control; the upper mechanism gradually relinquishes control over the lower mechanism. A person is increasingly determined by "adrenergic" factors.

The model of the triphasic response to prolonged stress proposed by Selye (e.g., 1956) implies an early alarm phase of lowered resistance, followed by increased resistance, and eventually exhaustion. However, this ignores the possible role of adaptation to adverse environments. Wilkinson (1969) summarizes a number of important studies demonstrating enhanced resistance or acclimatization to the effects of physical environments. For example, Balke and Wells (1958) used a psychomotor task and showed that adverse effects of altitude (15,000 ft) were reduced after 6 weeks but reappeared after 8 weeks at sea level. The time scale varies in different studies; Canfield et al. (1950) demonstrated adaptation to the effects of acceleration (5 g) within only 2 days of exposure.

The role of task factors as determinants of the degree of adaptation is emphasized, and previous task exposure appears to be as important as exposure to the particular stress. This has been indicated for low temperature (e.g., Clark & Jones 1962; Lockhart, 1968) as well as for acceleration (e.g., see Chambers 1963) and weightlessness (Wade, 1962). The original studies on heat effects by Mackworth (1950) showed that skilled operators show greater resistance to the effects of heat.

Duration factors are important aspects of concurrent state, likely to determine the impact of incoming events. In the case of long-term acclimatization, learning factors may be important in addition to changes in the way resources are mobilized. Incoming events must be thought of as acting against a background that is already patterned, and must be thought of as creating influences that change with duration of exposure and degree of work. The nature of the task and previous experience is a determining factor.

The Operation of Situational Factors in the Composite Model

Figure 5.6 illustrates the Composite Model of Stress and Performance. Although a number of potential modes of influence are illustrated, only two modes are operative (Mode 1, Mode 2) in this particular hypothetical situation. The task "gate" has attenuated the influence of Modes 2 and 4. A number of situation rules operate within the framework of this model:

1. The task is capable of acting as a gate device that allows some but not all potential modes to operate. Not all potential modes operate across all situations.
2. The task has features that will provide independently driven influences additive with stress influence.
3. The task has features that may interact with specified modes, such as arousal.
4. The concurrent state of arousal may be a pattern or balance of arousal systems. The stress influences may be compatible or incompatible. Individual dispositions and most recent previous experiences in relation to operative modes define compatibility.
5. The concurrent psychological state may determine which life history experiences are recalled, thus influencing response to a current situation. In addition, there may be prevailing mood states that lead a person to underemphasize over overemphasize his predicament.
6. The concurrent state of "data processing" may determine ways in which operative impact modes influence performance because of transient changes in load.
7. Disposition to externalize or internalize "control" will determine whether problem-solving modes of influence operate and may determine the features of catecholamine balance and prevailing 17-ACTH levels.

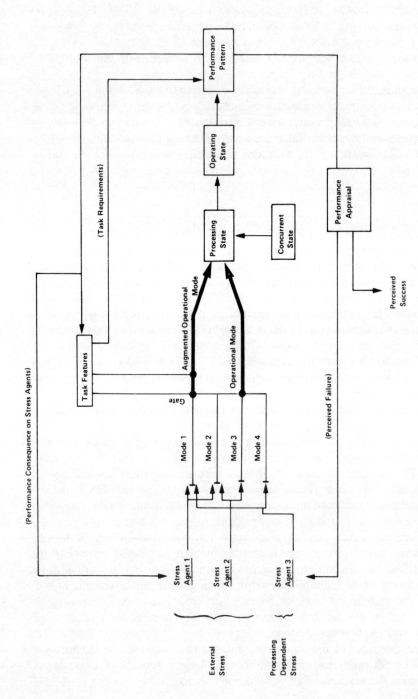

FIG. 5.6. The composite model of stress and performance: A hypothetical illustration of independently driven influences (modes) and the role of situational moderators.

8. Duration of stress exposure and work period will determine the magnitude of stress effect and the detail of performance.

The Locus of Action of Operational Modes

Irrespective of the number of modes of influence that are operative, there will be some integration at the level of arousal and mental resource mechanisms. It might be helpful to think of these major central mechanisms as providing control nodes. Changes in critical parameters that occur at this level will translate into the detail of performance because of the effect on timing, plan running features, and the data base from which plans are instigated. A person might be thought of as having a different functional characteristic and a different knowledge characteristic in conditions of stress. If these working features could be scanned, it should in theory be possible to obtain a digital pattern that represents risk. It is convenient to use the term "intrinsic risk" to describe the properties within a stressful scenario that changes the levels of negative or ineffective performance.

We have suggested that there are many sites of action for situational influences. Some will be effective in adding to or blocking modes implemented by the stress. In other cases there may be central influence at the control nodes. For example, we have argued that the compatibility of concurrent state of arousal in relation to incoming influences is a factor in deciding the arousal characteristics in processing state. It may be the case that compatibility of mental demand with existing resource levels should also be considered.

6

Stress and Plan Running

INTRODUCTION

This chapter and the following chapter are both concerned with ways in which stressful influences itemized previously might come to influence the detail of performance. The main additional interest concerns the implications for the assessment of personal control.

In this chapter the main concern is with small-scale lapses and inefficiencies that occur in performance. Although a person is capable of perfect performance, he occasionally fails. Equally, there are many occasions where he does maintain perfect performance even when tasks are quite complex. A model of the "rules" of the occurrence of lapses and inefficiencies must take both these aspects into account.

The occurrence of occasional lapses has implications for the assessment of control in that if a person notices the occurrence of an error, he is receiving evidence that suggests that his action was not effective. On a statistical model it might be argued that there will be a criterion for error tolerance before a person perceives loss of control. However, a person's attribution of the cause of the error might be a contributing factor; if a person believes that the cause of the error was a moment's inattentiveness, he can retain optimism about his capabilities; if he believes the error to arise from lack of knowledge or lack of capability, the outcome may be different.

A useful distinction is between "external control," which could be defined as the capability of exerting change in the desired direction, and "internal control," which is the extent to which on all trials a person can be sure that the response necessary for exerting external control is selected. Stresses may influence the latter independently of the former. A very tired driver may not necessarily attribute his poor driving to loss of skill but may conclude that because he is tired, he is not producing the right responses at the right time. One point to note is that the magnitude of the error does not relate to the magnitude of the consequences. On one occasion, an error may merely delay progress in the completion of the task; in another case, an error may result in a serious accident. Magnitude of consequences could contribute to estimates of control.

This chapter begins by considering the possibility that there might be changes in internal control due to the composite effects of stress on the timing of decision. First it is necessary to consider the experimental findings that provide the foundations for the model.

THE MICROSTRUCTURE OF PERFORMANCE EFFICIENCY: ERRORS AND BLOCKS

Central Decision and the Speed/Accuracy Trade-off

General speed and accuracy characteristics of performance are normally described by a trade-off or negative relationship in which faster speed is associated with lower accuracy levels (see Pachella, 1972, 1974; Pachella, Smith, & Stanovich, 1974). There are some exceptions to this general rule; on recognition tasks, responses that are faster are likely to be more accurate and associated with better confidence ratings (Norman & Wickelgren, 1969). However, on the majority of tasks studied, the negative relationship obtains.

One of the less quoted demonstrations of the speed/accuracy relationship was provided by Hick (1952), who varied the speed of responding in a choice reaction time task and calculated information transmission rates. When errors increased and therefore less information was transmitted, response speeds were faster. Thus a central foundation was provided for a speed/accuracy characteristic.

The same finding emerges from consideration of the relationship between speed and accuracy in programming responses onto target. Fitts' results (1954) showed that movement time between two targets in a logarithmic function of target width and movement amplitude:

$$\text{Movement time} = K \text{ Log} \left(\frac{A}{w} + .5 \right)$$

Where A is amplitude, w is target width, and K is an arbitrary constant.

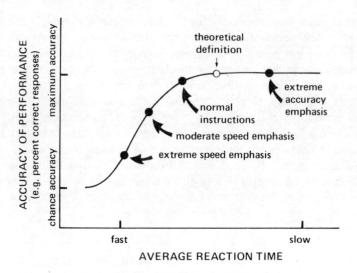

FIG. 6.1.   Ideal representation of speed/accuracy relationship with different speed/accuracy emphasis. (Redrawn from Pachella, 1974; reprinted by permission of the author and Laurence Erlbaum Associates.)

Welford, Norris, and Shock (1963) showed that a factor affecting departure from linearity in terms of the above function was the width of scatter of target hits. In other words, the error distribution was an intrinsic part of the equation for determining response speed; subjects could maintain higher movement time rates by being less accurate.

Figure 6.1 from Pachella (1974) provides an idealized representation of the speed/accuracy trade-off. The form of the function is such that at high response rates a further increase has greater consequence for error rates. Figure 6.2 from Hale (1968) illustrates that subjects are likely to have control over the speed/accuracy trade-off but also that setting for accuracy and setting for speed will produce different empirical relationships, which argues against a single central mechanism on which the balance depends. A sequential decision processes such as that of Wald (1947), which assumes that there is a speed-error factor in the decision mechanism for responses, would suggest that errors occur because of "noise in the system," and the distributions of correct and error RT should be similar. This is confirmed by an analysis by Fitts (1966), who reported no difference between error and correct RTs, but the weight of the empirical evidence is against this (e.g., see Egeth & Smith, 1967; Hale, 1968; Laming, 1968; Rabbitt, 1966; Schouten & Bekker, 1967). Data by Hale (1969) suggests that the effect of "speed set" is to cause an equivalent speeding of correct and error RTs. Error rates increased and subjects produced error rates of over 50% on some trials. Under "speed instructions," not only do correct and error responses both become faster, but subjects make more and faster errors.

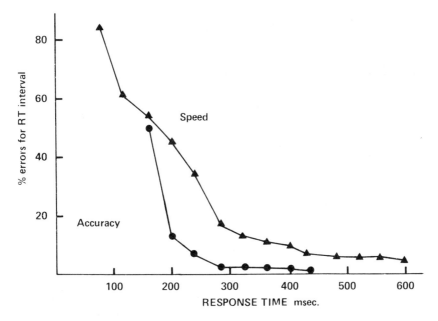

FIG. 6.2.   Speed and accuracy sets in terms of the proportion of errors to total number of responses for each 40 msec class interval. (Redrawn from Hale, 1968; reprinted by permission of the author and the American Psychological Association.)

The weight of the evidence supports the idea that subjects have a great deal of control over the speed/accuracy trade-off but that control is not necessarily exercised by change of a parameter in a single central mechanism. However, the consistent reporting of fast error rates and the association with speeded correct responses under "speed instructions" might suggest the operation of a decision criterion.

Studies by Conrad (1951, 1954 a & b) based on observations of the effects of speeded event rates in bobbin winding provided a convincing demonstration of the limitation in human ability to hold down error rates against increasing speed. As input rates rise, the incidence of omissions increases after about 130 to 140 signals per minute. One explanation is that a person advances the timing of his decision in order to cope with fast event rates, and thus response rate increases. However, if event rates exceed his ability to do this, some signals are omitted. The fact that omissions occur suggests that all input speeds cannot be accommodated by adjustments in timing; these data represent a very real limitation in processing ability of the sort described by Welford in his refractoriness experiments (e.g., see Welford, 1952).

Studies such as these raise the question of how much control a person has over his own performance. Firstly, it is apparent that he cannot avoid some errors; subjects typically produce 2–6% errors on a simple task such as naming a letter (Theios, 1973). However, it is also apparent that subjects can work slowly, making very few errors, or rapidly with numerous errors, or at a point between these extremes. Errors may need to occur in order that a person knows that he is near optimum levels (Rabbitt & Vyas, 1970). A person needs to perform slightly under the optimum operating point in order to be sure of optimizing his performance.

The demands of many experiments may affect not just speed or error, but may change the speed/error characteristic. This means that the latency may not be a measure of delays in internal processes but may represent a strategy. Posner et al. (1973) reported that the decrease in reaction time to shorter foreperiods may not necessarily be the result of alertness but of a change in speed/accuracy trade-off. Jennings, Wood, and Lawrence (1976) suggested that inconsistency in results concerning the effects of alcohol could be explained in terms of changes in speed/accuracy trade-off. Pachella (1972) argued that the equality of slopes for memory-scanning functions on "yes"/"no" responses might be lost if adjustment for error rate was made.

It is clear that on a large scale, when resources are overloaded, the form of performance reflects the use of strategies such as gating-out of irrelevant elements (e.g., see Miller, 1962). This implies control. However, what is unclear is the extent to which stressful conditions may reduce control. A study by Fisher (1980) suggested that control over time sharing may be reduced after one night's sleep loss.

There are three possibilities to consider. The first is the possibility that a person has the same level of control and changes the trade-off because, for example, he gives priority to speed of response; he might do this to finish the task quickly if he accepts a deadline or if conditions are uncongenial. The second is the possibility in that a person loses control and that stresses cause, for example, increased excitement, so that he responds more quickly. A third possibility is that stresses act on the rate of accumulation of evidence for decision, or the level of acceptable evidence, so that timing adjustment is required. If the timing adjustment is within the range of possibility and control is unimpaired, performance will be normally maintained. In order to consider these possibilities in greater detail, it is necessary to look at the microstructure of performance.

Timing of Decision and Speed/Accuracy Microstructure

In normal conditions, we might expect an irreducible minimum number of errors. This may be a built-in aspect of variable performance, which favors biological survival by aiding learning and adjustment. Figure 6.3 illustrates the evidence supporting the idea that errors are "fast-guess" responses. On

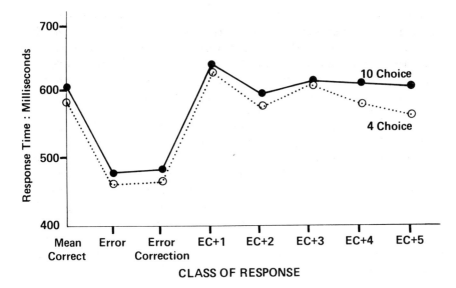

FIG. 6.3.   Profile of error and error correction latencies in a choice response task. (Redrawn from P. M. A. Rabbitt, Errors and error correction in choice response task. Reprinted from *Journal of Experimental Psychology*, 1966a, *71*, 2, 264–72. Copyright 1966 by the American Psychological Association. Adapted by permission of the author.)

a choice response task, error response times are faster than correct response times. Rabbitt (1966) showed that for both 4- and 10-choice serial response tasks, average error rates were 100–150 msec faster than correct responses. In the same study, the proportion of errors made was 1.4% for a 4-choice condition of a serial task and 3.7% for a 10-choice condition.

A model that makes sense of these findings is one that assumes that decisions have to be made with respect to incoming evidence and that it takes time for evidence to accumulate. Decision timing and evidence characteristics are both variables that determine the form of performance features.

Since reaction times are faster to more intense signals (e.g., McGill, 1963), we might assume that the rate of accumulation of evidence is a function of intensity. Equally, context and other priming effects alter the evidence requirement in that recognition latencies are generally lower for expected evidence (e.g., see Morton, 1969), therefore the level of evidence required for decision is also a variable.

When choice is involved, a straightforward evidence accumulation model assumes that decision is made on the basis of absolute levels of evidence. An alternative is that a cruder decision is taken as a function of relative levels. A more sophisticated version assumes that a "random walk" occurs from one alternative to the other as a function of evidence intake and subjective bias. Disposition to favor one decision rather than another is a function of decision bias at any one moment. The level of evidence required for decision may thus be reduced by the operation of bias.

A model that incorporates decision timing and involves the influence of evidence characteristics as determinants of performance detail is illustrated in Fig. 6.4. There are two independent variables: the level of evidence required for a correct decision, and the rate at which this evidence accumulates. Both these variables determine the optimum timing of decision. Responses made in advance of this are based on inadequate

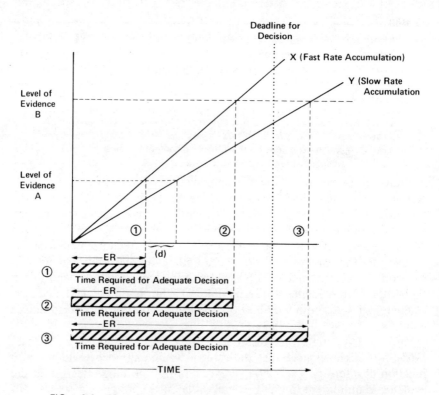

FIG. 6.4. Hypothetical illustration of the relationship between characteristics of evidence and decision as joint determinants of the likelihood of error. Fast guess errors (ER) in relation to level of evidence required for decision (A, B), rate of evidence accumulation (X, Y) and deadline for decision. In no. 3 fixed deadline anticipates adequate evidence for (B) because of slower evidence accumulation (Y) – therefore errors predominate.

evidence and, depending on choice available, will be errors on a specifiable proportion of occasions. Figure 6.4 illustrates how the "time zones" for errors effectively shift as a function of evidence characteristics because of changes in the position of optimum decision time. For level of evidence (A), and accumulation rate (X), in Fig. 6.4, only very fast responses will fall into the error zone (1), and response rates will be fast anyway. Conversely, for a higher evidence requirement (B) and slow-rate accumulation (Y), there is a slower optimum decision timing and a greater zone for the occurrence of errors (3).

If the task is externally paced, a deadline may be imposed, such that if a subject does not respond within a fixed time, the signal disappears. Thus the timing of externally paced events in relation to the above variables will be a critical factor in determining the microstructure of speed and accuracy.

If an externally paced change is not imposed, the task is self-paced and the subject has the possibility of exercising control over timing. To the extent that accuracy has priority, he should move toward optimum decision position for the task. To the extent that speed has priority, one would expect him to advance the timing of decision.

Yellott (1971) proposed that for a given set of conditions two "strategies" are possible; the first is to maintain rapid response times by fast guessing, and the second is to delay responding and wait for adequate evidence. The first strategy will result in a proportion of errors that will vary as a function of the degree of choice, the second in delays in responding the size of which may vary as a function of the degree of interruption distortion or delay of evidence.

The question then is whether the timing of decision is fixed and inflexible throughout the task, or whether the subject makes constant adjustments. A view proposed by Swensson (1972) assumed that a deadline was self-determined in self-paced conditions and that if the evidence was inadequate, a response would be made anyway. An explanation by Broadbent (1971) of the occurrence of errors in high noise on the 5-choice serial reaction task has similar assumptions: The subject has a disposition to respond in some conditions even if the evidence is incomplete. If noise causes interruption in the perception of evidence, he will go ahead and respond anyway.

However, there are a number of examples where fine adjustments do appear to be made to performance during a task. Experiments on the effects of bursts of noise on the same 5-choice serial response task (Fisher, 1972) suggested that cycles of fluctuating effort occurred during a task as a function of events that occurred within it. Just after the occurrence of a 2-sec burst of noise, performance was enhanced, but it slowed gradually again until the next burst occurred. Error occurrence was enhanced during the speeding-up of responses. Thus what could be happening is a change in decision timing while the task is in progress.

There are a number of ways in which conditions might effectively change the proportions of errors and response delays. Firstly, in self-paced conditions, a person may advance the timing of decisions relative to optimum, thus increasing the risk of error, or retard the decision, thus increasing the likelihood of blocks. If the task is externally paced, the deadline for response is determined by the task; if it is advanced relative to optimum, a person is forced to respond or "miss" a trial, perhaps causing an error; if it is retarded, then a person has more personal control over decision timing as in self-paced tasks. If the evidence on which decision is dependent is retarded or interrupted, a person may be forced to retard his decision, which, on a self-paced task, will cause a delay in responding (block), or may proceed normally and thus incur error. If the task is externally paced, again this option may not be open to him; if he does not respond he misses a trial and may score an error. Thus the advance/retard decision may be under personal control or effectively determined by operating conditions.

The issue of the degree of personal control is important. It has been assumed so far that the advance/retard decision is the result of decisions about timing made by a person. Speed/accuracy trade-offs that change under different instructions support the view that control is possible. It might be assumed that in stressful conditions a conscious decision is made by a person to change the timing relative to optimum. He may do this because he considers that successful avoidance behavior requires speeded activity, or that the cost of error would be high. He may compensate for what he believes stresses may do to his performance. If he believes a highly complex environment distracts him, he may speed up the rate at which he responds.

Equally plausible is that arousing or nonarousing conditions may change the timing of decision without personal control over the change. A person may be very "wound up" and tense, thus ready to respond rather than do nothing. Equally, he may be too tired to respond quickly, and so his behavior is sluggish. In these cases, internal states will translate into the detail of performance by producing operating conditions conducive to automatic advance or retard. These internal states may be changed by drugs or by external conditions such as noise or excessive stimulation.

Stresses may also cause a comparable advance/retard change by the "overload" mode of influence. A person who is mentally preoccupied or has too much to do already may shift toward advance timing in order to maintain performance or toward retard when too many other "internal" or "external" sources of information intrude. These shifts may not always be under personal control.

Stress and Degraded Evidence

Stressful conditions may have other effects, which will contribute to effective advance/retard decision position by changing the location of optimum. In the case of weakened, masked, or degraded evidence, the rate at which evidence accumulation occurs will be slowed. Thus, as shown in Fig. 6.4, the position of optimum evidence level is retarded. Therefore if a person maintains the same advance/retard position, since optimum has shifted, a different pattern of errors and blocks will ensue. Personal decision may be required to adjust to slower accumulation rates of evidence, but internal states also created by stresses may act against this. A person may know he ought to slow down in responding to degraded evidence produced by noise, but because of the stimulating properties of noise may be rather more aroused than normal and may tend to respond rather than wait.

Other factors may operate to advance effective optimum. If a person is "primed" to recognize a particular set of signals, rather less evidence will be required, and the position of optimum timing can be advanced. In theory, this could counteract the effect of degraded evidence as far as the operation of advance/retard decisions is concerned.

Error Types and Criterion Placement

The account so far supposes that when errors occur as the result of "guesses," they are randomly distributed across all possible likelihoods. However, there are now a number of different models proposed to explain the nonrandom distribution of guesses. Luce's model implies a fixed bias toward one category of response with little elementary processing (e.g., see Luce, 1963), whereas both Townsend's "activation" model (Townsend, 1971) and Broadbent's "sophisticated guess model" (Broadbent, 1967) allow for a greater degree of processing and presumably within-task adjustment. There are three possible outcomes of either paced timing of decision or distortions in evidence; one is to wait for adequate evidence, another to "fast guess," and the third to make an informed guess based on what is likely. A sophisticated guessing model assumes that there is bias in the set of possible stimuli but that a given stimulus acts to delete the unlikely set.

If we consider that forced guessing might in a simple formulation produce false positives and omissions, as described in the vigilance discussion in Chapter 4, criterion change will alter the proportion of both error types. When more complex situations are considered, informed guessing models are needed because the probability of a guess is not randomly distributed across response categories.

In simple situations, the signal detection formulation is useful; criterion position on no-signal/signal distributions determines bias in guessing. The hypothesis is that adverse circumstances move the criterion to increase or decrease certain reports. A person may make a more definite decision on weaker evidence (e.g., see Broadbent & Gregory, 1965). Alternatively, arousal change might shift the total signal and signal-plus-noise distributions, thus resulting in an effective criterion shift (Welford, 1973).

In situations where a number of different possibilities exist, we might imagine response bias to be represented as a value on the likelihood of stimuli. The value will then prime the system so that rather less evidence is required for decision. We might therefore imagine sets of signal/no-signal distributions for each possible alternative; criterion position will represent both the disposition to report one kind of signal and not to report the others. If a person has a consistent matrix, criterion positions should roughly represent response likelihoods.

In summary, there are three ways in which error and response delay will be influenced by stress conditions. Firstly, stresses may degrade data, thus requiring an effective change in speed of response in order to maintain stable error rates. Secondly, stresses may automatically advance or retard decision timing: a person becomes tense with anxiety or slowed with fatigue. Thirdly, stresses may operate via cognitive routes to change the way a person perceives the task; he may perform to compensate for expected changes associated with stress or perceive completing the task quickly as a way of controlling stress. The advance/retard model will provide the basis for an inverted U relationship between arousal and performance if it is assumed that as arousal increases, timing of decision approaches optimum and is further advanced in hyperarousal. Thus at low levels of arousal, responses are slow and subject to delays, whereas at high levels responses are fast, but fast-guess errors occur. The finding that noise appears to increase the proportion of errors with increasing task duration, whereas sleep loss tends to increase the proportion of gaps (Broadbent, 1971) is accounted for on the assumption that arousal levels build up with duration of exposure to noise so that decision timing becomes advanced, whereas in sleep loss arousal diminishes and decision timing is retarded.

However, there are difficulties with the generality of the negative trade-off assumption of the advance/retard model. Studies of blocking by Bills (1931) showed that blocks are associated with high speed as well as with slowed responding and monotonous conditions. Equally, errors may accompany slow inert patterns of behavior in adverse conditions (e.g., see Davis, 1948). The translation of arousal into "running speed" may not be that simple; anxiety commonly has the effect of slowing performance on complex tasks such as intelligence tests (see Levitt, 1968). An experiment by Siegman (1956) varied the speed instruction on an intelligence task and found that highly anxious subjects performed less effectively than normals on timed subtests of WAIS and more effectively on untimed tasks.

Error and Slowness within the Context of Plans

Since plans are hierarchically organized and involve the transmission of evidence down through successive levels of decision, a slip arising from faulty timing may produce errors that differ according to level of slip. A timing slip at a superordinate level may mean that a false intention is made; a slip at a subordinate level may merely result in a mistarget. So timing slips could account for some of the variety in error form.

There are implications for researchers wishing to analyze errors in terms of origins: A typist may type "TEH" because he was intending to write "TEHRAN" but failed to complete the word or because he was supposed to write "THE" and ordered the letters wrongly. "Context" enables us to guess at the intention of the typist and to assign a probability to the location of the error. For example, if he is typing a text about Iran and it is clear that he is referring to a city, then we would assume that the lapse was a failure to complete the letter sequence "RAN." Because of the difficulties attached to locating the source of an error from its characteristics, Ellis (1979) argued in favor of self-analysis of handwriting errors.

On simpler tasks, the error location may be inferred from knowledge of the correct response alone. Rabbitt (1966) analyzed error occurrence on a serial task; adjacent errors defined as touching the adjoining keys were found to be more likely when a movement across five or more grids was required (a reach of 8 in. or more) and were found to consist of roughly equal numbers of overshoots (47%) and undershoots (53%). Nonadjacent errors took the form of repeated responses and bounces. Although it appeared that these errors had origins at the level in which target-hitting was programmed and the "superordinate" intention was good, it remains possible that the circumstantial evidence is misleading. In the case of repeated presses, Rabbitt points out that a possible cause is uncertainty about whether a contact has been made, which results in checks; this would imply that a superordinate intention governs some of the mistarget errors.

Error Detection and the Origin of Errors

If the perception of control depends on noting and representing data about the degree of relatedness between action and outcome, the occurrence and detection of error will be of importance. If the error is not detected, there will be an unexplained noncontingency. If it is detected, the error-outcome pair could continue to contribute toward a hypothesis of relatedness, because the logic is of the form (not $A \rightarrow$ not X), as compared with ($A \rightarrow X$) for normal trials (where A represents action and X is a form of outcome). If undetected, the logic is of the form ($A \rightarrow$ not X), and this could weaken the relatedness hypothesis. Moreover, if a person notes lack of progress or regression of progress but does not detect the error, he may lower his estimates concerning the perception of control.

Early studies by Rabbitt (1966) showed that not only were errors on a serial-choice task fast latency responses (see Fig. 6.3), but correction responses were equally fast and so accurate that error rates were as low as .001%, compared with 2.5% for normal responses. This would imply that complete information is available to the error correction system and that the initiation of the correction response can proceed in parallel.

One way to make sense of the short error latency followed by the short correction latency illustrated in Fig. 6.3 is to assume that a subject acts in advance of adequate evidence in producing his response initially, but that inadequate evidence continues to accrue so that the correction response occupies the same temporal position as a normal response would occupy. In other words, relevant evidence is not terminated by the production of a response but continues to provide a code for monitoring.

Despite the proficiency of error detection devices in some cases, people do not detect all errors made. Rabbitt's studies showed that on simple keyboard tasks most errors are detected; subjects are faster when required to produce a correction response rather than a common response (Rabbitt, 1968), but even in these circumstances only 74.1% of errors were detected, and one false identification was made.

Errors that arise because of faulty timing should be easier to detect and correct than errors that arise from a superordinate level of the plan because of attention or memory failures. Rabbitt and Vyas (1981) examined data from each of 154 subjects tested during experiments on a self-paced response task and reported no relationship between error latencies, the probability of correction, and correction time. The authors point out that subjects are responding to "easy discriminable signals by selecting easy and compatible responses to them" (p. 227).

The evidence accumulation model would thus appear to be applicable to simple discriminations where slips are fast, evidence continues to accumulate, and corrections are both fast and accurate. Even so there is up to 26% loss on detection efficiency; it may be that the "internal signal" produced by the error monitor is treated rather like an infrequently occurring event, thus producing a "vigilance effect" with increasing task duration.

Rabbitt and Vyas (1981) provided a difficult tone discrimination task in which pairs of tones 25 Hz apart had to be discriminated. In a control "easy" condition, in which the tones were 200 Hz apart, 3% errors were made and 85.2% were corrected. In the difficult discrimination 11.38% errors were made and only 24.1% were corrected. Correct responses were slower for difficult discriminations, and errors that were corrected were fast responses as compared with those that were not. What is important is that subjects corrected the same absolute numbers of errors in both easy and difficult discriminations. Therefore, the extra errors made in the case of difficult discriminations might have been different in origin; they were slower errors and could have been due to perceptual or memory failures. An alternative explanation considered by Rabbitt and Vyas is that the faster a response, the more can a subject extend the time for gaining additional evidence with which to assess its accuracy. If discriminations are so difficult that subjects are slow in producing a response, they will have little extended time. This latter explanation assumes that the speed of response is controlled overall, or that a subject has an internal "deadline" and will not deliberate beyond that time.

In a second experiment based on discrimination of line length in which random chequerboard masks reduced discriminability, thus effectively curtailing the time available for deliberation, results showed that subjects could correct perceptual errors as well as motor errors. There are a number of findings of importance. Firstly, as line length discrimination difficulty increased, there were more errors. Although the percentage of detections was reduced, the absolute number of corrected errors increased: Thus some perceptual errors were corrected. Secondly, error correction times actually increased with the difficulty of discrimination and became shorter as exposure controlled by the mask became shorter. Thirdly, uncorrected errors were as slow as correct responses. Fourthly, for the most difficult discriminations, false error corrections increased for exposure durations of 200 msec or longer.

Rabbitt and Vyas believe that these findings support the hypothesis that perceptual errors can be detected by extension of evidence collection beyond the period defined by the response. Overall average for error correction responses was increasingly weighted by slow detection errors in the case of difficult line discriminations.

The assumption must be that the decision to respond is still advanced relative to the optimum for adequate evidence, but that the evidence continues to be available and is used to initiate a slow correction response. This is prevented when short exposure durations are imposed and correction times are reduced. Presumably this would indicate that subjects cannot continue to process evidence in the form of a visual trace in memory.

The "Committee Decision Model" favored by Rabbitt and Vyas assumed that at signal onset a number of parallel decision processes (likened to committee members) begin to accumulate evidence, but the decision time required by each is a variable. A decision about the nature of the signal is the result of a "vote" taken. A rapid decision will have less votes to count than a slow decision. An impulsive decision even for a difficult task can be followed by a consensus later with a greater probability of being right. In the case of fast accurate correction times for simple tasks (Rabbitt, 1966), the assumption is that all committee members have the same limited probability of accuracy, independent of voting speed.

Daily Lapses

Before taking some of these ideas further in terms of their importance in the perception of control, it is important to consider some of the features of the variety and form of errors people produce in their daily lives. These errors are less easily explained by changes in decision timing. Information concerning detection of these errors provides information about the likely effects of stress on "plan running."

One of the earliest attempts to collect details of error occurrence is provided by Jastrow (1905), who itemized lapses such as "placing the coffee strainer on the tray whilst leaving the cup in the kitchen." Jastrow's study was useful in identifying the likely conditions of error occurrence. The first condition, referred to by Jastrow as the "subconscious element," involved the confusion or transposition of concurrent activities. An example given by Jastrow of a lapse that involves transposition of activities is as follows: "A young lady upon receiving a letter whilst she is engaged in putting her hat away, tosses the perused sheets in the hat box and places the hat in the waster paper basket" (p. 487). Additionally, Jastrow noted that activities regularly repeated were vulnerable because the individual would have no knowledge as to whether or when he had performed the action. In the latter case the detection of the omitted action depends on circumstances that favor detection. Jastrow noted too the vulnerability of automatic activity—the highly skilled individual who can perform a number of actions with minimal involvement of consciousness may actually be vulnerable to daily lapses.

A fundamental modern contribution to the understanding of the occurrence and characteristics of errors has been provided by Reason (1976, 1977) from diary studies that required the detection of errors for a period of two weeks. Results indicated the importance of overload conditions and also the vulnerability of automated skills. Basic data on error rates collected from diary studies (Reason, 1976) indicate that error rates are surprisingly low, averaging out at less than one per day. A theory of errors must take note of what then appears to be surprising *lack of vulnerability*. If we compare these findings with laboratory research on errors and these lapses are assumed to arise from a mechanism that produces errors at fixed rates of between 2 and 6%, the average daily activity level per day would be between 100 and 600 responses! This would hardly seem plausible as an indication of human daily response frequencies. Thus lapses in daily life as reported by subjects must either be different or there must be some negative bias so that a great number of daily errors are either not detected or not reported.

The kind of model that might take account of the occurrence of lapses and the high rate of failure to produce lapses might be one in which there is a basic fixed rate of error production as part of the variability of human behavior; increasing the rate of activity increases the likelihood of a lapse. A "fruit machine" analogy provides a useful basis for comparison; given a fixed probability of obtaining "lemons" by pulling the lever more quickly, there is an increased chance of obtaining "all lemons." This model merely supposes that as activities are speeded, there are more activities, resulting in increased chances of error. The conditions associated with overload and time pressure would thus by raising activity levels increase the probability of error. Automatic activity would have to be assumed to be performed more fluently and quickly, thus incurring the same ultimate penalty.

A recent useful approach to the understanding of the production of errors in everyday life has been made by Broadbent et al. (1981), who introduced a questionnaire measure designed to investigate self-reported failures in perception, memory, and motor function. The most interesting finding was that responses to all questions tend to be positively correlated, and, over-all, responses are correlated with ratings given by a spouse and are stable over long periods of time. A study by Weeks looked at retest correlations over a period of 21 weeks and 65 weeks, which produced correlations of $r = .824$ and $r = .803$, respectively (quoted by Broadbent et al., 1981).

There are reported positive correlations between the cognitive failure questionnaire and a modified version of the Middlesex Hospital Question-naire (Crown & Crisp, 1966), which involves self-report of affective symptoms. Broadbent reports correlations between CFQ and anxiety, depression, and somatic symptoms for groups of males and females on the subject panel, a management group, female laundry workers, and student nurses. In each case, the total CFQ score and the total MHQ is significant at beyond .01 level. The only negative correlations with CFQ occurred for the obsessional personality scale.

A study by Parkes (1980a & b, 1981, quoted by Broadbent et al., 1981) of nurses working on different wards provided data that suggested that CFQ did not change significantly as a function of stress incurred on the ward, whereas MHQ did reflect the difference. This would suggest that CFQ is a measure of a stable set of error production tendencies that do not appear to change as a function of stress levels experienced.

This approach raises the possibility that the mechanism responsible for the production of errors differs in the level of its output for different individuals, and that output should be constant across different working conditions. The problem with the CFQ measure is that subjects make an abstraction that transcends specific situations. Some element of attribution is likely to be involved. A person may make allowances for the fact that for the last few weeks he has been working under pressure and base his perceptions on long-term evidence from his qualities across a broader spectrum of his own life history.

A possibility not so far considered is that certain conditions favor the occurrence of errors because the rules of plan running are violated. Just as it is possible to argue that for a fixed probability mechanism, increasing activity levels increase the frequency of error, so it could be argued that by general disorganization in life style a person is more vulnerable to error.

Table 6.1 provides a short synopsis from a diary maintained by a mature student in Dundee. It seems reasonable to conclude that the presence of so many dogs and cats in a small flat leads the subject to live a life full of potential hazards. Equally, a person without an adequate filing system may constantly lose his papers. The decision that might be important is the initial one to allow too many animals in a small space, or not to spend time evolving a filing system.

It is therefore possible that some people might be more vulnerable to stress effects on their daily lives precisely because they have created a spatial and temporal format for living that increases hazards.

Stress and Fundamental Planning Failures

Lapses and the Detection of Lapses in Daily Life

Both Jastrow and recently Reason noted that overload is a likely condition for error. Stressful conditions may be situations in which there is too much concurrent activity. The possible reasons for this have already been described in Chapter 4. Alternatively, conditions in which the density of activity is high may be perceived by a person as stressful. Support for this is provided by the study by Friedman, Rosenman, and Carroll (1958), in which serum cholesterol levels in U.S. tax accountants rose as a function both of objective and perceived work load produced by the need to meet tax deadlines.

In an attempt to look at the profile of events preceding the occurrence of error, Fisher has recently completed a study that required subjects to record the activities during a period of 6 minutes preceding a previously specified error (in this case the third error made). Control conditions were obtained by requiring the same information to be obtained in relation to a telephone call. Subjects were given paper with horizontal lines, each of which could be used to record a particular activity; there was a marked time scale in minutes across the horizontal axis.

Figures 6.5 and 6.6 illustrate the records of patterns of preceding activity associated with two "transposition" lapses. In the first case (Fig. 6.5), the subject who was poaching eggs and listening to the radio attempted to grill the radio set. In the second case (Fig. 6.6), the subject who was preparing for a bath threw his towel into the bath instead of climbing in himself. In both cases there is a build-up of concurrent activity that is partly externally

TABLE 6.1.
Note from Subject Who Took Part in Diary Study and Reported High
Error Rates

"I have a husband, 8 cats and 3 dogs. That is a lot of animals and people to inhabit a one-bedroomed flat. The animals all cluster on and around the bed at night and they follow us about from room to room during the day, especially if they are hungry or we are preparing food, etc. So they very definitely "get under your feet". I stand on them so often, not because I am clumsy, but because often there is very few bits of floor left unoccupied for me to walk on. Very often it's like an obstacle course in our house, especially at feeding time!"

Sample from diary:

Wed 14th   Tripped over cat.
            Forgot to put chair in front of fridge to stop animals getting in and eating contents.

Thur 15th   Stood on Dillan's ear (One of the dogs).
            Forgot to get milk.

Fri 16th   I had just put dogs back on lead after a run. Instead of giving them a biscuit I let them all off the lead by mistake.

Mon 19th   Tripped over cat.
            Stood on Zippy (One of the dogs)
            Stood on Dillan's ear (He has very large ears).
            Banged knee against dressing table.

Wed 21st   Bought six items in shop, only put five in bag.

Thur 22nd   Tied dogs outside shop, went in shop and bought a few things, left shop and went up the road without dogs.
            Tripped over Zippy.
            Forgot to wind clock.

Fri 23rd   Forgot to get butter.

Sat 24th   Stood on Zippy when I got out of bed.

Mon 26th   Tripped over cat.
            Forgot to switch immersion heater off.

            etc....

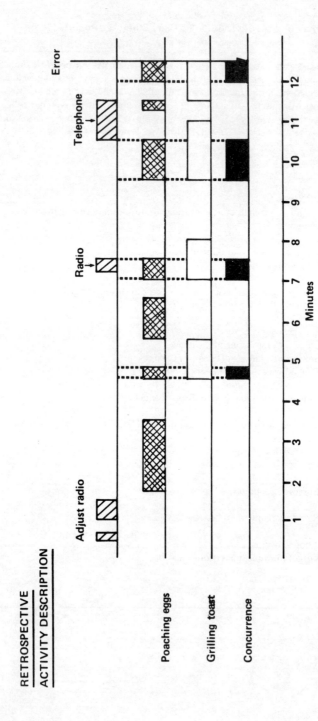

FIG. 6.5. Retrospective analysis of overlap of activity in conditions leading to transposition lapse (error = trying to grill radio set.)

RETROSPECTIVE
ACTIVITY DESCRIPTION

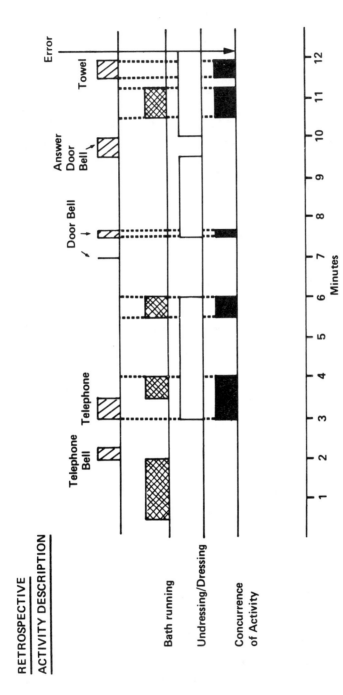

FIG. 6.6.   Retrospective analysis of overlap of activity in conditions leading to transposition lapse (error = throwing towel into bath.)

paced, and in each case there is an interrupting event. The reported levels of concurrent activity were 80% greater than control conditions and 69% greater than for other reported motor slips such as falling or dropping an object.

Studies by Fisher (1975a, 1975b, 1977, 1980) investigated switching of attention on concurrent tasks but in conditions where the motor response was single and did not require the execution of chains of activity. The orderly nature of time sharing in quite complex dual task situations was a main finding; people do seem to be able to cope with concurrent activities, but usually by assigning priority to one "data stream." Also it was noted that an increase in task load tended to cause a change in priority structure, and that sleep deprivation caused a tendency to persist with the task in hand at the time of the intruding event. The most important finding from the point of view of discussions here was that increasing task load did not cause a breakdown in the orderly nature of attention switching.

In earlier considerations of laboratory studies on errors and the detection of errors it was found that some rather simple tasks such as choice response tasks are characterized by fast error responses and equally fast corrections (Rabbitt, 1966), whereas difficult discrimination tasks were characterized by slower response times, more errors, and slower correction times (Rabbitt & Vyas, 1981); the important point is that the extra errors made on difficult discrimination tasks could be detected because although the percentages were reduced, the absolute number corrected rose.

In the case of the detection of errors that do not depend on discriminations of existing evidence but involve not sampling signals or forgetting items or actions, it is likely that the codes necessary for detecting the error will not be present. The occurrence of the error could be totally missed unless circumstances remind a person.

An opportunity arose to sample self-assessments of anxiety and degree of work pressure during an energy and resources conference in Houston, Texas. Individuals were asked to indicate the degree of self-perceived anxiety on a five-category scale from "not anxious" through to "very-anxious," and to rate degree of work load from "not busy" through to "very busy." An anxious group, who rated in the highest category of anxiety but rated in the "not busy" category on the other scale, was selected and asked to keep two-week diaries, as well as a "busy" group, who rated high on the "busy" scale but low on anxiety, and a control group, who rated low on both scales. Both groups also kept two-week diaries of daily lapses.

Table 6.2 shows the main results of interest. Those subjects who self-reported high anxiety showed a slightly greater proportion of errors over the two-week period than did controls ($p < .01$), although there was not the same level of errors as for "busy" people ($p < .001$). Error rates for

TABLE 6.2.
Table of Error Detection Details for Different Self-selected Subject
Populations

Subject groups	Mean errors per day	Median detection time in minutes	Proportion of immediate detections
"Busy" subjects (N = 12)	3.51	149.63	31.3%
Anxious subjects (N = 14)	1.59	7580.81	12.1%
Controls (N = 15)	.98	173.65	35.1%

the control group averaged out at less than one per day and appeared consistent with the error levels reported by Reason (1976). An important difference was among the data on error detection for the three groups. "Busy" subjects with high error rates actually behaved like controls as regards the detail of error detection. There was no increase either in the proportion of errors not detected immediately or in the speed of detection for those not detected immediately. By comparison, the anxious group was characterized by an increased proportion of errors not immediately detected ($p < .001$), and even when using the median as a measure of central tendency in order to avoid the problems caused by occasional very large scores (some detection lags were over a week), the anxious group had slower detection rates than the control group ($p < .001$).

The first obvious possibility was that anxious subjects produced different kinds of errors from controls or from busy subjects. Dividing the detail of errors made into "attentional errors," "memory errors," "motor errors," "situational errors" (where a particular environment causes a subject to produce a strongly associated set of behaviors inappropriate at the time), and "transposition errors" (where elements of concurrent activity are switched), there are no evident differences between the subject groups. Equally, use of judges to rate errors in terms of the degree to which a particular error "would have had consequences that should have been obvious to a subject," produced no significant differences. As far as it is possible to tell using these data, the kinds of errors did not differ; the change must have resulted from differences in error detection.

There are obvious methodological difficulties with reported lapses. The frequency of activity may determine error levels. There may be criterion effects in the reporting of lapses. It is difficult to classify errors in terms of their characteristics or in terms of perceived consequences for the subject.

Despite these difficulties, the result does suggest a need to examine further differences in error detection for different mental states or working conditions. There are two possible explanations of the difference in error detection for anxious people in the Houston study. Firstly, it is possible that in anxiety conditions, the errors arise from cognitive failures, so that the codes available for detection of errors are not present; only circumstance will tell a person whether he has produced a lapse. The point about this explanation is that error differences did not appear on the classification used to categorize errors. A second possibility is that the monitoring system fails to operate effectively; thus, even though the codes and the evidence for detection are available, the monitoring system does not operate. As a result, one effect of anxiety might be to make a subject less aware of his own behavior and the consequences it produces. A "double lapse" hypothesis might account for this behavior; a person lapses twice, first in producing the slip and then in failing to detect it. Being "absent-minded" might imply not only that a sweater is worn inside out but that a person fails to detect it!

There are some grounds for supposing that both arousal increase and the demands of intrusive material in thinking could have the effect of reducing the role of supervisory activity required for the effective monitoring of behavior. High arousal may change the way information is processed, but in addition may provide a source of information to be monitored, thus reducing capacity available for the taks. In addition, the content of daily "worry work" may demand capacity and reduce the available resources for monitoring efficiency. These explanations are conjectural—research is needed involving studies of lapse and lapse detection in people with problems or people who are anxious. At least part of the research must be laboratory-based, so that the relationship of detection to error characteristics can be established.

Stressful Conditions and Planning Operations

One possibility that might account for the relationship between overload conditions and the occurrence of transposition lapses is that the rules that control the combination of activities are violated. Thus, for the most part people do switch activities in daily tasks without making errors; only occasionally does the skill break down. High states of overload, conditions requiring switching of actions causing preoccupation, seem most likely to create a sudden transposition error. These might be conditions in which a supervisory system that switches dominant and subordinate plans in and out operates inefficiently.

Similarly, if states such as self-rated high anxiety are associated with less effective detection of errors as well as with an increase in the number of them, it might be true that there are changes in function of a mechanism that monitors performance, as well as a change in the availability of codes on which detection depends.

In addition, we have to cover the fact that automatic activity seems to increase vulnerability to error, even though these errors are not frequent. It is not the level of activity that itself creates error; automatic activity proceeds along acceptable levels of efficiency normally. It therefore appears that the problem must lie with perhaps a higher-level system that supervises automatic function, or perhaps with the preparation of responses at a lower level.

Reason's studies suggest that 40% of errors are associated with "situational pull" (Reason, 1982). It is not known how often these habit tendencies are prevented by the operation of a supervisory or monitoring system. An interesting question would be how long a person persists in performing a situationally determined inappropriate action before he realizes that the action is inappropriate. If there is a monitoring failure, the sequence of activity might reach completion before there is realization that the whole sequence is inappropriate.

There are therefore two possible ways in which a format for the production of errors may be created by stress conditions. Firstly, there are conditions where too many actions have to be completed; this is common in overload situations or when deadlines have to be met. Secondly, stresses may create a failure in supervisory activity—monitoring, checking, or counting. A normally functioning supervisory system could reduce the vulnerability associated with strong habit intrusions and automaticity by implementing monitoring checks.

The main question is what function a supervisory system might have in the context of planned activity. Preserving the notion that planned activity is organized hierarchically and in such a way that some activities are embedded in others, one fundamental problem could be too many potential "blueprints" lying around at the same time. A supervisory system that could switch activities in and out of focus would be a useful prerequisite. It may be that there will be constraints on the rate of switching, so that too many embedded plans or too great a rate of change will cause problems. Equally, we need a model that will handle the idea of long- and short-term blueprints. Long-term plans may contain specifications for short-term activities and must be held in some kind of working memory for a long time.

Thus, there is good reason for proposing a working memory for plans addressed by intentions. There may be limitations on this memory, so that some plans brought into focus may "fade out" and not be implemented. Equally, some plans may be held in focus for lengthy periods and dominate behavior.

If we now assume that the stacking of plans in focus is guided by a supervisory system, it is possible that this activity itself requires capacity and that reduction of resources will impair this orderly process. Korchin (1964) quotes a statement by Rioch (1955), which implies that troops in battle may not be able to think ahead and plan activity. Their behavior is very much "here-and-now."

We have been assuming that the supervisory activity continues to provide a monitoring service. If a plan is in focus, the intention it generates can be registered and the actual change in behavior can be checked against it. A malfunction in supervisory activity may then mean that the plan is held in focus, the intention is clear, but that the execution of action is not correctly monitored.

The Capture of Existing Inefficiences

A completely different way of considering inefficiencies in stress is that they are artifacts, *"captured"* by randomly occurring accidental events. The basis for this possibility is that—as shown by Feller (1966)—an event occurring at random with respect to time during an on-going time series is more likely to select a long time interval in which to occur. The only assumption needed is that moments of inaccuracy are usually long time intervals. As far as the occurrence of response delays is concerned, this will be the case; in the case of errors, although they are fast responses, the total time of error, plus error correction, plus post-error slowness, may together provide a long time interval during which a subject is likely to be less ready for incoming events. There are some grounds for arguing that inefficiency periods may be long enough to attract random "accidental" events.

Running State and Performance Patterns on Complex Tasks

A question of importance for this chapter is whether "running state" is likely to determine more than just an increased proportion of small lapses and blocks in performance. There are good logical grounds for supposing this might be the case. If either by conscious decision or increased arousal response timing is speeded, there would be less time to inspect stimulus sources, and less time to do the necessary memory work in forming a long-term store of the structure of the task. Merely by increasing speed of response, a person may form an unrealistic cognitive model of the task. This may be particularly evident in the case of complex tasks, where, as will be described in the next chapter, planning of how to sample a task might be critical. Some of these points can be illustrated with respect to the results of an experiment on search and memory in loud noise (Fisher, 1983b). The task required that a subject sampled sequentially a face-down array of 52 playing cards. Inspecting each card one at a time, using one hand, subjects were required to detect and report confidence levels from "high" through "medium" to "low" associated with the detection of matched pairs.

The main features of the findings are shown in Table 6.3. In the presence of loud noise, subjects were reliably faster to complete the task but inspected more cards in order to do so. They could be compensating for expected or perceived memory loss in noise by working harder. Alternatively, subjects might by inspecting cards more rapidly reduce efficient recall of the occurrence and position of cards.

Subjects in noise did not show any increase in the selection of wrong pairs, but there was a change in confidence levels about correct and error pairs. In loud noise, subjects were less confident relative to quiet about pairs that turned out to be incorrectly chosen and more confident about pairs that turned out to be correct. One explanation is that noise makes subjects more definite about relatively weaker evidence. An alternative is that because of speeded search rates in noise, there is less time to consider the evidence and therefore a subject bases his decision on early impressions and opts for one of the two extreme confidence levels.

TABLE 6.3.
Performance Patterns in Quiet and Noise on a Memory and Search Task

Basic memory and search variables		Quiet (55 dBA)	Noise (100 dBA)
$\overline{X}$ number of cards sampled		132.3	151.5
$\overline{X}$ inspection time per card (in secs)		5.19	4.24
$\overline{X}$ number of error pairs		14.2	12.0
$\overline{X}$ number of samples to first correct pair		8.44	16.5
$\overline{X}$ total time taken (in secs)		686.64	642.36
Confidence estimates			
% Correct pairs	"high"	59.61	71.79
	"medium"	12.39	10.83
	"low"	28.0	15.98
% Error pairs	"high"	38.3	26.38
	"medium"	8.6	12.32
	"low"	53.1	61.0

Finally, an additional reliable result was that for the first 30 cards sampled, a greater proportion were from the central rather than the peripheral segments of the array of cards. One explanation is that noise has caused narrowing of attention (see Easterbrook, 1959). However, attentional focusing on central aspects of a spatial array is not easily explained, for there is no reason why central items should be more salient or pairs more probable. An alternative, different explanation is that increased speed of response favors a strategy of selecting centrally located cards because movement is reduced and cards can be rapidly inspected. The advantage of this explanation is that central inspections are determined by expediency as part of an adjustment to speeded responding, rather than resulting from any perceived probability advantage to centrally available sources.

Taken collectively, these results suggest a picture of performance in noise characterized by increased speed, decreased memory efficiency, increased confidence about decisions, and increased attentional selectivity. It remains plausible that speeded response rates provide the single causal factor: Subjects, because they respond faster in noise, may allow themselves less time to register the information in memory than they need. This is illustrated by:

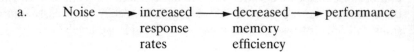

a.   Noise ⟶ increased ⟶ decreased ⟶ performance
                  response   memory
                  rates   efficiency

Alternatively, increased response rates and decreased memory efficiency may be conjoint responses to stress, which combine to determine the character of performance. This is illustrated by:

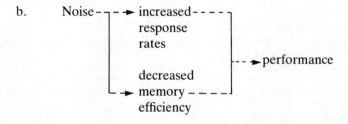

b.   Noise ⟶ increased
                  response
                  rates
                                          ⟶ performance
                  decreased
                  ⟶ memory
                  efficiency

As far as the "running state" notion described in this chapter is concerned, the casual sequence illustrated in (a) provides a basis for the argument that running speed may have a specific effect on the detail of performance accuracy, but it may also have a profound effect on the higher mental process on which the main character of performance ultimately depends.

RUNNING STATE, PERFORMANCE COMPETENCE, AND CONTROL

There are a number of ways in which stressful conditions could translate into the detail of performance. The first, considered at length in this chapter, is decision timing. By advancing or retarding decision time relative to optimum, a person can change the speed accuracy balance of his performance. The same effective change can be induced if the task imposes a deadline for decision. Equally, a person may advance or retard timing because of arousal change; if tension levels are high, he may have a disposition to respond quickly.

There are a number of ways in which stressful conditions may influence the variables in the evidence accumulation model. Firstly, there may be degraded evidence that will in effect change the temporal position of optimum. Secondly, there may be expectancies that change the "priming" levels associated with certain kinds of events, thus effectively changing the position of optimum decision timing.

The model allows for character and variety in lapses, if it is assumed that the formulation applies to any point in the plan where evidence is transmitted. Thus, from intention to action, from action to response sequencing, and from sequencing to targeting of response, there are points at which decisions must be made and the above considerations on timing are important. An error can occur because there was a fast guess in the translation from intention to action, or because of a fast guess in the programming of response onto target. The form of the error may vary.

Additionally, stresses may create conditions that make planning difficult. New plans may be required, too many plans may be pushed into focus, resulting in the occurrence of planning anomalies. There may be failures in the monitoring of plan running, so that errors that would normally be detected escape and remain undetected.

Evidence for the Assessment of Control

The model of the perception of control presented in earlier chapters suggested that control might be assessed by means of the statistical representation of evidence about action and outcome. This would be particularly important in a situation not encountered before, where a person could not call upon a store of previous expectancies.

If this is the case, then detection and tolerance of error are likely to be important. If a person produces errors, these are trials where the action and outcome are not as expected. If a person produces a "not response" and achieves a "not" result, this does not challenge the contingency between response and outcome in the way that it does if he produces an appropriate response and achieves a "not" result. In the latter case the evidence suggests the right course of action but an unpredicted result.

If a person does not detect his error, he does not know he has made a "not" response; therefore he thinks he has made an appropriate response, and yet he notes consequences that indicate a "not" result. In other words, he thinks he has done the right thing but sees reality as behaving unexpectedly. From evidence of performance on simple tasks in the laboratory, it would seem that about 20–25% of errors may be undetected and could lead to this assessment. However, it would also be the case that if the person does not even note the unpredicted change in consequences as well as not detecting his error, his perception of control may be unchanged. A pilot who is so absentminded that he does not notice his error but also does not notice the extraordinary drop of the aircraft may be similar to the perfect pilot as far as the perception of control is concerned.

The point was made earlier that the perception of control must involve not only the perception of contingency between response and outcome, but the perception that the change is in the desired direction. If a person misrepresents his errors, he may begin to feel that the situation is being externally controlled. In the case of the pilot who does not notice his error, if he does notice the change in flight path he may also begin to think that he is incapable of controlling the system. If he does detect his own error, he can retain the previous assessments of objective control.

Even if the contingency assessment model is thought of as a "straw man," so that in practice a person simply notes change in reality as an indication of his progress in achieving control, many of the above considerations apply. As far as the subjective assessment of control is concerned, a person who makes many errors but detects few of them and detects few of the changes in reality that result might be in the same position as the person who makes few errors. What is different is that in the case of the former the person's assessment of control is distorted with respect to what is actually true.

Stress, Error Detection, and Control

This chapter has been concerned with slips that arise from changes in the timing of decision, or possibly from the violation of rules of planning. For the most part, the codes on which error detection depends remain available; studies suggest that 50–75% of these errors are detected. If error rates increase in stress and detections decrease in proportion, a person may need to attribute the cause. Also, since error data reduces the number of obvious contingency pairings, there may be less hard evidence on which to base estimates of control.

A point made in a quite different context by Jones and Davis (1965) is that negative features often provide more information than positive features in "normatively positive information environments." If an individual believes that "people are sincere," then it is of more interest to him if he finds an individual who is not sincere.

If we apply this principle to errors, we would suppose that since error rates are normally not high, errors will provide a person with more important information about his performance than normal responses. So, if a person operates a rule-of-thumb strategy for assessing control, we might expect him to be more interested in his errors. From arguments developed in the previous chapter, we might also expect that internalizers would seek more information of this kind.

The above considerations rest to some extent on the assumption that control assessment is a computation from the frequency of events. In fact, work by Howell and Burnett (1978) suggests that people are poor estimators of the frequency of events. Knowledge of the system or "generator knowledge" will influence the global estimate of different event frequencies. People might have expectancies about how they will perform under certain working conditions. If so, these expectancies might bias the way "error" and "correct" frequencies are represented globally. There is evidence by Fisher (1983a, e) to suggest that stresses increase the expectancy of poor performance in noise; thus a person under stress may overrepresent his errors.

These considerations are important because a person may maintain optimism about his level of perceived control if he attributes the cause of perceived less efficient performance to the presence of stress. Seligman's treatment of dogs designed to produce helplessness equated with depression was to shock the animals first in conditions where escape was impossible because of the restraining harness. One way to look at his result is to argue that the animals failed to attribute their helplessness to the presence of a harness and the absence of response facility; helplessness therefore became a generalized assumption about all future occasions. A person who notices his performance deterioration in stressful conditions may retain optimism for the future if he makes allowances for himself because he was working under stress.

A study by Fisher (1983e) involved requiring subjects to assess the quality of typing performance on a 5-point scale from "very poor" (1) through to "very good" (5) for a hypothetical typist. Information about the conditions the typist was working under was given to the subjects. One group of subjects judged the hypothetical typists to be working in "quiet conditions," and one group in "noise conditions." There were 4 objective levels of errors, as shown in Table 6.4. Each subject was shown a

TABLE 6.4.
Ranking Assessments by Normal Subjects on the Quality of
Performance of a Hypothetical Typist Allegedly Working in either Quiet
or Noise (Experiment 3. Fisher, 1983e)

	Objective level of error	$\overline{X}$ ratings[1]
Mean category ratings for working in quiet	2%	1.41
	5%	1.92
	10%	3.93
	15%	4.34
		2.89
Mean category ratings for working in noise	2%	1.23 NS
	5%	1.46 *
	10%	2.88 **
	15%	3.10 **
		$\overline{X}$ 2.16 (Experiment 3 from Fisher, 1983g)

TABLE 6.5.
Ranking Assessments by Normal and Depressed Subjects on the
Quality of Performance of a Hypothetical Typist Allegedly Working in
either Quiet or Noise (Experiment 4, Fisher, 1983e)

	Objective level of error	Nondepressed $\overline{X}$ ratings[1] BDI < 8	Depressed $\overline{X}$ ratings BDI < 9
Mean category ratings for working in quiet	2%	1.34	2.50
	5%	1.49	3.61
	10%	3.71	4.39
	15%	4.01	4.81
		$\overline{X}$ 2.64	3.83
Mean category ratings for working in noise	2%	1.29 NS	2.91 NS
	5%	1.31 NS	3.89 NS
	10%	2.95 **	4.35 NS
	15%	3.04 ***	4.79 NS
		$\overline{X}$ 2.15	3.99

Mann Whitney test comparisons—Quiet and Noise:
* = $p<.05$ ** = $p<.01$ *** = $p<.001$ NS = not significant
[1] 1 = very good
  5 = very poor

typescript. The errors were all letter transposition errors fabricated and ringed in red. The percentage of errors was summarized at the end. The subjects looked at a typescript and then made a judgment.

Table 6.4 shows that, with the exception of the 2% condition, there were significant differences in the assessments made for those assumed to be working in noise as compared with quiet. Greater allowances were made for errors in judging the quality of performance. When comparable material was presented to a group of students with scores greater than 9 on the Beck Depression Inventory, one of the findings of interest illustrated in Table 6.5 was that less allowance was made by subjects for the performance of the (hypothetical) typist believed to have been working in high noise. Results might be taken to suggest that depressed students are hard on people. If this is true, it follows that lowered self-esteem might gradually arise from constantly applying hard judgments to all observed behaviors, including self-produced behavior, and therefore constantly accepting the responsibility for failure.

7

Stress and Plan Ingredients

INTRODUCTION

In the previous chapter the main concern was with a source of errors arising because of factors influencing the running of plans; it was assumed that a person could in theory produce perfect performance but simply failed to do so on all occasions. Stressful conditions were argued to be likely to raise the frequency of these incidental slips. Since most of them can be detected immediately, the question of importance is how tolerant a person can be expected to be of his slips before he revises his opinion in favor of loss of control on the task.

In this chapter, the effects are studied of stressful conditions on more fundamental planning processes concerned with the representation and utilization of knowledge about the task. If a person does not form a representational data base, he operates with a distorted impression of the structure of events. Systematic bias may be evident in the pattern of errors he produces, since he acts under false hypotheses. In these conditions he will not have the codes necessary to detect his errors. He might therefore be expected to misrepresent his lack of competence.

However, the above formulation depends on the assumption that processes such as memory and attention, on which the foundation of task knowledge ultimately depends, are adversely affected by stress. This is a simplistic view; there are conditions where both memory and—independently—attention have been shown to improve in stressful conditions. It seems generally true that only at severe levels of stress, perhaps where life itself is at risk, is it likely that these fundamental cognitive processes will necessarily be impaired.

152

Before discussing the effects of stressful conditions on higher processes in greater detail, it is useful to consider in wider perspective the possible demands made on the planning of performance in stressful conditions. A person may need to do a great deal more than just continue to produce successful actions. He may have to make decisions about how much effort he is prepared to make and how much cost there will be in biological terms. Equally, a person may need to make economies in conditions of overload, so that he does not waste resources. If there is high cost attached to error, precautions against the consequence of error may have to be taken in advance; a man who plans to walk through a snake-infested desert should prepare for error by wearing snake boots and implementing checking procedures by avoiding jumping large stones or walking into caves and crevasses.

Experimentally, there is little information about how these decisions are made. In some cases there may be rules of conduct, such as, for example, how to prepare for a trek through snake country. On other occasions new plans may be required. In these cases the elements may have factors in common with the main features of TOTE units described for basic skills by Miller, Galanter, and Pribram (1960). Firstly, a discrepancy is noted (the nail is not flush with the wood), then an operation is implemented (hit the nail). However, the source of the discrepancy may differ in more complex cases. For example, a person may note the discrepancy between the level of effort required for the task and the level of effort it is reasonable to devote to it. Cost-effectiveness decisions are also part of overall planning decisions.

Economy of Effort

Economy of effort occurs whenever it can be inferred that a person has made some adjustment in order to reach the same goal, but with less total energy expenditure. An individual engaged in running a marathon would be expected to be slower for the first mile than the individual who is running a total distance of a mile. Although on "first mile" performance measures the marathon runner could be argued to be demonstrating lowered efficiency, given the total context of the race he is behaving efficiently by conserving energy, thus ensuring that he will complete the race with the fastest time overall.

The concept of economy of activity is an interesting one, with a long history in psychology. In the 1920s there were a number of attempts to consider the question of economy of effort in terms of strategies. For example, Waters (1937) working with rats believed that the "least effort principle" was evident in terms of strategies used to achieve the goal. "Our rats found that by sticking to the outside path they more readily achieved the goal" (p. 17). The "outside path" may require more activity initially but it is more likely to be successful. A rather different approach was chosen by Hull (1943), who assumed that "least work" was more likely to be a determinant of choice; whenever two behavior sequences are possible, the one requiring least work will be selected. The notions of "best strategy" and "least work" as determinants of economy were partly reconciled by Zipf (1949; revised, 1965), who formulated the notion of the "least probable rate of work"; the best strategy is assumed to involve the "least work" in the "long term."

If the individual is assumed to be able to "set" his performance levels in terms of these considerations, then there must be available mental representations of cost and consequences attached to likely courses of action. Decisions may depend on the outcome of anticipatory process, and there must be sufficient control to ensure that the decision is carried out.

Cognitive Economies

Zipf assumed that the "least effort principle" is biologically adaptive. He evaluated economy of effort in terms of mental operations involved. Reduction in the number of operations is the basis of cognitive economy, as was illustrated with respect to the analogy of an artisan and his tools. The minimum equation of the arrangement of the tools is

$$W_r = f \times m \times d$$

where W_r = tool's total work range; d = distance of tool to artisan's lap; f = relative frequency with which a given total (r) is used; and m = mass of tool.

Each tool represents a cognitive operation and is assumed to be specifiable by a value that indexes the effort required. In the case of minimum effort, the $f \times m \times d$ operation is at its smallest value. For example, by reducing the size of all the tools ("close packing"), the value of d is reduced. Equally, tools that are most frequently used are assumed to be given a position that represents least distance. As the number of tools to be used increases, the law of diminishing returns operates, since the distance of the last tool increases. Therefore, by analogy, cognitive operations may be made more efficient by increasing the versatility of each tool ("Principle of Economical Versatility"). Similarly, by using two well-placed tools instead of one expensive tool ("Principle of the Economical Permutation of Tools"), the number of tools may be kept to a minimum. Finally, simplification through the use of a single highly specialized tool will have a rather similar result.

By means of these illustrations, Zipf introduced the notion that economy of effort is specifiable in terms of mental operations. The most efficient performance is that which achieves the given result with the fewest possible intervening transformations. Zipf illustrates his laws of economy with reference to empirical work on speech units, showing a negative correlation between word length and word frequency and by illustrations of the way in which words become amalgamated to make economic units, as in "brother-in-law."

Efficient Allocation of Energy and Information Resources

It seems reasonable to think of the gross character of performances as being the result of the operation of a number of trade-offs, some of which may depend on decision. Firstly, there is the energy/performance trade-off. An individual may have to decide how much physiological cost he is prepared to incur in order to maintain performance. He may "keep going" at the expense of energy transfer systems. A man who is highly fatigued or sleep-deprived may expend extra effort to sustain performance. Secondly, there is the possibility of allocating resources in different ways as a function of task demands. By trading off time for performance adequacy a subject may sustain an acceptable level of performance but require extra time in order to do so. If time is unimportant and the task is self-paced, this may be an acceptable strategy.

If we assume that at least some of these trade-offs may be determined by decision, then we assume that control is available and that reference codes available in knowledge must contribute. Navon and Gopher (1979) propose allocation of resources according to a "utility" principle. The allocation principle is likely to involve high-order decision processes and to be capable of infinite revisions and change; the resultant performance profile reflects decision as to allocation policy. This results in the "performance operating characteristic" (POC); capacity, far from being fixed, is an abstraction from "the stable level of what the system can supply in circumstances of heavy load" (Navon & Gopher, 1979).

Efficient allocation of energy and information resources requires that control must be possible; there must be a mental representation of the demands of various competing tasks and the goal requirement. In cases where conditions are so uncertain that the individual has no idea what demands are likely to occur, then allocation policy is unlikely to be efficient and may be determined by instructions, by random decision as to priority, or by whatever event happens first.

Economies and the Reduction of Effective Demand

An obvious logical distinction to make is between objective and subjective demand. It was implicit in Zipf's thesis that cognitive economies save resources. However, it is plausible that for a given level of objective demand, processing economies will dictate the available resources and will change the POC.

A number of economies have been proposed by researchers working in slightly different areas. In skilled performance, perhaps the best-known although possibly the least understood phenomenon is that of "automatization." With increasing practice, components of a task come to be organized into smooth coordinated units, with apparent reduction of demand on higher information processing centers and decreased conscious monitoring. As argued by Bahrick and Shelley (1958), automatization frees higher systems for time-sharing between other inputs. The obvious interpretation of automatization is that there is an effective reduction of resource demand because of the operation of cognitive economies.

In addition, there are ways in which data may be compressed or monitored more efficiently. If any individual learns rules or heuristics, then he need not process information in such depth. Given a representative "model of the task world," including an accurate representation of probability structure, uncertainty is reduced.

Posner (1964) proposed a taxonomy of information processing tasks based on possible economies in processing. For example, some tasks favored "gating," because only a certain proportion of the available information is relevant. Once the subject has learned the rule, gating greatly reduces the demands of the task. Efficiency and reduction of resource demand may be assumed to be synonymous.

In a recent paper investigating the processes of language development, Wolff (1982) considered the evolutionary importance of economies in data processing. He argued that selection pressures will favor techniques that reduce redundancy in data, so that the volume of information is lessened. Wolff proposes five major principles of data compression and considers the possible implications of each for language learning. The labeling of repeating patterns by simple codes and the coding of patterns that share common contexts provide basic methods of reducing input. When the pattern is represented by a sequence of repeating symbols, then the "run length" may additionally be reduced. Choosing the most representative group in situations where there is conflict or ignoring part of the data will serve to compress data. Compression techniques may occasionally lead to error. Wolff notes the occasional occurrence of run-on errors (Wolf, 1982), in which a particular structure when present leads the individual to misconstrue the final outcome.

Stress and Strategy

Stress may provide conditions in which planning decisions about how to allocate resources are essential. Firstly, there may be a need to decide the amount of effort to be allocated. Secondly, there may be a need to decide how to allocate resources across two sets of demands when a dual task paradigm is created. Thirdly, there may be a need to decide the allocation of resources across various elements of a complex task. Increased arousal or increased information processing demand could both have this effect. In some cases it might be helpful to think of a "stress performance operating characteristic" in which, as with the "performance operating characteristic" described by Gopher and North (1979), utility principles determine the trade-off.

Research on sleep deprivation and performance has provided evidence of reversal points; after a period of time, a parameter changes level. At least one interpretation is that a person abandons the plan to cooperate, expend effort, and stay awake in favor of disengaging and drifting toward sleep (see Murray, Schein, Erikson, Hill, & Cohen, 1959).

Research on the effects of noise bursts on a serial response task (Fisher, 1972), and more recently on the effects of continuous noise on a dual task design set up on a microcomputer (Fisher, 1983c), has shown that there appear to be within-task speed adjustments that might be symptomatic of cycles of fluctuating effort. This implies the operation of a strategy to maintain speed in the presence of adverse noise conditions.

In the previous chapter, the operation of a strategy on a memory and search task was described (Fisher, 1982); the effect of loud noise was to speed up the rate at which subjects detected matched pairs in a search task, but the effect was due not to enhanced memory efficiency but to increased inspection effort. This could be explained as being the result of a considered strategy to maintain performance or even improve it in conditions of loud noise. However, it might also be the result of an unavoidable pattern brought about by increased arousal raising activity levels, thus speeding search time.

In some cases, strategies can only be effectively selected if there is a prior data base from previous experience. A number of laboratories have described stress effects that are order-dependent in within-group designs (e.g. see Millar, 1980; Poulton & Edwards, 1979); at least one explanation is that when an inexperienced person first works in stressful conditions, learning is reduced and he does not have an adequate data base for the implementation of strategies for maximizing efficiency.

Taken collectively, all the trade-offs that have been described may be subsumed under the general heading of "policy decisions." Policy decisions are dependent on ingredients of higher cognitive process and as such will reflect the data-base or model of "how the world is," the major aim or intention, and performance features. It is reasonable to envisage a process in which a decision criterion is set so that performance is directed with respect to biases in one direction rather than another. A subject who has decided to stay awake or complete an arduous race may set a criterion based on persistent behavior and depletion of resources. This is an aspect of planned behavior not often considered in an experimental setting. A study by Fisher (unpublished) investigated how long a subject would persist in trying to find a missing number in a series when the number was actually random. Loud noise (100 dB) was delivered via earphones. A between-group design was used. The experiment is similar to the experiment described in Chapter 4 on the effects of flashing lights. As illustrated by Table 7.1, noise reduces the period a person will spend on a difficult problem ($p < .001$). There are a number of alternative hypotheses: An obvious suggestion is that the unpleasant environment created by loud noise leads to an advance strategy of "early disengagement." Subjects could escape from the noise by giving up with the problem; in this context, lack of persistence may be a means of exerting control over adverse conditions rather than representing a "helplessness" response.

TABLE 7.1.
Period Spent Solving a Problem in Noise and
Quiet in Self-paced Conditions

	Quiet (60 dB)	Noise (100 dB)
Average persistence in minutes	20.8	8.1*
S.D.	5.1	2.0

* $p < .001$

PLAN INGREDIENTS IN STRESSFUL CONDITIONS

An important distinction noted earlier is between knowledge that is acquired prior to a particular situation being encountered and knowledge acquired during the situation. In the former case, compensatory or "economic" strategies may be put into effect immediately; in the latter, some type of trial-and-error adjustment must be made, unless a person is able to extrapolate from a previous experience perceived as relevant. The distinction is important because if stresses have influence capable of distorting the data base, only those individuals able to call on previous task experience will be able to generate accurate responses and have the codes necessary for the detection of errors and the accurate assessment of control.

Two interdependent processes, attention and memory, have been shown to exhibit functional changes in stressful conditions. The change is not necessarily detrimental but is capable of distorting the data base on which planning depends.

Changes in Attention Deployment

One of the most interesting issues to develop in the last 20 years concerns the deployment of attention across an array of sources that are spatially or temporally separated. There are two fundamental aspects to attention deployment: how a structure for deploying attention is made available and how internal control is maintained over the structure. In the former case it is important to distinguish the use of a preexisting structure, because the task is familiar to the subject, from conditions of novelty where a structure must be simultaneously acquired.

One of the strongest statements suggesting that in dual task designs people can hold and maintain a "priority structure" came from Kahneman (1970), who presented evidence suggesting that capacity may be allocated efficiently. Subjects can maintain performance on a primary task, allowing deterioration to occur on a secondary task as difficulty levels increase. Kantowitz and Knight (1974, 1976) found some contradictions; although secondary task performance declined with increasing task difficulty, the extent of the decline did not relate as clearly as might be expected to level of primary task difficulty. They assumed that the lack of interaction between primary and secondary task difficulty refuted the basic Kahneman view. In fact, Lane (1977) argues that the interaction is not essential to the Kahneman view because whether the two variables interact will depend on the shape of the function relating task difficulty and capacity to performance as well as to the difficulty of each task. Nevertheless, there are other objections to the view that the priority structure is clear. Although instructions have been found to influence significantly the time sharing process (Fisher 1975b), there are also cases where a change in the load on one task changes the apparent priority structure (Fisher 1977), and also a case where the priority structure was not well retained in a particular control group as compared with previous control groups in previous identical studies (see Fisher, 1980). The latter finding suggests that although subjects can preserve a clear dual task structure assigning priority to the "primary" or "main" task, they do not always do so.

Learning may be a factor that changes the way two tasks are combined. A useful idea by Gopher and North (1977) was to present subjects with a sequence of single and dual task trials. Tracking was one of the tasks; digit cancelation was the other. As single task performance improved, task difficulty levels were increased. In spite of this, dual task performance continued to improve. The explanation could not be that the independent tasks were becoming more automated but it could be argued that it is an illustration of an improvement in the actual time-sharing process.

There are cases, particularly in the areas of sleep loss and in overload, where a person may not be able to preserve attentional structure. In sleep loss, the saw-tooth curve of performance decline suggest stops and starts arising from loss of control (e.g., see Wilkinson, 1965), and there is evidence of perseveration of responses on one task at the expense of the other, which does not occur in control conditions (Fisher, 1980). Equally, experiments have indicated that there may be underresponse to lack of stimulation and overresponse to its presence (see Burch & Greiner, 1958). In cases of overload, a person can only operate effective strategies if he has time in advance, or if load levels are not excessive. After that responses are more likely to be ad hoc (e.g., see Miller, 1962).

Attentional Selectivity on Multisource Tasks

An aspect of many complex tasks is the existence of a number of different elements requiring either spatial or temporal distribution of attention for adequate performance. The vulnerability of multisource tasks to arousing conditions such as loud noise has been demonstrated (Broadbent, 1951, 1953; Jerison, 1957); the addition of more sources of information increases the probability of performance deterioration. At least one possible explanation is that it is not the increased uncertainty that is important, but the requirement to deploy attentional resources effectively under conditions where limitations are unavoidable.

However, if anything, work on multisource monitoring tasks has indicated that the limitation in attentional resource is not some naturally occurring inhibitory process but the result of a cognitively driven process, perhaps similar to the operation of a strategy.

The research that first drew attention to this possibility was by Hockey (1970a, 1970b). Using a task designed originally by Bursill (1958), in which a subject was required to track a central display change and at the same time monitor a semicircular array of six lamps for the occurrence of signals, he compared performance changes on both tasks for biased and unbiased signal conditions in quiet and noise.

He reported an improvement on the error score of the tracking task and on centrally placed signal sources in the biased condition, relative to peripherally situated sources. The effect of unequal detection times in the biased condition was true for quiet, but more evident in noise; thus noise had the effect of enhancing the biasing of attention.

Unfortunately, there have been a number of difficulties with dual task design in noise, which have weakened the confidence that might have been attached to the result. Firstly, Poulton (1976) pointed out that the apparent channeling effect towards central sources could be explained in terms of the masking effect of noise on peripheral switches likely to produce less certain responses. Secondly, in a series of four experiments designed to replicate the main Hockey findings, Forster and Grierson (1978) failed to

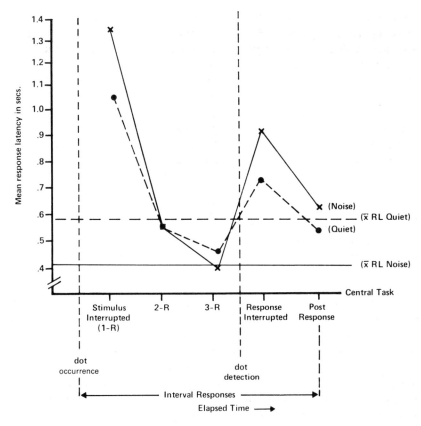

FIG. 7.1.   Average interval during central task performance, showing effect of occurrence of secondary task signal and response, in quiet and noise conditions.

find any evidence to support the selectivity phenomena. A later replication by Hartley (1981b) provided some support for the selectivity hypothesis in reporting an interaction between central and peripheral locations reliable at the 5% level. Although Hartley sees his results as roughly comparable with the Hockey effect, Poulton (1981b) points out that two of the results for the tracking task are in the wrong direction, and overall tracking is reliably worse in noise.

Fisher (1983c) tested the selectivity hypothesis using a comparable dual task design set up on an Apple microprocessor.[1] Results show that when the two tasks are combined in loud noise, there is increased rate of responding between dual task intervals on the central 4-choice task, but depressed response speed in the actual intervals, as illustrated in Fig. 7.1.

---

[1] With the assistance of John Cason, who wrote the original version of the program.

This result, which is reliable, is consistent with the notion of fluctuating effort and gives support both to the hypothesis that the main task is given priority and to the opposite view. Monitoring task efficiency is depressed in the dual -task conditions both for quiet and for noise, but the effect is reliably worse for noise. There is no evidence of a change in the detection speed across the six spatial sources in a condition where signals are equally probable. However, as shown in Table 7.2, when response position on the central tasks at the time of occurrence of the secondary signal is taken into account, there is attenuation of detection of dots in extreme peripheral positions for contralateral combinations (PCL in Table 7.2).

This can be taken to suggest a "moving-window" attention process that can cope with all combinations except the contralateral extremes. The results would at least indicate that a "basic constraint" limitation on attentional flexibility is tenable.

Experiments are currently under way to introduce bias into the frequency of the distribution of signals across sources on the monitoring task, and to vary the duration of the occurrence of the dot. It appears from the results so far that a short duration dot has a markedly different effect on the interaction of the two tasks; the tendency to interrupt all responses on the secondary task is increased.

There is other evidence that supports the notion of a cognitively driven attentional limitation. Attentional restriction in high arousal towards perceived high-priority rather than low-priority elements of the task was observed by Bacon (1974). Priority differences imply cognitive involvement. Using a task involving the monitoring of three sources for faults, Hamilton (1967) measured observing responses to the three sources and found that when the rate at which observing responses were made was slowed by pacing, there was increased sampling of the high probability source. This effect was subsequently found by Hockey (1973) to be augmented in noise, and the double-checking of sources was reduced.

The selectivity hypothesis has also been investigated on versions of the Stroop Test (Stroop, 1935), in which the color indicated by a word normally interferes with the naming of the color of the ink in which it is written (see Jensen & Rohwer, 1966). Interference produced by the word-color and the color of the ink will be reduced if attention is more selective, and there should be less delay in naming the ink color. Thus Callaway and his coworkers showed that amphetamine reduces the level of interference (see Callaway & Dembo, 1958; Callaway & Stone, 1960), although the difficulty is that the effect is apparent in terms of overall speed and may not represent resistance to the confusion produced by word naming (e.g., see Jensen & Rohwer, 1966; Venables, 1964). An investigation of the effects of noise on the level of interference on the Stroop test produced some further complexity: Hartley and Adams (1974) found that

TABLE 7.2.
Dot Detection Latencies in Relation to Spatial Separation of Dot and
Current Central Response (In Secs)

			Quiet	Noise
Peripheral lateral	D1:C1	X̄	.636	.905
		S.D.	.210	.413
	D6:C4	X̄	.534	.839
		S.D.	.106	.302
		Mean	.585	.872
Central	D3:C2	X̄	.629	.862
		S.D.	.301	.309
	D4:C3	X̄	.601	.816
		S.D.	.210	.301
		Mean	.615	.839
Peripheral contralateral	D1:C4	X̄	.760	1.201
		S.D.	.106	.412
	D6:C1	X̄	.733	.902
		S.D.	.109	.401
		Mean	.746	1.052

Schematic representation of codes used in table

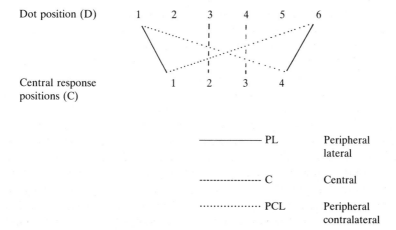

Dot position (D)   1   2   3   4   5   6

Central response   1   2   3   4
positions (C)

——————— PL   Peripheral
                                       lateral

----------------- C   Central

················· PCL   Peripheral
                                       contralateral

when the Stroop color words were presented on playing cards that were required to be sorted, noise increased the time it took to sort the "Stroop effect" pack by about 3%, which would suggest interference to be greater. In a second experiment, where the material was presented in written form on sheets of paper and noise exposure was varied, subjects showed less interference in the combined condition for 10-minute noise exposure. These findings would argue against the view that increased arousal reduces interference at the central level, because the phenomenon depends on presentation conditions.

Explanations of Attentional Selectivity

Firstly, it must be emphasized that using a comparable dual task design, experimenters have not produced consistent results to demonstrate either increased priority toward the main task or a difference between peripheral as compared with centrally located sources in the monitoring tasks.

Given the evidence that attentional deployment does change in favor of high-priority task elements, at least for noise, there remains the possibility that this is an artifact of masking of feedback, as suggested by Poulton.

Accepting the basic idea of cognitively driven attentional restriction, the need is then to understand why. Although most research mentioned so far has assumed that selectivity results from arousal increase associated with stress, it remains equally plausible that mental overload properties of stresses could have the same effect: If there is too much to do, a person may concentrate on what seems to him to have the greatest priority.

There are a number of interpretations that do depend on the assumption that arousal is responsible. The best known is the hypothesis by Easterbrook (1959), which supposes that there is increased cue restriction with increased arousal. This is beneficial at first in limiting input to what is essential, but not later, in that relevant signals are missed. The restricted cue utilization motion carries the assumption of a single monotonic relationship between arousal and a key variable in accounting for the inverted U relationship between arousal and performance.

The Easterbrook hypothesis is not clear as to why the monotonic relationship should exist or how restricted cue utilization favors performance in the early stages. A model that does tackle the logic of relationships between arousal and attention deployment but seems, if anything, to increase complexity is that of Callaway and Stone (1960), based on their own experiments on the effects of amphetamine in reducing the Stroop effect. These authors propose a reduction in probabilistic coding of environmental events because of high arousal. The effect of this is increased load on a person and greater need for attentional restriction. However, the basis for attention deployment in favor of high-priority elements benefiting performance initially is removed.

Some attempt has been made by Teichner (1968) to link attentional selectivity to speed of processing. This might provide the basis of an explanation of the relationship with arousal. However, Teichner's attentional bandwidth hypothesis proposes increased speed of response as a result—not a cause—of narrowed attention; as bandwidth narrows, there is greater rate of change of activity and greater response speed.

An interpretation by Broen and Storms (1962) of the possible relationship between arousal and apparent attentional narrowing is based on the notion of response competition provided for in the learning theory models of Hull (1943) and Spence (1956). The main point is that any situation defines a set of dominant and nondominant responses. As drive level increases, since it is multiplicative with habit strength, the propensity for behavior to be governed by dominant responses is increased. As drive level increases further, a limitation is reached. This ceiling means that dominant responses have maximal influence, but nondominant responses can continue to increase until behavior is governed by less important responses.

None of these models provides an account of the fragmented, disorganized behavior evident in very high levels of anxiety. Behavior is not merely characterized by narrowed attention, which produces inadequate performance. There is a new element that appears to relate to control of attention. Wachtel (1967) uses the analogy of a beam of light and argues that attention at very high levels of arousal is described by a beam with narrow width and unstable scanning characteristic. As a result, the perceptual world appears fragmented and the individual is a "slave to minor variations." The inexperienced individual in this state would have an inadequate data base and poor control over sampling. Behavior would appear energetic but be disorganized and random.

The point made by Wachtel is that there may be important differences between "broadening" and "narrowing." Two logically distinct dimensions are "scanning" (or how quickly the beam moves across the field), and "focusing" (or the width of the beam). Wachtel cites an example of an obsessive personality who, on clinical observations, appears to create great breadth of scanning but uses a "narrow beam." Thus intellectually there is a great deal of material available, but concern is with details, and the material is poorly integrated. Wachtel criticizes the view that at moderately high arousal levels, attention is narrowed, whereas at high levels there is general breakdown, because this suggests that there is a sudden point of breakdown: Two specifiable locations on the relationship between arousal and performance are required. Wachtel actually argues that when behavior is disorganized and any event captures attention, width could be argued to have increased and performance should improve again. This gives a "two-humped camel curve" (p. 420) not actually found in practice.

Wachtel believes that the problem can be resolved on the assumption that at very high levels of arousal, although there is narrowing, the beam begins to move in a rapid and unstable way. Thus the anxious person is slave to minor variations in the field, is unable to concentrate, and is hyperdistract-able. A possibility raised by this is that a mediating speed factor is involved; at very high levels of arousal, scanning speed is raised to the point beyond which information can be properly processed. Under these circumstances control of scanning might also break down, because the data base becomes inadequate and unrepresentative.

It is worth noting at this point that arousal may not be the only cause of disorganized attention; an individual who is anxious may be under mental pressure from the information he is processing. Under conditions of overload we might expect the breakdown of supervisory systems that control sampling behavior. Also, the system is self-maintaining in that poorly coded task structure will lead to overload because a person has no system for giving priorities.

Changes in Learning and Memory

In the case of the learning of material, attention and memory are inextricably linked in that although looking does not necessarily imply seeing, it is at least a precondition. Storage and retrieval of information provide the basic processes on which an adequate model depends, yet treatment of this source of internal information may involve "internal attention"; information may be present but only easily retrieved. It might be appropriate to think of a person sampling between different sources of "memory material," rather in the way he might sample the spatial sources of a task.

Intentional Learning

It is useful to consider, if only briefly, possible effects of arousal or anxiety on the intentional learning of material. In the basic development of the inverted U arousal/performance hypothesis, research was concerned pri-marily with learning and memory tasks paired against increasing degrees of anxiety or levels of arousal. For example, Courts (1942) showed an inverted U relationship between mean memory score on the learning of nonsense syllables and assumed the U curve to be typical of the rela-tionship between learning and the degree of experimentally induced tension. An experiment by Wood and Hokanson (1965) is interesting in that Courts' procedure was replicated, but the task used was less depen-dent on learning. Even at maximum induced tension, performance was not actually below normal, although a U curve was obtained.

Korchin and Levine (1957) demonstrated that in the learning of false arithmetical equations, anxious subjects showed poorer learning of incorrect pairs and increased omission of responses. The authors argued that this might suggest cautious decision making. One possible explanation that follows from the idea that memory material has to be sampled is that anxiety might favor the recall of dominant overlearned (correct) pairs of sums but make the storage and recall of odd (incorrect) pairs difficult.

Incidental Learning

One of the interesting aspects of learning is the apparent capacity to acquire information incidentally. Levitt (1968) argues that incidental learning may be more significant in human life than formal learning. A problem for all studies of incidental learning is that what is "incidental" is defined not objectively but subjectively, in terms of the priority structure as perceived by the subject.

In the laboratory it is possible to manipulate what is objectively incidental by presenting the subject with a formal central task and later asking for recall of incidental material. Silverman (1954) showed the effects of anxiety on an incidental learning task. The main task involved making a response to a display consisting of the appearance of a line of appropriate length. At the same time, 20 two-syllable words were recited in the background at a muted level; this was not presented as part of the experimental situation. The stressed subjects, continuously threatened by electric shock during main task performance, recalled about half as much of the incidental material as the control group.

The close association of learning and attention is illustrated by these studies. It is impossible to say for certain that the effects are the result of learning rather than of the sampling process on which learning depends. If the subject does not see an event, he cannot be expected to have any recall of it. In terms of the attention models considered earlier, it is possible that at high levels of stress, attention limitations operate, and incidental material is not sampled. The difference between central and incidental aspects of performance increases with increasing age (e.g., see Lane, 1979), suggesting perhaps that the balance reflects capacity level.

Stress and Memory Efficiency

There is now a great deal of research from different areas of experimental psychology that leads to the conclusion that memory processes are different in stress. There is evidence from different conditions of arousal to suggest (1) that short- and long-term recall are differentially affected, (2) that recall of information from long-term memory is differentially affected by condition of arousal, and (3) that the degree of order in presentation and recall may interact with stressful conditions.

Recall Interval and Arousal. A direct relationship between memory change and arousal level is supported by physiological findings of Warren and Harris (1975), using a paradigm that involved presentation of a single-trial free recall task. Phasic changes in EEG alpha and skin potential were found to be positively related to recall at immediate retention interval (2 min), but not after a delay of 45 minutes. However, there have been a number of studies that have not replicated enhanced long-term recall after learning in noise (e.g., Farley, 1969; Haveman & Farley, 1969). In a review of the research in this area, Craik and Blankstein (1975) are more accepting of the interaction with long-term recall but are clear that the relationship with short-term retention is confused.

A study by Kleinsmith and Kaplan (1963) involving the association of shock with certain paired associate items presented under high states of arousal (indexed by skin resistance measures) were better recalled after a day or even a week had elapsed, whereas the same items presented in low states of arousal were better recalled within 45 minutes of presentation. Poor immediate recall of high-arousal-learned words is explained by Kleinsmith and Kaplan in terms of reverberation of the memory trace; during the early perseveration phase, the trace is assumed to be relatively unavailable, and therefore immediate recall is impaired. Using 75-dB noise, Berlyne et al. (1965) presented paired associates and reported that in comparison with quiet conditons, noise improved recall after 24 hours, but immediate recall was impaired. Berlyne et al. (1966) subsequently confirmed that high noise facilitated long-term recall but did not impair short-term recall.

All these findings fit roughly with the proposal developed by Walker (1958) that there is greater temporary inhibition during arousal. In the case of the Kleinsmith and Kaplan result, there is the added difficulty of possible unexplored effects of suppression or caution or perceptual defence. In the case of experiments that have been concerned with noise, it is worth commenting that on a masking hypothesis, rehearsal might be expected to be so depressed that facilitation of long-term recall would also be impaired. On a temporary inhibition hypothesis, it is only accessibility that should be altered, and therefore the material remains available for recall at a later time.

Poulton (1979) is quite specific about the likely changes in memory function consequent on masking; he argues that noise may interfere with the duration of the storage of items. More frequent rehearsal is then required, and a consequence of this is capacity reduction, which will slow down the rate of additional processing and produce memory errors. Poulton later claims that the lowest level of continuous noise found to produce deterioration through masking is 72.5 dB A or 75 dB (flat) and cites in support an experiment by Frankenhaeuser and Lundberg (1977).

There is relatively little discussion of the nature of impairment. The normal characteristic of memory performance in noise is depression of recall rather than total "knockout." In addition, recall may be facilitated later. If a person was unable to complete the processes necessary for storage, we would expect loss rather than attenuation, and we would not expect subsequent improvement when a person is later asked to recall. For this reason, it might be better to consider masking to depress retrieval at the time, rather than producing total interference.

On a strong version of the masking hypothesis, evidence that shows that changing the acoustic character of noise does not change the impairment features of recall is relevant. Equally relevant is evidence that shows that suppression of rehearsal by other means reduces the difference between quiet and noise. Recently, Millar (1979) attempted to suppress rehearsal by use of an articulatory task. On the masking hypothesis, quiet/noise differences should be reduced. Unfortunately, Millar's results are equivocal. Firstly, consistent with the masking hypothesis, where articulation suppresses rehearsal, noise and quiet groups have almost identical recall but only on the performance of the first day. On the second day, recall reliably improves in noise: Millar suggests that a factor might be reduced novelty, leading to boredom and fatigue on the second day, which causes deterioration in quiet. Acoustic confusions and ommission errors were reduced in noise in all conditions, which argues against masking.

There is some evidence from Baddeley (1968) to suggest that rehearsal might involve articulatory rather than auditory processes, because 70 dB noise impairs perception but not retention of items. Broadbent (1978) has questioned involvement of auditory encoding: deaf children produce acoustic errors in memory for letters. Folkhard and Greeman (1974) propose that high muscle tension associated with increased arousal damages subvocal processes needed for short-term rehearsal.

A comparable technique for inducing suppression of subvocal rehearsal was developed by Wilding and Mohindra (1980), who required subjects to repeat the word "the" continuously during list presentation and until recall. Subjects were required to reproduce in order a sequence of five letters. Some lists were acoustically confusable; others were not. In the presence of 85 dBC white noise, there was *no* suppression. Suppression therefore was an important determinant of the effect of noise in improving recall.

Recall from Long-Term Memory.   If a person is to benefit from experience, it is important that stress does not change the recall of information from long-term memory. Research on arousal at the time of recall has generally provided confusing evidence. Pascal (1949) found that relaxation instructions prior to recall enhanced performance. In contrast,

Uehling and Sprinkle (1968) reported improved recall in arousal. Both studies support the idea that arousal is a relevant factor in recall. Investigations by M. Eysenck (1974, 1975) involving personality factors rated activation levels and white noise as means of manipulating arousal. The first finding of interest is that a retrieval U curve was obtained; extraverts (assumed to be low-arousal) who were activated produced better retrieval levels than those who were not, but they still performed worse than introverts (assumed to be high-arousal). Equally, introverts who were low on activation did better than those who were high. The second important feature is that both arousal as measured by introversion/extraversion and activation (Thayer's Activation–Deactivation Check List, 1967, 1970) interactively determined recall latency for both category and item recall.

Both Eysenck and independently Millar (1980) confirmed that items that are dominant in semantic memory have faster retrieval in conditions of high arousal. Millar's results were, however, concerned with recognition of words rather than recall. His results differed from Eysenck's not only in that recognition was affected, but there was no evidence of suppression of nondominant items.

A suggestion considered by Eysenck (1975), and also independently by Millar (1980), is that retrieval from memory could be likened to "internal attention": there is an internal ensemble of stored items that have value or priority attached to them, and high-priority or dominant sources would be favored by selectivity of internal attention. An experiment by Cohen and Lezak (1977) is in keeping with this hypothesis; they reported that exposure to loud noise of 95 dBA, administered on a random intermittent schedule, did not impair the recall of task-relevant information, but significantly reduced the recall of less relevant and irrelevant cues. Both "social cues" and "nonsocial cues" are depressed in the same way. Posner and Rossman (1965) argue that attention is required for the rehearsal of items in short-term memory; in line with this view, it could be argued that the Cohen and Lezak result occurred because attentional resources were deployed maximally on the rehearsal of nonsense syllables.

A result of comparable interest is that certain aspects of evidence may be better recalled under stressful conditions. Working with loud noise, Schwartz (1974) showed that when subjects heard short meaningful stories, common names were better recalled in both quiet and noise. However, signal detection theory analysis showed that in quiet conditions subjects showed a criterion shift; a risky criterion was used for common names and a cautious criterion for rare names. In noise, the criterion was unchanged, but sensitivity increased for common names. Schwartz suggests that arousal affects the accessibility of information for retrieval.

Features in the Structure of Material.   An important aspect of memory in stressful conditions concerns the structure of the material presented. On the hypothesis that stresses limit attentional sampling, it might be expected that a person would be less likely to notice the structure of material. Equally, on a superficial processing hypothesis, which supposes that in stress there is less capacity available for context-dependent processing (e.g., see Weinstein, 1974), the same conclusions would follow.

However, some experiments have demonstrated that conditions of high noise or high incentives improve recall of ordered material when the same ordering of material is permitted (Hockey & Hamilton, 1970; Hamilton, Hockey, & Quinn, 1972; Daee & Wilding, 1977; Millar, 1979). Incentives and noise appear to act differently in this respect, because evidence suggests that whereas noise aids recall of order, it does not aid recall of spatial cues; incentives do appear to increase the efficiency of both (see Davies & Jones, 1975; Fowler & Wilding, 1979; Hockey & Hamilton, 1970). There are also experiments that have failed to show an effect of noise on ordered recall (e.g. Murray, 1965; Sloboda & Smith, 1968; Haveman & Farley, 1969; Davies & Jones, 1975). Equally, there is some evidence that suggests that recall is actually impaired (Wilkinson, 1975; Salame & Wittersheim, 1979). It is worth noting that there could be a relationship with task difficulty level; Dornic (1974) showed that category clustering in recall was reduced by the addition of a secondary task; however, although this effect was comparable in some ways with the effect of alcohol, item information was affected, but order information was not.

STRESS AND THE DATA BASE FOR PERCEPTION OF CONTROL

Objective Changes in the Locus of Control

The previous considerations are relevant to the ideas developed in this book in two principal ways. Firstly, all plans, including plans to cope with stressful conditions, are dependent on an adequate representative data base. Distortions arising from attention and memory changes are likely to render a person ill equipped to perform effectively. Just when he needs to do well, he may underperform. The result of this could be a shift in locus of control, so that more of what happens will be decided by external agents. In cases where a person is dealing with animate sources of stress, as in social situations, accidents, and assaults, decisions will be taken by the other agent. It is possible, from all that has been said, that the previously experienced person will be less vulnerable in this respect, because he will have an intact data base of knowledge to draw on. Even so, there may be changes in the retrieval of information. Dominant habits would be expected to prevail, because ease of retrieval of memory may be facilitated. To the extent that previous habits are going to provide the right information, a shift in the locus of control may be prevented.

The less experienced person is more likely to acquire a data base that is distorted relative to what is actually true. His attention may be captured by what he sees as salient; but what he sees as salient may be fortuitous.

Figure 7.2 conceptualizes the focusing of a number of different modes of stress influence on the fundamental process that determine the "model of the world." In effect, the changes act directly on knowledge, part of which is concerned with the cost of actions and the economies that may offset

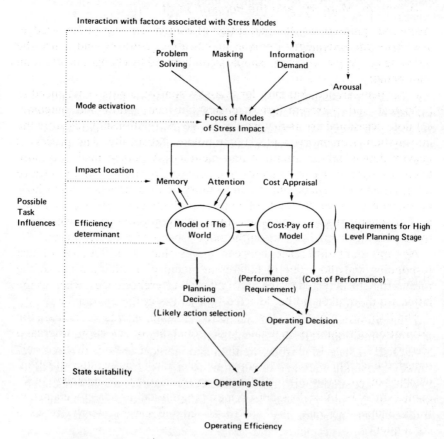

FIG. 7.2.   Conceptualization of the effects of stress on the fundamental basis of plans.

them. It is this knowledge store that contains the eventual ingredient of action selection and the codes for assessing the levels of control obtained. On the left side of Fig. 7.2, additional task factors are indicated. For example, the nature of the task determines precisely which aspect of memory and attention are involved ("impact location"). Also, the criterion for judging efficiency ("efficiency determinant") is set. Finally, compatiability of task features determines the degree to which the final operating state characteristics are suitable ("state suitability"); a person may be making the wrong decisions about cost, so that he may oversacrifice his resources for the task, or persist with inappropriate actions.

Changes in the Perception of Control in Stress

Attention, Memory, and the Perception of Control

As already pointed out, the perception of control depends on knowledge. Therefore the judgments a person makes about control—and hence the outcome of a stress scenario—should be influenced by changes in attention and memory.

It has been argued that in order to assess control, a person may need to (1) detect and represent contingencies between action and outcome, (2) note occasional errors that would change the relationship, (3) store the information in memory, and (4) extrapolate statistically. The process is heavily dependent on attention and memory. A person might be more likely to overrepresent "salient" happenings in stress and to retrieve information with high dominance in memory. If we assume a person who is pessimistic is faster to think of unpleasant outcomes, then errors may appear salient. If stress causes selectivity of attention, a person who tends to be pessimistic might focus on the poor aspects of his performance.

An important difference between errors that occur because of fast responding and those due to failures in memory or attention is that the former may be detected by means of internal reference codes, whereas the latter are more likely to be detected by changes in the environment.

The implication of this is that one effect of stress may be to increase the proportion of small slips that have high probability of detection, whereas a second effect may be to increase the proportion of failures that are only detected if circumstances are compelling. Moreover, in the latter situation, changes of attention might mean that even relatively compelling consequences may be missed. A person may not only fail to detect a change in traffic lights, but may also fail to notice the car he nearly hit as a consequence.

If a person detects his errors accurately, perception of control represents his own level of performance efficiency. Thus if he performs badly and he cannot explain away the errors, he should assume he is incompetent. A person who is oblivious of his errors may live dangerously, but if compelling circumstances do not occur, he may never be aware of his own shortcomings and might overrepresent his level of competence.

From what has been said previously, it seems reasonable to conclude that both types of error (cognitive failures and execution slips), may arise in stress. The issue of importance is the balance between these error types for a particular person or a particular situation. However, an added factor is that a person may develop bias in the perspectives for viewing his own performance. His perceived level of control may be discrepant with actual achievement.

Pessimistic "Generator Bias" in Stress

More detailed consideration of what is likely to be involved in the perception of control suggests that at some stage a person must summarize the trials of his own performance even if only crudely in order to assess control. Inevitably he will be involved in assessing subjectively the frequency of different classes of events. This process is likely to be subject to bias of various kinds.

Work by Kahneman and Tversky (1972, 1973) and Tversky and Kahneman (1974) has shown how subjective probability is influenced by factors such as the class of events to which an item belongs and its availability in memory. The authors suggest that estimates are made on the basis of heuristics. Howell and Burnett (1978) distinguish frequency knowledge and "internal–external causality" as important elements of probability judgments. In the case of frequency, it is assumed that appraisal of a repetitive series of events generated by a stationary process will gradually lead to a representation of objective value. In cases where there is no stable generator of events and no historical profile on which to base an opinion, prior beliefs are likely determinants of subjective behavior. The accuracy of the model the subject builds of his task will depend on the exposure profile—that is how many events an individual experiences before a decision is made. In the case of really complex tasks, he may have to rely on heuristics. These situations allow prior knowledge to dominate.

What is unknown is the relative balance between prior knowledge and data obtained from the task as a determinant or moderator of the data base. Marques and Howell (1979) propose that specific processing is required for transformation of "multiple impressions," and that the degree of specific processing required is reduced by prior knowledge. Having conducted a series of four experiments involving manipulation of prior knowledge, the authors concluded that prior beliefs about frequency generators play a major part in the allocation of attentional resources, particularly in the absence of task-related cues, indicating a need to process frequency data more deeply. Subjects actually proved rather insensitive to frequency shifts; in the first experiment, a 20% shift in frequency data only resulted in small amounts of processing of discrepant evidence. The authors contest the assumption that frequency data is coded automatically. What appears to be likely is that a subject codes frequency data in accordance with "generator bias" or bias resulting from what he expects to be likely.

An important finding in this respect is that stresses are associated in the minds of many people with deteriorations in performance. If this operates in the form of a "generator bias," we might expect that a person working in stress would overrepresent the degree to which his performance deteriorates.

An experiment by Fisher (1983a) has shown that estimates of reaction latency produced under either quiet or loud noise conditions reflects a "pessimistic" bias. The experiment involved the completion of 100 2-choice reaction times in either quiet (55 dBA headphone noise) or loud noise (100 dBA headphone noise). As illustrated by Fig. 7.3, subjects produced each reaction time that required a decision about whether a number was "odd" or "even" and then judged the reaction times on a 4-category scale from "very fast" through to "very slow." In a second phase, those *same* reaction times were presented again, under instructions that lead the subject to believe they were merely random time intervals. As part of the design, one group of subjects produced and judged their performance in noise, and one group produced and judged performance in quiet. Noise levels were 100 dB; quiet levels were 55 dB. In the second phase of judgments we further subdivided those two main subject groups into two subgroups each. One judged the so-called random time intervals in quiet and one in noise. Thus if noise affected the process of judging time intervals per se, then there should be judgment differences in the second phase between the noise and quiet subgroups.

The main result of interest is shown in Figs. 7.4 and 7.5. Although reaction times produced in noise were significantly faster than those produced in quiet, subjects described them as slow a greater percentage of times on the 4-category judgment scale. Thus, in comparison with the data for the group who produced their reaction times and judged them in quiet, subjects in noise were producing significantly *faster* reaction times but perceiving them as *slower*. The effect disappeared when performance was compared in the second phase across the four subgroups, who all believed they were judging random time intervals. Logically the only way this effect can be established is by comparing the shift in rating behavior between noise-produced and quiet-produced conditions, from the first to the second phase of the test. As shown in Fig. 7.6, the shift is evident for those who first produced and rated reaction times in noise; in Phase 1, more slow

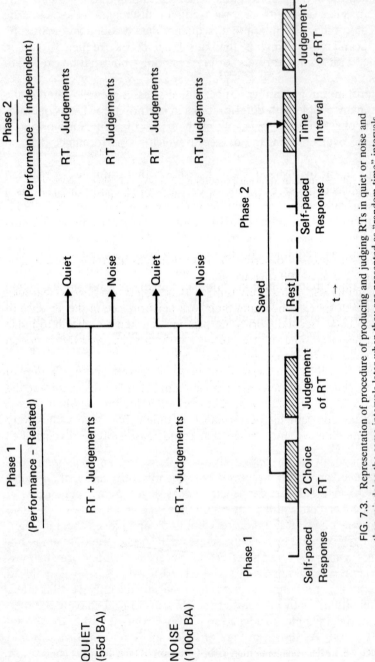

FIG. 7.3. Representation of procedure of producing and judging RTs in quiet or noise and then rejudging the same intervals later when they are presented as "random time" intervals. (Reprinted from S. Fisher, Pessimistic noise effects: The perception of reaction times in noise. *Canadian Journal of Psychology*, 1983a, 37(2), 258–71. Reprinted by permission.)

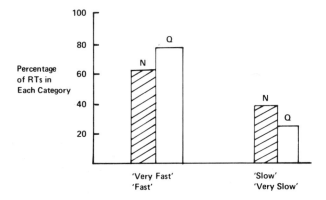

FIG. 7.4. Histogram showing proportion of "fast" and "slow" category ratings for self-produced (performance related) RTs in quiet and noise (Phase 1 condition.)

categories were used to describe the data, whereas in Phase 2 fewer slow categories were used, relative to quiet.

The main interest in this study is firstly that subjects do have a clear idea of the detail of speed concerning their own performance in the absence of explicit feedback. Secondly, they are pessimistic when they begin to judge their own response times in the presence of high noise, and this is *not* an effect of noise on the judgment process per se.

In order to check the pessimistic bias, we asked another group of subjects to generate an average reaction time that would represent the performance of a hypothetical subject working in loud noise when given a value said to represent his performance in quiet. Two base values were chosen at random within a range that could reasonably be expected to

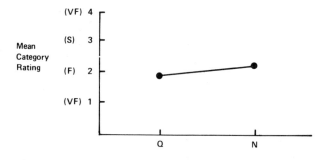

FIG. 7.5. Mean category rating for self-produced RTs in quiet and noise.

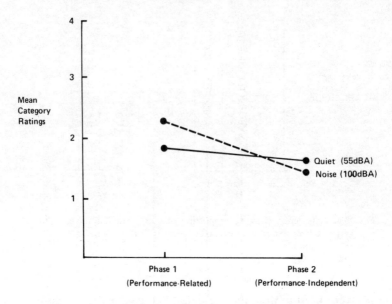

FIG. 7.6.   Phase 1–Phase 2 shift in mean category ratings for noise and quiet groups.

represent average reaction time under normal conditions. Figure 7.7 shows the result: All subjects generated a value that demonstrated a belief of increased slowness in noise ($p < 4.001$). Controls who generated a value believed to represent average reaction time when a hypothetical subject worked on a second test in quiet conditions, generated a value near to or slightly less than the original base value.

Thus subjects who are uninformed about noise do expect "worse" performance in noise, and their expectancies translate into increased slowness when they consider reaction times. From the main experiment we would suggest that subjects do have knowledge about their own performance in the absence of explicit feedback, but that pessimistic expectancies might have led subjects to suppose that their performance is likely to be slower.

This raises the possibility that the unexpected faster performance in noise is in some way a compensation, perhaps resulting from increased effort (Kahneman, 1973). Figure 7.8 illustrates a number of alternative explanations: The idea that speed and rating behavior are independently influenced is illustrated by (1), the possibility of compensatory activity by (2) and (3). Further research is needed to establish which is valid.

A subsequent investigation was carried out concerning expectancies for uninformed subjects in a number of different stressful conditions. Using a

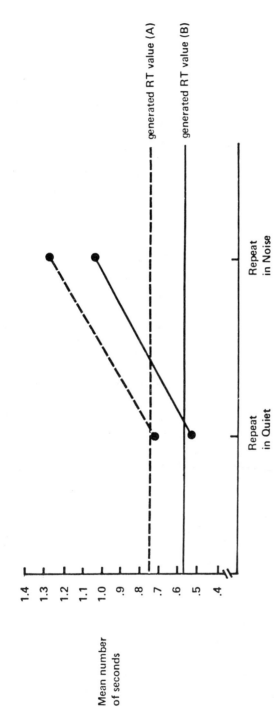

FIG. 7.7. Predictions of response times by subjects for a hypothetical person asked to work at a task in

1. Repeat conditions or
2. Noise.

(Reprinted from *Canadian Journal of Psychology*, 1983a, 37(2), 258–271. Reprinted by permission.)

(1) Independent or Parallel. [Ratings and performance features are independent]

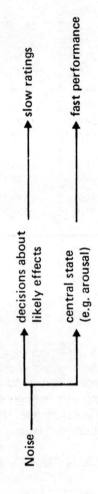

Noise

decisions about
likely effects → slow ratings

central state
(e.g. arousal) → fast performance

(2) Compensatory Performance

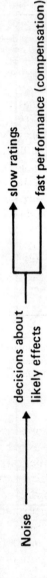

Noise → decisions about
likely effects → slow ratings
→ fast performance (compensation)

(3) Compensatory Judgements

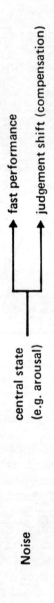

Noise

central state
(e.g. arousal) → fast performance
→ judgement shift (compensation)

FIG. 7.8. Schematic representation of possible explanations of shift in the use of the category system for self-produced RTs in noise, from Phase 1 to Phase 2.

TABLE 7.3.
Estimates Given by Uninformed Subjects Asked to Assess the Performance of a Hypothetical Person Working Firstly in Normal Conditions—base value—and in One of a Number of Repeat or Stressful Conditions—predicted value (from Fisher, 1983e).

	Nondepressed (BDI < 9)[1]		Depressed (DBI > 9)[1]	
Presented base value	3.6% errors	5.6 sec	3.6% errors	5.6 sec
Repeat condition	$\overline{X}$ 3.50% (NS) S.D. 0.61	5.00 sec (NS) 1.00	$\overline{X}$ 3.9% (NS) S.D. 0.82	5.81 sec (NS) 1.01
Noise	$\overline{X}$ 14.25*** S.D. 3.19	7.03*** 1.86	$\overline{X}$ 14.29*** S.D. 3.15	8.09*** 2.81
Sleep deprivation (1 night)	$\overline{X}$ 23.54*** S.D. 6.91	9.75*** 2.01	$\overline{X}$ 22.59*** S.D. 7.03	9.90*** 3.91
Sleep deprivation (2 nights)	$\overline{X}$ 48.51*** S.D. 12.90	11.50*** 2.31	$\overline{X}$ 49.80*** S.D. 20.30	12.90*** 3.81
Physical fatigue (from 1 day's work)	$\overline{X}$ 23.20*** S.D. 5.10	9.87*** 2.01	$\overline{X}$ 29.30*** S.D. 6.81	10.83*** 2.08
Incentives	$\overline{X}$ 1.50** S.D. 0.10	3.39** 0.40	$\overline{X}$ 14.96** 4.98	10.39** 5.10
Social stress (being watched by other people)	$\overline{X}$ 10.40*** S.D. 3.10	6.77** 2.14	$\overline{X}$ 31.31*** S.D. 10.00	15.80*** 4.89

Wilcoxon Test Comparisons

 * Comparison with base value, significant $p < .05$
 ** Comparison with base value, significant $p < .01$
 *** Comparison with base value, significant $p < .001$

[1] BDI = Beck Depression Inventory (Beck, Ward, Mendelson, Mock, & Erlbaugh.)

between-group design and either percentage error estimates or response time estimates, subjects were asked to generate a value to represent average performance of a (hypothetical) subject working in one of a number of stressful conditions. Table 7.3 shows the results: Not only do subjects expect slower and more error-prone performance generally, but there are specific predictions of worse performance in conditions of fatigue than in conditions of noise or social stress.

The effect was true for both nondepressed students (Beck Depression Inventory, Beck et al., 1967). A main difference, which was statistically significant, was that depressed students gave estimates suggesting poor performance in incentive and social stress conditions, whereas normals were less pessimistic about social stress and tended to see incentives as beneficial to performance.

TABLE 7.4.

Estimates Given by Uninformed Nondepressed and Depressed Subjects of
Self-produced Performance in Repeat and Stressful Conditions.

	Nondepressed (BDI < 8)[1]		Depressed (BDI > 9)[1]	
Presented base value	3.6% errors	5.6 sec	3.6% errors	5.6 sec
Repeat condition	$\overline{X}$ 2.90**	5.00*	$\overline{X}$ 4.6**	6.60**
	S.D. 1.22	1.59	S.D. 1.39	2.31
Noise	$\overline{X}$ 5.81	7.10*	$\overline{X}$ 25.32***	10.01***
	S.D. 1.31	0.85	S.D. 4.01	3.10
Physical fatigue	$\overline{X}$ 6.41***	7.15*	$\overline{X}$ 29.81***	12.98***
	S.D. 1.81	2.06	S.D. 9.01	4.01
Incentives	$\overline{X}$ 1.90***	3.00**	$\overline{X}$ 10.91***	10.51***
	S.D. 0.09	0.91	S.D. 2.83	3.50
Social stress	$\overline{X}$ 4.4 (NS)	3.01*	$\overline{X}$ 36.60***	20.80***
	S.D. 1.8	1.21	S.D. 9.4	5.12

Wilcoxon Test Comparisons

   * Comparison with base value, significant $p < .05$
  ** Comparison with base value, significant $p < .01$
 *** Comparison with base value, significant $p < .001$

[1] BDI = Beck Depression Inventory (Beck, Ward, Mendelson, Mock, & Erlbaugh.)

An interesting question is the extent to which subjects make the same
estimates when assessing *their own* likely performance, knowing that they
will be asked to undertake the task. Figure 7.4 shows that nondepressed
students give more favorable estimates in this condition, whereas depressed students remain pessimistic.

Thus normals may resist being pessimistic about their own skills. The
finding is of interest in view of the finding that a negativity bias exists when
people make judgments; losses are greater than gains in influence (Kogan
& Wallach, 1967). Normals may also resist evidence about "losses" when
assessing their own likely competence. Perhaps when normals expect the
worst, they rise to the challenge, whereas depressed individuals expect the
worst and confirm it.

BASIC PREMISES OF THE STRESS/PERFORMANCE
RELATIONSHIP

The following hypotheses are proposed from information presented in this
and preceding chapters:-

1. A number of conditions will be stressful only on a proportion of occasions and for a proportion of individuals; the more intense the hazard and the greater the consequence, the greater the probability that it is perceived and reacted to by all individuals.
2. Any stress condition has a number of potential *modes* or ways in which it can influence performance. There are specific influences on task input and general influences on arousal and capacity, which influence the processing of information.
3. At any one time, situational factors determine which operating modes are implemented. On some occasions a stress may impose problem solving demand, on others it may not.
4. The greater the intensity and duration of the stress, the greater the probability that one or more impact modes may operate.
5. Modes operate via three major control centers in causing changes in performance. The influence may be via any one or all three of these control centers. Control centers are (a) decision timing, (b) planning rules, (c) knowledge.
6. Changes can be described in terms of the risk of poor performance. Although performance may be improved under certain circumstances, generally the greater the number of influences operating and the greater the intensity and duration of influence, the greater the risk of poor performance.
7. The locus of control is likely to shift whenever there are changes in performance in the direction of increased inadequacy. This is more likely to occur because of a systematic change or distortion in performance produced by a change in knowledge than because of an increase in the proportion of slips and small inefficiences.
8. The evidence on which successful control assessment depends may be influenced by certain stress conditions. Again, the evidence will be more distorted when a person cannot detect his own inefficiencies. This is more likely to occur when the data base is influenced by stress, so that a person has no knowledge to use in detecting inefficiency.
9. Pessimistic bias occurs about performance in stress in uninformed subjects. This may alert them to negative features, such as failures or errors, and cause them to underrepresent control.

8

Loss of Control in Stress

INTRODUCTION

In the previous four chapters we were concerned with the origins of inefficiency in performance in stress. The second part of this book is concerned with the consequences of depressed efficiency levels. A logical outcome is a shift in the locus of control from the individual. A state of total inefficiency is a state of helplessness. It is also a state where a person accepts punishment because he cannot avoid the stress. Because he has lost control, critical factors such as the intensity and duration of stress exposure are externally dictated. Loss of prestige may be part of the punishing consequences.

We begin by considering how even mild inefficiencies may lead to a worsening of conditions and to a state of incompetence. There are a number of feedback loops that can be identified that, once operative, will ensure that the situation worsens.

THE IMPLEMENTATION OF STRESS LOOPS

Primary Feedback Loops

As illustrated in Fig. 8.1 a and b, a secondary feedback loop can be set up when ineffective performance occurs. If a person makes too many slips, or the timing of his action is wrong, or he simply does not have the capacity for effective response, the result may be the same. A primary feedback loop is a condition in which action either is irrelevant or ineffective; it thus

PRIMARY FEEDBACK LOOP

a. TRANSIENT DEPRESSION IN POSITIVE INFLUENCE ON STRESS VARIABLE DUE TO ERROR

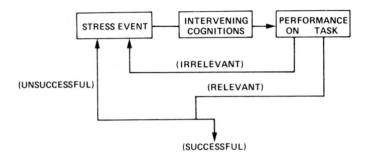

b. POTENTIAL FOR INFLUENCING STRESS VARIABLE DEPENDS ON RESOURCE ALLOCATION
(DUAL TASK CONDITION)

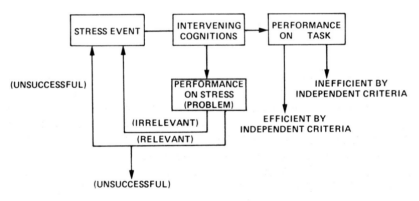

FIG. 8.1.   Flow diagrams illustrating how conditions of transient inefficiency or resource allocation may lead to positive feedback loop producing reduced control.

fails to ameliorate the stressful condition. If the stress factors are not self-limiting, then failure to produce effective action will mean that the problem continues or even escalates, imposing further pressures as a consequence. As shown in Fig. 8.1a, successful, relevant performance provides an exit from the loop. In Fig. 8.1b, a dual task situation is illustrated: One loop may operate if performance is inefficient with respect to the problem of the stress; another may build up if performance is inefficient on a daily task. Inefficient daily performance provides an additional source of stress.

Augmented loops occur when stresses impose problem-solving demand, but also create conditions unconducive to successful performance. This

2 AUGMENTED PRIMARY FEEDBACK LOOP

a ACTIVATION OF IMPACT MODES

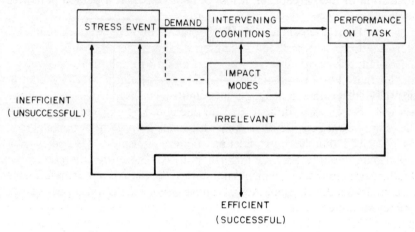

b. CAPTURE

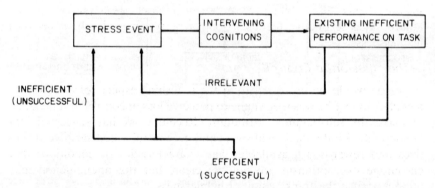

FIG. 8.2. Flow diagrams illustrating conditions in which stress augments positive feedback loops by promoting inefficiency.

could be because, as illustrated in Fig. 8.2a, stress modes operate to reduce efficiency. Equally, as illustrated in Fig. 8.2b, stresses may *capture* a moment of inefficiency, or arrive at a time when a person is already coping with another problem. In both cases, efficient performance will cause an exit from the loop but, given the prevailing conditions, will be unlikely.

Secondary Feedback Loops

A secondary loop will be implemented when a person perceives that his action is ineffective. The question of interest is how he decides about this.

Irrespective of whether a person persists with different courses of action or makes the decision impulsively on the basis of just a few trials, an implication of the perception of loss of control is that a person perceives helplessness.

The extent to which a secondary loop is implemented depends on interpretation. As described in Chapter 3, failure can be part of the plan; fear-of-failure individuals typically select either a simple task, or a task so difficult that failure is inevitable. The important point is that in the latter case they are protected against blame and social disapproval because the task will be seen as so difficult that no one could be expected to succeed. This is important because a secondary feedback loop occurs when a person has perceived that he fails and finds failure punishing. The perception provides an important source of further stress. Therefore, the perception of failure or helplessness, which is not part of the plan, is a precondition for a secondary feedback loop. Actual failure is not necessary; a person may see himself quite wrongly as having failed and still the secondary loop will operate. The mental processes involved may be centered on exploring the reasons for failure. Conditions that favor the loop occur when others are shown to succeed or when an authority admonishes a person for the failure. In a secondary feedback loop a person worries about his own helplessness.

The "Illusion of Control"

A person would be protected from the punishing aspects of a secondary feedback loop if he was less willing to perceive loss of control or if he failed to make the self-blaming attribution. Recent work has suggested that nondepressed individuals will overestimate control when positive incentives and rewards are available. The characteristics of conditions that encourage overoptimism are not yet clear, but the phenomenon may protect against the transmission of helplessness.

A study initiated by Jenkins and Ward (1965) defined degree of control as the degree of perceived contingencies between response and outcome and demonstrated that representations of contingencies are not isomorphic with objective contingencies. In very simple tasks, where a subject makes one of two possible responses and receives one of two possible outcomes, control ratings tend to correlate with the number of successful outcome trials.

As shown in Fig. 8.3, results from Alloy and Abramson (1979) show that in a paradigm similar in most respects to the one used by Jenkins and Ward, a large number of "hits," or conditions where financial incentives are given for "wins," cause normal subjects to overestimate the degree of control objectively present. Depressed students acting as subjects were found not to do this; they went on "getting it right" and providing a

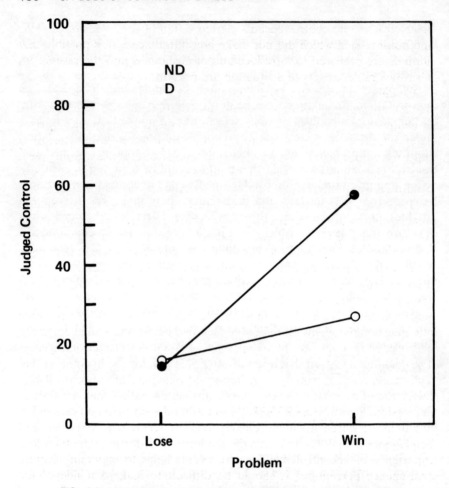

FIG. 8.3. Judged control for depressed (D) and nodepressed (ND) students as a function of problem type. (Redrawn from Alloy and Abramson, 1979, with the permission of the authors and the American Psychological Association.)

realistic estimate of control levels. This led the authors to conclude that depressed subjects were "sadder but wiser." If depressed people are shown to be so accurate, this presents a difficulty for any model that assumes that depression is transmitted as a state of learned helplessness. The one problem is that assessment of personal skill is not required in these experiments.

Although the experiments demonstrated an asymmetrical relationship between motivational factors and control assessment, introspective reports from subjects suggested that the assessment itself was empirically based: "I believed I had no control because I tried different sequences of pressing and non-pressing which did not make any difference." It is possible that normals are prepared to introduce an optimistic bias into the assessment when favorable aspects of a situation are present.

A number of points emerged from this study. Firstly, the data suggested that lack of contingency may be more difficult to detect than the presence of contingency. Secondly, outcome valence and frequency are important determinants of perceived control. Thirdly, there was greater illusion of control when an active as compared with a passive response was involved. Finally, the appraisal is subject to differences in mental state. This is confirmed by an interesting experiment by Alloy, Abramson, and Viscusi (1981), who used a technique developed by Velten (1968) to induce simulated moods in depressed and normal subjects. Normal women subjects, induced to be depressed, gave accurate judgments of control in the noncontingent condition when "wins" occurred, whereas depressed women, induced to be normal, showed the "illusion of control." Thus, transient mood states simulated by subjects appear to be as important as enduring dispositions.

Schwartz (1981) actually argues that the Alloy and Abramson results call into question the relationship between learned helplessness and depression because, as he points out, nondepressives cannot detect noncontingency. The data might suggest that normals can never develop the hypotheses that lead to depression, namely, that important outcomes are uncontrollable. Detection of noncontingency has to be a symptom rather than a source of depression. Schwartz assumes that normals tend to form hypotheses of the 'if x then y' nature and are more likely to be subject to bias. Experience of helplessness actually counteracts the tendency to distortion, and therefore experience of uncontrollable aversive events helps to maintain accurate contingency perception. It should be difficult to make a nondepressed person transmit the disposition to be helpless through experience of uncontrollable events.

Therefore, we might imagine that the illusion of control is actually a healthy depression-resistant process. Langer (1975) actually suggests that the illusion of control is the inverse of learned helplessness. Normals might be armed with a robust self-serving approach in which internal attributions are made for success and external attributions are made for the lack of it. Perceiving control in conditions where it does not exist may be a very healthy process, which helps a person to resist helplessness in negative-outcome conditions. Ward and Jenkins (1965) actually showed that even in the complete absence of contingency, normal subjects will perceive control: Subjects presented with facts about cloud seeding and rainfall were asked to judge contingency; when information was presented in the form of pairs of events and outcome across time, subjects reported contingency, even though chance was implied by the experiment.

The possibility that normals may resist helplessness by overestimating control is interesting in the context of this chapter because if stresses do change the locus of control, helplessness and depression may be a specific result and not a permanent change. We need them to try to understand resistance, or lack of resistance, as a function of decisions about control. An experiment by Alloy and Abramson (1981) involved giving normal subjects a pretreatment of controllable noise, uncontrollable noise, or no noise. Subjects were then required to judge the amount of control in a noncontingent situation where there was either success or failure present. Contrary to the predictions of learned helplessness theory, normal subjects exposed to a prior treatment of uncontrollable noise showed a robust illusion of control when success was present. Depressed subjects remained accurate, irrespective of prior treatment. However, the illusion of control was not shown by those normals who had previously experienced controllable noise treatment. This latter result presents a difficulty for a helplessness resistance hypothesis in that normals *are* clearly affected in some way by prior treatment and do not merely overestimate when success is present.

In spite of this, the resistance hypothesis has some credibility. It appears that a number of factors may encourage the illusion of control and may enable a person to resist negative outcomes to situations of helplessness. Wartman (1975) argues that factors such as knowledge of goal or personal involvement may strengthen the illusion of control. Langer (1975) also confirms that factors from skill situations such as competition, choice, familiarity, and involvement could all act to strengthen expectancy of personal success probability. In six studies the introduction of these elements strengthened the illusion for normal subjects. Langer and Roth (1975) argue that early successes strengthen the illusion.

The Rules of Optimism

From the evidence quoted so far, it appears that even if the conditions are so set that a person is objectively helpless with regard to changing a negative experience, there may still be resistance to the learning of loss of control. In this chapter we have argued that stresses may bring about a change in the locus of control, either because of stress-related influences or because a person is already prepared and not in the right mental state for effective action. However, if the resistance hypothesis developed above is valid, a proportion of people experiencing these situations will not expect to remain helpless or to be helpless in other similar situations. They will seek out and find control and will resist depression. In an account of his experiences in various prisons in the Soviet Union under Stalin's regime, Dolgun (1965) reports establishing control over small aspects of daily life despite the deprivation stresses and interrogation stresses he experienced; this, he claims, enabled him to resist the punishment he experienced, and to survive. The questions of importance are how he thought of exercising control by other means and to what extent obtaining some control may be protective even in cases where it is largely irrelevant with respect to the main factors in a situation.

Even if a person recognizes loss of control and perceives himself to be helpless, he may retain optimism if he does not blame himself excessively or if he continues to note "special circumstances" that describe the conditions in which he is helpless. The dogs studied by Seligman presumably never actually noted that they were only helpless in the treatment condition where there was no escape possible; perhaps they did not make the discriminations necessary to distinguish the two experimental situations because they were under the stress of pain at the time the discrimination needed to be made.

A person who produces and detects errors in stressful conditions could preserve optimism for the future if he notes the differences between a previous and a present condition. Work quoted in the previous chapter showing that people expect to perform poorly in stress may be important; if a person expects that stresses have adverse effects, he may make the attribution that he has not coped because of the effects of stress and thus experience helplessness without becoming pessimistic about the future.

The evidence reviewed so far also indicates that negative expectancies associated with depression are not likely to result in underestimation of control. The depressed students in the Alloy and Abramson study did not underestimate the contingency between action and outcome; they continued to give meaningful estimates even when normals showed the illusion of control. A useful definition of pessimism is the repeated failure to be optimistic.

A question of importance is the precondition for optimism in normals. Apparently, depressed students do not respond to the special incentive conditions in the way normals do; they continue to see them as irrelevant. The transmission of helplessness might depend on a failure to sample the environment for positive factors, or alternatively it might arise because of a failure to think illogically and perceive positive conditions as relevant to the perception of control.

In the Alloy and Abramson experiments, incentive and monetary reward were manipulated. It is possible that depressed students failed to note these critical features. However, this interpretation does not fit well with findings such as that by Loeb, Beck, and Diggory (1971), which showed that depressed subjects were sensitive to reward and failure factors; performance on a subsequent different task was differentially influenced by success or failure on a first task.

Incentive is a complex treatment because incentives are both arousing and informative. An attempt was made by Fisher and Ledwith (1983) to see whether a condition primarily associated with arousal increase could produce the illusion of control in normal subjects. If so, this would suggest that information is not a necessary condition of the effect.

There were three possible reasons for predicting a change on contingency estimation in loud noise: Firstly, the arousing properties of noise could create conditions for optimism; secondly, since, as outlined in the previous chapter, normal people expect to have lowered control in stress, there might be evidence of weakened estimates of contingency; finally, because stresses such as noise are frequently associated with changes in attentional deployment and with depression of short-term memory, evidence on which assessment of contingency depends may be distorted or unavailable.

The experiment involved a very simple design. Subjects depressed one of two keys on an Apple Micropressor and received on the display either a blue or an orange signal in the corresponding position on the screen. The task was to sample the task for 40 trials and then assess the degree of control over outcome. There were 3 objective levels of contingency—25%, 50%, and 75%—defined by conditions where response A led to event A and response B led to event B. A total of 48 students were assigned at random either to work in noise levels of 95 dB or in levels of 55 dB (quiet). The experimental arrangement was so basic that in effect a subject was sorting out two sets of frequencies, and a straight counting strategy should have provided the answer.

The sequence was preprogrammed so that on a series of randomly determined occasions irrespective of the subject's choice (left or right response), he would always receive the compatible display event. It was thought desirable to have the same sequence of events for all those in the 25, 50, and 75% conditions respectively. For this reason the trials of objective contingency were predetermined, and the remainder were random trails; on half the occasions some of the trials would appear to the subject as if they were random. As a result of this design, a totally different unpredicted effect occured and led to some further interesting results.

Figure 8.4 provides an illustration of contingency estimates given by subjects in the three different objective contingency groups, in quiet and noise. Since half the random trials should be indistinguishable, by the subject, from contingent trials, a straight count of R–R and L–L event should give the subject an estimate close to the equation

$$\frac{100 - \text{objective contingency}}{2} + \text{objective contingency}$$

As shown in Fig. 8.4, estimates were close to this. In both noise and quiet conditions there were significant positive correlations between objective contingency and estimated control ($p < .001$).

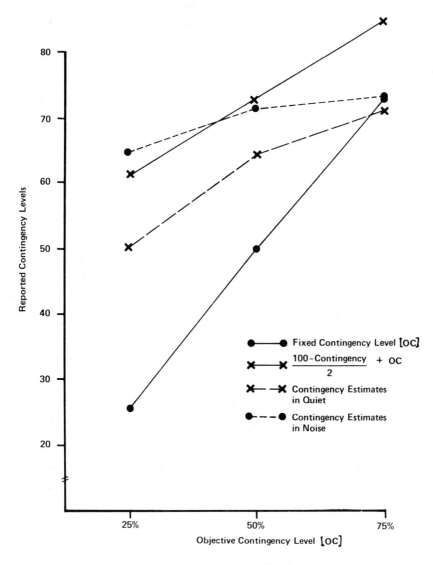

FIG. 8.4.   Subjective estimates of control against objective levels of contingency in conditions of quiet and noise. (Reproduced from Fisher & Ledwith, 1983.)

TABLE 8.1.
Achieved Success and Estimated Control for 3 Categories of Objective
Contingency in Quiet and Noise Conditions

	Quiet (55 dB)			Noise (95 dB)		
Objective contingency	25%	50%	75%	25%	50%	75%
Actual 'success'	58.6%	74.88%	84.75%	66.0%	76.88%	87.25%
Estimated control	50.13%	68.75%	73.12%	69.0%	73.13%	75.38%
Difference between estimated control and success	−8.47	−6.13	−11.63	+3.0	−3.75	−11.87
Difference between objective contingency and estimated control	+25.13	+18.75	+1.88	+44.0	+23.13	+.38

Table 8.1 indicates that subjects in noise appear to overestimate the level of control in noise relative to quiet conditions. The effect was only significant, however, for the 25% and 50% contingency conditions ($p < .01$ and $p < .05$ respectively). Nevertheless, this was sufficient evidence to suggest that subjects in noise were actually overoptimistic about control levels. However, an important assumption was that success, defined in terms of the frequency of contingent action outcomes, did not differ between the two groups. This is where we made an astonishing discovery: Success was actually higher for subjects working in 95-dB noise than for those working in quiet. This result seemed impossible because there was a fixed proportion of trials, and then the remainder were generated by means of reference to a random sequence. Thus no subject should have been able to improve his success rates; each subject's success should be defined by

$$\frac{100 - OC}{2} + OC$$

where OC is the objective contingency level. Analysis showed that success in terms of contingent trials differed significantly for the 25% condition. It seemed that subjects in noise had been sufficiently motivated to try to predict occasional runs in the sequence. Although the sequence was random and there was no response bias, subjects in noise had managed to increase the number of successes by up to 5 by making predictions. The difference scores between actual successes and control estimates for subjects working in noise were more discrepant than for subjects in quiet who had fewer contingencies. The results raise a number of interesting hypotheses. Perhaps subjects in noise were more motivated to predict the sequence and, as it turned out, some prediction was possible. As discussed in the previous chapter, noise does appear to favor the ordered recall of material; perhaps subjects in noise simply found it easier to find sequential dependencies in a series of randomly presented alternations. However, as far as the question of the effects of noise on the perception of control is concerned, there is a serious difficulty. Those subjects in noise actually received more contingent trials because of prediction, and therefore the base level of control estimation data is different.

The noise effect is itself intriguing; it could be argued that normal subjects do seek out and maximize the chances of success under conditions that enable them to do so and when there is positive incentive to do so. A self-serving strategy may be operative. A question of interest was whether depressed students would behave like this. Using exactly the same design, with the same predetermined random sequences of 40 trials in each of the 3 objective conditions, 12 depressed subjects (scoring 9 or above on the Beck Depression Inventory) were assigned at random to either quiet or noise conditions.

Table 8.2 shows, firstly, that the effects described previously were replicated for the nondepressed group; subjects in noise increased success rates and therefore raised the evidence for contingency assessment; actual assessments overestimated success for the 25% and 50% conditions. This was not true for depressed subjects. There was no evidence of increased success or increased overestimation in describing the data in noise as compared with quiet. This still leaves open the question of whether the increased accuracy in assessing received contingency data in noise is a function of higher levels of data received.

Both depressed and nondepressed groups gave estimates of control that correlated positively with actual objective levels of data received on the issue of accuracy of control assessments. There was evidence that noise induced the illusion of control, moreover it did appear to be associated with an attempt to make the most of evidence about control. The study with depressed subjects was less discrepant for the noise condition. An obvious conclusion is that depressed subjects in noise were not motivated, or not able to maximize success in obtaining and assessing control evidence in the same way as normals.

The results lend support to the hypothesis that normals may operate self-serving optimistic strategies in stress. On the level of "collection of

TABLE 8.2.
Achieved Success and Estimated Control for 3 Categories of Objective
Contingency in Quiet and Noise Conditions for Depressed and Normal
Subjects

		Quiet (55 dB)			Noise (95 dB)		
	Objective Contingency	25%	50%	75%	25%	50%	75%
$\overline{X}$ Actual	Normals	59.1%	70.8%	82.1%	68.2%	78.1%	87.0%
success	Depressed	57.8%	72.1%	83.5%	59.3%	72.3%	81.3%
$\overline{X}$ Estimated	Normals	49.1%	64.8%	73.1%	69.5%	77.9%	85.4%
control	Depressed	50.7%	65.1%	71.8%	51.9%	63.1%	69.8%
$\overline{X}$ Difference	Normals	−10.0	−6.0	−9.0	+1.3	+1.8	−1.6
between	Depressed	−7.1	7.0	−11.7	−7.4	−9.2	−11.6
estimated control and success							
$\overline{X}$ Difference	Normals	+24.1	+14.8	+1.9	+44.5	+27.0	+10.4
between	Depressed	+25.7	+15.1	−3.2	+26.9	+13.1	−5.2
objective contingency and estimated control							

evidence" a person may increase his successes where possible, take more careful note of the evidence, and produce estimates positively biased when rewards do appear. All these may be ways of resisting helplessness and maintaining or raising self-esteem.

A point of importance is that in this case the effect of noise-induced stress on normal subjects appears to be to raise the motivation for attention to detail. This is a different result from that reported by Dittes (1961) on failure-induced threat, which suggested that individuals might attempt to raise self-esteem by imposing "closure." The operation of closure was defined as an attempt to provide meaning in a meaningless section of text, or to provide impressions of another person on the basis of more prominent traits without noting inconsistency.

Tertiary Feedback Loops

Studies that index states by means of self-report on questionnaires and diagnostic procedures have the common property of assuming that information about biological state is available to a subject. In fact, major issues in theories of emotion have been concerned with whether perceived state of physiological change is a sufficient condition for an emotional experience (James, 1884; Cannon, 1936, Schacter & Singer, 1962). There is actually little research that makes clear what aspects of biological state a person is aware of. States of high muscle tension, stomach discomfort, or heart palpitations may be more readily evident than changes in blood sugar level or in adrenal function.

There are two questions of interest. Firstly, there is the question of whether the information has directional properties or whether it consists of a train of signals indicating merely a change in general energy level. Secondly, there is the question of how much information of this kind is monitored and what proportion of mental "work space" must be given over to such monitoring. A simple cognitive economy would be to monitor information only when some critical level of function has been exceeded. There might be no basic awareness of heart rate until violent physical exercise conditions or shock cause heart rate changes.

Not enough information exists on the perception of biological changes in order for any definite conclusions to be reached concerning the amount of detail available to a subject. The objection raised by some of the early physiological theorists, that in general visceral systems are poorly inner-vated and therefore unlikely to provide a rich source of information (e.g., Cannon, 1932, 1936), is implicitly confirmed by biofeedback studies, which assume that the individual is unable to make use of information concerning changes indicated by falsified feedback. However, since studies have also made available as analogue or digital information on a display.

Studies of falsified heart rate information (e.g., Stern, Botto, and Herrick, 1972) have shown that changes in actual heart rate accompany changes in physiological function unless the information is specifically shown that GSR may also change as an accompaniment of falsified information indicating heart rate change (e.g., see Hirschman, 1975), there is the possibility that what is changed is not specific but represents a change in general level of arousal. The importance of information available concerning biological responses is emphasized in an experiment by Valins and Ray (1967), who showed that if falsified heart rate information lead subjects to believe there was no change in heart rate during the presenta-tion of slides of snakes, subsequent ability to handle a live boa constrictor was improved. Unfortunately, Valins and Ray did not record actual heart rate; thus there is no way of knowing whether physiological change accompanied feedback indicating change, or whether the effect should be explained exclusively in cognitive terms. The authors favor a cognitive explanation, arguing that cognitions about internal reactions are important modifiers of behavior. According to this view, the subjects believed themselves to be relaxed while seeing slides of snakes, and so fear concerning the handling of a live snake was reduced. This was seen to be consistent with earlier findings by Valins (1966), which showed that males who were given evidence to suggest change in heart rate accompanying slides of seminude females subsequently rated these slides as more attractive. This was irrespective of whether the change had been in the direction of increased or decreased heart rate, which could be taken to suggest that direction of change is less important than magnitude. This could be taken to favor general arousal change or to suggest that any change in intensity has implications for cognitive awareness.

High levels of internal states could create a further feedback loop, which promotes further deterioration within a stress scenario. The perception of a high level of bodily tension and physiological activity not only provides a source of further distress but causes a change toward using up capacity by mental preoccupation or worry work concerned with states of biological discomfort.

Work by Tompkins (1970) has suggested that negative emotions are more likely to be associated with a high density of neural firing. The negative emotions are predominantly fear, distress, and anger, and they are likely responses to extreme levels of stress. If this information is presented for processing, escalation of deterioration in performance would be expected.

A tertiary loop is implemented when a person worries about the state he perceives himself to be in and the feelings it provokes. Curiously, it may be these states that lead a person to seek help.

TOTAL INCOMPETENCE AND CRISIS

The point made so far is that there is likely to be an orderly progression of deterioration that characterizes life stress scenarios when a person is unable to exert control and it is important that he does so. This could in theory occur because the world behaves unjustly; a person makes all the right responses but cannot gain control. Equally, the same could be true when there is in reality no solution to the problem. The ultimate stage is where a person is totally incompetent to change or control the world around him. This is a state of complete control breakdown and will have implications for mental well-being.

Crisis and Models of Mental Disorder

Phenomenological states that accompany intense stress experiences are often similar in many respects to states of mental disorder. It would be wrong to conclude that such similarity implies a common causal process, but the indications for research are to search for evidence of a "stress connection" in the background of mentally disordered people.

One major problem is the lack of rigorous criteria for defining matching similarity in such complex states. There are well-recognized symptoms that accompany response to intense stress and are commonly present in clinical states of anxiety, such as changes in breathing, swallowing, faintness, dizziness, and irritability. Marks and Lader (1973) emphasize that anxiety states feature in 2 to 5% of the nonclinical population, compared with 27% in clinical patients. There is no clear criterion for distinguishing these conditions. Korchin (1964) recognizes problems presented by distinctions between normal and neurotic anxiety and proposes a continuum in which differences in intensity, degree of debilitation, and duration are critical. The distinction between what is clinical and what is within the distribution of normality may actually be a function of a number of factors, including availability of medical resources and the nature of the condition itself. Depression, for example, may be a state of response reduction not conducive to help-seeking (Davis, 1970); this has recently been borne out by the cases of severe depression encountered by Brown and Harris (1978) in their door-to-door surveys in Camberwell, London. Depressed patients may be a self-selected subset; help-seeking may itself represent an attempt to establish some control.

Perhaps more convincing are the attempts to build experimental models in the laboratory. Here, conditions of specific stress are created and the resultant states likened to states of clinical disorder. Thus, Masserman (1943) modeled anxiety neurosis in laboratory experiments with cats. Seligman (1975) modeled depression in laboratory experiments with dogs. Davis (1948) produced experimental depression in pilots by introducing fatigue and increased task difficulty levels.

In the 1960s it was thought that certain extreme levels of stress produced states that modeled psychosis, particularly schizophrenia (see Hollister, 1962). Luby and Gottlieb (1966) described the effects of sensory deprivation, sleep deprivation, and LSD-25 as producing states that were "transient reversible psychoses," but the criterion for comparison was not clearly established. There are a number of experiments that report phenomena that resemble specific symptoms reported for schizophrenic conditions. Thus, Fisher (1980) reported response perseveration in sleep-deprived subjects who had been one night without sleep. Flavell et al. (1958) showed that on a word association test increased time pressure produced a tendency to perseverate in the production of words and to make clang associations. On a similar kind of task, Usdansky and Chapman (1960) have shown that, in normal subjects, time pressure increases the probability of associative interference when distracting stimuli are present.

SPC-O

These studies do at least demonstrate that similar symptoms can be produced as transient reversible conditions in normal subjects within the boundaries of normal processes: It is not necessary to introduce the idea of biological or psychological pathology. An important distinguishing feature in patients appears to be persistence of states beyond what is seen to be an appropriate context by observers.

Exactly the same considerations apply to naturalistic observations following losses and disasters, which also appear to demonstrate clinical phenomena as transient reversible states. For example, Parkes (1965, 1978) traces the progression of behaviors forming part of the reaction to severe loss. Anxious, searching behavior predominates initially and is then more likely to be replaced by reduction in responsivity and withdrawal. Fried's study of the reaction of Boston slum dwellers to relocation showed a comparable depressed response (see Fried, 1962). Price (1967), basing his remarks on the results of the observation of bird behavior, points out that changes in rank order in relationships are accompanied by a number of behavioral and mood changes. The movement upward is accompanied by signs of elation, the move downward by behavioral signs characteristic of depression. Price argues that these differences may be functional in preserving harmony in groups, since depression in the loser means that the winner will not be challenged.

These and related studies demonstrate that it is possible to produce "pseudoclinical" states in normal people in natural unpleasant conditions. The existence of unpleasant conditions may, however, depend both on meaning given to an event and on the acceptability of the meaning to other observers. If a person is likely to be attacked by an intruder, any panic or disturbance he shows may be acceptable. If he believes he will be attacked by trees, his panic behavior is likely to be regarded quite differently. There are some interesting grey zones in this respect: A nonreligious person may accept more readily that a religious man fears the devil than that a man fears trees. The tolerance area of what it is reasonable to believe may determine the degree to which behavior is seen as persisting out of context.

Crisis and Different Aspects of Control

An hypothesis worth considering is that decision making about control provides the flavor of the disorder. Thus, mental disorders of various kinds may be adaptive aspects of attempts to establish or regain control. There are really three aspects to decisions about control that might be important determinants of symptomatology. Firstly, there is *disengagement, or* "*quitting.*" This is one response to perceived loss of control and is best likened to a state of helplessness. Experiments by Seligman have indicated how this state could be engendered out of context by prior treatments of uncontrollable shock in his experimental dogs (Seligman, 1975). Disengagement or quitting must involve some punishment. In the case of the Seligman dogs the punishment is to accept shocks that could be avoided. In the case of a human being, the punishment could be basic, as in accepting poverty or isolation, or more complex, as when a person accepts damage to his prestige and accepts failure.

Secondly, there is *attempting to achieve control when the odds are against success*. A person receives feedback about his ability to control the situation that suggests that he is losing, but he continues to struggle. Persistence in the face of uncompromising odds is likely to be accompanied by high levels of anxiety and is deviant when the evidence shows success is unlikely. Pathological bereavement may be of this nature, when a person refuses to accept the death of a loved relative. Persistence with any problem when it cannot logically be solved is as pathological as premature disengagement and helplessness. The question that we should try to answer concerns the rules that govern persistence; we need to know what governs persistence/disengagement as a feature of behavior.

For those who engage the problem, an influential factor is likely to be the nature of the problem scenario. Some problems will have much in common with the paradigm of hitting a nail on the head. There is a knock-on effect of progress, and occasional failures do no damage to this progress. A student struggling to write up his thesis may be in just this position. Every acceptable action he produces contributes to the end product; failure and "bad days" do not detract from progress. This can be compared with other sorts of problems, in which failure cannot be so easily tolerated. A person attending an important interview cannot afford to make errors, because the period he has for impressing the interviewer is limited. This situation can be compared with a condition in which the nail actually rises back out of the wood when there is a miss! These differences may be very important moderators of the flavor of mental state in a struggle for control. In one condition a person may note gradual progress, in another he may detect that setbacks resulting from failures and errors put him back to zero progress.

Finally, there is control by avoidance; despite superficial behavioral similarities, it should not be confused with a passive helpless state. Withdrawal may be a form of passive resistance or avoidance. A person in effect produces a "no response" in order to resist an approach or avoid an encounter. Equally, of course, he may produce a positive avoidance response, as in many conditions of phobic fear. The important point about these situations, as far as the control model is concerned, is that a person will have to maintain vigilance, since one successful avoidance does not mean that another encounter may not be forthcoming. Equally, he may not ever receive the information he needs in order to know that his evasive action was successful. He cannot build up the contingency data required for stable perceptions about control.

Various clinical symptomatologies could have evolved as ways of exerting control by avoidance. Schizophrenic thinking and talking may be adjustments to the desire to avoid social encounters. There would be nothing more off-putting to a participant than a respondent who talks with strange phrases or strange logic. These mechanisms, if successful, would be preserved and eventually develop into a response style: Politicians appear to evolve techniques for not answering key questions by using material that is relevant but not to the point. Meichenbaum (1979) has considered the possibility that schizophrenic speech is functional in this respect.

These considerations, admittedly speculative, raise issues concerned with mental and physical illness as outcomes of decisions taken in stress scenarios. The issues are developed further in the final two chapters.

9 Control Decisions and Vulnerability

INTRODUCTION

Development of ideas about the role played by the perception of control in stress would be incomplete without consideration of the concept of vulnerability. It is apparent that the stress factors that impose on a person during a particular encounter do not completely determine outcome. Some individuals appear to encounter severe disrupting influences and yet appear to cope; others appear to reach a state of crisis of one kind or another.

One of the important differences between clinical cases and cases of normals under stress may turn out to be the persistence of symptoms. Vulnerable individuals may be those who remain affected for a long time by an unpleasant experience. A risk model provides a useful description but fails to provide an explanation of how vulnerability is represented. Using an analogy with heart disease, conditions of overweight, experiencing stress, lack of exercise, and age increase the risk of an attack. An explanation is available in terms of changes in the structure and function of the cardiovascular system. In the case of the risk of mental disorder, it is now possible to identify a number of genetic and environmental factors that change the risk. The representation of risk in psychological structure still needs to be made explicit.

The main approach to be developed in this chapter is that vulnerability to life events is represented in knowledge, an important aspect of which is concerned with control. Thus vulnerability is argued to be a form of metamemory.

Firstly, we will consider some of the evidence that demonstrates the relationship between precipitants and psychological disorder. What is clear is that variance is high and correlations are generally low. It is then possible to examine the possibility of preparing influences in the environment that increase the risk for precipitants to have a negative outcome. We concentrate on two influences: social circumstance and early trauma or deprivation. Finally, the last part of this chapter is concerned with trying to interpret these risk factors in terms of decisions about control. The hypothesis pursued is that adverse life experiences with negative outcomes may prepare a person to change expectancies about control in a subsequent situation. In other words, the main concern is with life history sequential dependencies.

The reader will appreciate that it is not possible to do justice to the large volume of research relevant to the issue of vulnerability or to issues such as the definition and diagnosis of mental conditions. There are excellent clinical texts that cover some of those important issues (e.g., Mayer-Gross, Slater, & Roth, 1960; Henderson & Gillespie, 1962; Becker, 1974; Beck, 1967; Lundin, 1965). As far as this chapter is concerned, selectivity is essential, and we apologize to those who may feel that their research has been neglected.

A dictionary definition of vulnerability normally involves the term "susceptibility" and implies that the individual who is vulnerable will succumb to certain situations. It remains possible that vulnerability is very general, so that a person is at risk for a number of different precipitants, or very specific, so that only certain configurations will be relevant. In the latter case, we would expect an even smaller proportion of crisis outcomes to precipitants than in the former case; using a lock-and-key analogy, vulnerability may be so specific that only certain keys will turn the lock.

Before considering these issues, it is necessary to deal with some of the important features of predisposing and precipitating factors in relation to personal crisis and mental disorder. One important aspect is the problem of establishing the evidence. Almost all the available evidence consists of cases where a person already in crisis of some kind provides the evidence or where a particular precipitant (e.g., bereavement) is investigated in relation to outcome across a population of sufferers.

PREDISPOSING AND PRECIPITATING FACTORS AND RISK

Difficulties in Definition

At least one of the problems encountered by almost any attempt to relate events in life history to subsequent outcomes and states is that of precise definitions. The literature on background factors in mental disorder frequently refers to precipitant stresses in the aetiology of psychological reactions and physical health. On some occasions, the outcome is not expected; crisis is acute, rather as when a particular blend of chemicals suddenly becomes volatile. On other occasions, the condition appears to be predictable, suggesting a slowly evolving change. Breakdown is chronic rather than acute, and there may be only a very loose relationship to a precipitant, as if material is being soaked in a particular dye so that color begins to increase gradually toward the point of total color saturation. The difference may be determined by the dynamics of stress scenarios within life histories. For example, control by avoidance as a response to social stress might involve progressive elaboration of strategies, whereas transmitted helplessness might have more definite associations with precipitants. These differences are important because they affect the relationship with a precipitant as perceived by external observers. As will be evident later, schizophrenic-like states appear to have very unclear relationships with precipitants. This may be because the symptoms represent a slowly evolving pattern of control by avoidance, which only appears as a state of crisis when control becomes ineffective or when other people increase the pressure because they see the avoidance strategies as strange behaviors.

A methodological problem of importance is that those who actually become patients are self-selected. Acute crisis may be a cry for help; admission to hospital may be a form of control by avoidance. Brown and Harris (1978) showed the prevalence of "clinical-like" states of depression in working-class women at home, which illustrates that, particularly for depression, the nature of the condition may predispose against help-seeking (Davis, 1970). A further point from the Brown and Harris study is that not only does the mental condition predispose against help-seeking, but the factors that help to precipitate and maintain the condition may themselves dispose against it. Having little money, poor opportunity, and low mobility are additional factors that prevent help-seeking, particularly when there are young children at home.

A further difficulty is that in cases of elaborate control by avoidance the precipitant may not be easily elicited from the patient. Medical personnel impose the same if not more pressures on patients who respond with alarm to social encounters. The desire to remain solitary in quiet surroundings is violated by busy wards and constant assessment or treatment, and these conditions may act as potential precipitants. Not only does the patient seek to avoid the conditions, but "private meanings" may dictate particular aspects he seeks to avoid.

Finally, difficulties arise from the technique of retrospective reporting of life events. A study of 76 neurotically depressed patients by Schless et al. (1974), using the 43-item list of events on the Holmes and Rahe scale

(Holmes and Rahe, 1967), showed that uniformly higher rating was given to the life events by the depressed group. Differences were 5 to 6 times greater than the standard error of the mean weight of an item in many cases. By comparing ratings on admission and discharge, any changes could be attributable to treatment and changes in symptomatology. The results confirmed that the tendency to rate life events more highly appeared to be an enduring feature, because ratings were as high on remission. The authors see depression as characterized by a general alarm response. It is important if the change influences the account given of a personal life history, because information about the precipitant and disorder is less reliable. The problem is worsened if there are selective effects on memory. Normal subjects have been shown to recall pleasant experiences readily (Beebe-Center, 1932); depressed subjects show some evidence of increased speed and intensity in the recall of unpleasant memories (Lloyd & Lishman, 1975). The authors of the latter study suggest that depression is associated with a "hedonic set" that directs recall toward unpleasant experiences. These findings fit with the model of negative cognitions emphasized by Beck as being central to depression (e.g., see Beck, 1967, 1970) and clearly renders suspect any account a depressed individual may give of his life history profile. To some extent, the problem of patient reporting can be alleviated by requiring patients' accounts to be corroborated by a relative. There remains the problem that the relatives' impressions may themselves be affected by being exposed to patients' negative accounts of life events.

Even supposing that these problems can be solved, there remains the difficulty that correlations do not necessarily imply causation. The relationship of a disorder to a precipitant may be fortuitous, or there may be self-selection processes involved.

The Effect of Immediate Stress

A precipitant is generally defined as an event occurring in close proximity to a state of abnormal functioning and is normally considered to be causally related. There are two difficulties. Firstly, as mentioned previously, retrospective studies may be contaminated because of the subjects' knowledge of the disorder. Secondly, there is an indirect form of contamination in that there is a common process that relates to the precipitant and the disorder. The investigator may be the common process; he may take more detailed recordings when the subject appears anxious or depressed on interview.

A finding that is consistent is that the meaning of an event for an individual is a critical factor. This suggests that there will be idiosyncracies and that common denominators will be difficult to find. Clinical depression is not related in any clear-cut way to preceding environmental circumstances. Loss of a "significant other" is rated high on stress scales (e.g., see Holmes & Rahe, 1967), yet only about 3% of bereaved people are likely to be treated for depression (see Parkes, 1965, 1978). Investigations of the occurrence of precipitants 6 months prior to disorders have produced a number of rather different findings, indicative perhaps of the difficulties of these kinds of studies. For example, Hudgens, Morrison, and Barchha (1967) reported little evidence of events prior to the onset of depression. By contrast, Paykel et al. (1969) gave 185 patients from outpatients and emergency treatment groups a modified list of the Holmes and Rahe scale and reported increased frequencies of occurrence of a life event in the 6 months prior to symptoms; depressed subjects reported a total of 313 events in 6 months (mean: 1.69 per subject); controls reported 109 events (mean: .69 per subject). The results indicated that there was an increase in the reported frequency of events such as arguments with spouse, marital separation, change of work or in conditions of work, serious personal illness, death of immediate family member, family member leaving home. Depressed subjects reported a greater proportion of undesirable events in which "exits" or losses of one kind or another were more important than "entrances." The authors recognize the importance of *meaning* in accounting for the diverse pattern of results. They acknowledge that the fundamental question is why some individuals become depressed and others do not, because the results indicate a difference in frequency and undesirability, not the presence or absence of variables. Most of the events reported were "everyday" events, not catastrophic occurrences. Elements argued to be important were personality, previous experience, and capacity to adapt and cope.

A study by Beck and Worthen (1972) compared depressed patients with a schizophrenic group and showed that in the former case there *was* evidence of a clear precipitant 6 months prior to a disorder. Out of 21 depressed patients, 95% provided evidence of a precipitant; in half the cases this involved the loss of a "significant other person." By comparison, only about half of the group of schizophrenic patients provided evidence of a clear precipitant. In addition, the weight given to the stressful quality of the reported experience was greater in the depressive group. This latter finding is difficult to interpret because, as shown by Schless, Schwartz, Goetz, and Mendels (1974), depressed individuals tend to give greater weight to experiences they have not themselves encountered.

As indicated above, there are good reasons for supposing that the precipitant should be less evident as a clear factor in the life history of schizophrenics. Firstly, phobic withdrawal might limit the number of events encountered. Secondly, private meanings that evolve as elaborate means of control could provide new precipitants. In a study by Brown and Birley (1968) investigating events in the lives of a group of schizophrenic patients in which onset of symptoms had occurred within 13 weeks of admission, the main comparison was with the frequency of unpleasant events occurring in the three weeks before onset. The main result was that patients, as compared with normal population controls, experienced nearly double the number of events (1.74% as compared with .96% for controls). In fact, 46% of the patients had undergone at least one event in the three-week period prior to onset, and 12% had been subject to events in preceding intervals. In conclusion, the authors believe that the precipitant alone is *not* a sufficient condition for the disorder and locate a background pattern of tension in the home as an important consideration.

Beck and Worthen (1972) point out that a number of the hazards reported by Brown and Birley were not clear hazards at all, and many of them involved events that could be assumed to have positive qualities. Thus the problem of unclear precipitants and private meanings raises particular difficulties for the investigation of schizophrenia as a response to stress.

Many studies have led to conclusions that indicate that *vulnerability at the time of occurrence of a precipitant* is the important factor (see Clayton, Halikas, & Maurice, 1972; Hudgens, Morrison, & Barchha, 1967); precipitants lead to a worsening of conditions already underway or trigger admission to the hospital. Hudgens (1974) argues that there has been little convincing demonstration that intense stresses can cause these disorders in "previously sound individuals." A study of a group of adolescents showed that for 20 out of 22 patients with depression, onset was preceded by stress that was objectively serious and meaningful for the patient. A key factor distinguishing the depressed patients from those who were well was a significantly higher incidence of psychiatric disorder in the histories of the biological parents; but there were also more severe nonpsychiatric illnesses preceding the onset of depression. This suggests that general vulnerability might result from an accumulation of preparing influences in determining reaction to severe events.

The literature on the effects of stressful life events in terms of reaction produced in those exposed suggests that there are two elements: *desirability* and the *degree of change*. Relationships have been established between various measures of psychological distress and both physical and mental illness in terms of these measures. Many situations involve both factors combined. A study by Sheatsley and Feldman (1964) showed that on a checklist of 15 symptoms used to assess mental health in general populations (Langer, 1962), the effect of the assassination of President Kennedy produced one or more negative symptoms in 89% of a randomly selected normal population during the four days following the assassination.

Studies such as those conducted by Brown and Birley in relation to schizophrenia (1968) or depression (1970) have largely involved undesira-

bility as the key factor. However, there has been more recent concentration on *change* as a main feature. Dohrenwend and Dohrenwend (1970)
defined stressful events as those that "disrupt or threaten to disrupt the
individual's usual activities" (p. 115). Holmes and Rahe (1967) introduced
a technique in which the *degree of readjustment* required by change was
given greater importance. Good prediction was obtained by summing the
readjustment scores yielded by the experience of an individual during an
observation period, and Theorell and Rahe (1970) associated high readjustment scores with coronary heart disease.

Dohrenwend (1973) attempted to separate desirability and change as
factors in stress and reported that generally the two were confounded;
individuals with low life-change scores reported more positive categories
than did those who scored high. Analysis suggested that life change is most
highly correlated with stress and may be a more important variable than
undesirability.

Crisis Theory and the Role of Precipitants

The theory that chronic conditions differ from acute reactions in previously
normal individuals is inherent in the formal development of crisis theory by
Caplan (1964). However, Caplan also argued that the effect of the
precipitant should not be separated from previous life history; old problems successfully resolved were assumed to be beneficial, but when
unsuccessfully resolved they were detrimental.

The view proposed by Beck and Worthen (1972) is that crisis theory is
only applicable for normals under threat. They propose a continuum based
on parthenogenic characteristics. At one end there are healthy people who
suffer a precipitous loss, where crisis theory is seen as giving an accurate
account of behavior. In the center are those who have some character
disturbance and who react strongly to precipitants rated as stressful by
normals. The authors argue that the crisis model appears to fit well with
these depressed groups. At the other end of the continuum are the
schizophrenic groups, who are seen as those with profound character
disturbance and whose reactions are poorly predicted by the crisis model.
The greater the departure from the norm of healthy intact personality, the
less the relevance of crisis theory as a predictor of mental disorder.

A probabilisitic model developed by Schulberg and Sheldon (1968)
assumes that the probability that a hazardous event will occur, that the
individual will be exposed to the event, and of counterharm resources
combine multiplicatively to determine outcome. The implicit assumption is
of a reciprocal relationship between vulnerability determined by previous
factors and the characteristics of a particular current situation. Thus the
normal individual and the previously disturbed individual could, in theory,
appear similar in phenomenology, but the state will be expected to affect a

high proportion of individuals. Less intense experiences would affect those already vulnerable. A useful distinction is between two sets of risk factors: A particular stress scenario could be described in terms of the risk of poor performance and crisis (intrinsic risk). Genetic factors and life history experience moderate the risk of a negative outcome (extrinsic risk).

Predisposing Factors and Vulnerability

Nearly all theories of behavior allow for past influences to determine present reactions. The basis of Freudian theory was the role played by infant experiences as determinants of functional relationships between unconscious elements of behavior. Jung emphasized the role played by the ancestral past—a theme that has been revived by the concept of "preparedness" (see Chapter 1). Learning theories of all types are at least united in the assumption that each new experience combines in some way with previous experiences as a determinant of behavior. Whereas there are few theories that deny the importance of early life, some give a philosophical bias toward determinism.

There are a number of important questions that must eventually be tackled by research. There is a need to know whether stressful experiences are different from normal experiences in preparing the individual for a subsequent encounter. We might hypothesize that stressful encounters afford protracted and intense learning periods; equally, we might hypothesize that learning under stress will be impoverished, and therefore carryover would not be strong. Finally, there might be "state-dependent" learning features, so that previous encounters permit learning of responses specific to that encounter.

There are two basic kinds of predisposing environment: One is associated with experience of high frequency of change or unpleasantness, the other with early deprivation and trauma. The former situation might be described by an "obstacle model"; life is full of unpleasant events, and these summate in determining vulnerability. The latter might be described by the "big bang" theory; an early trauma changes the whole nature of the subsequent course of events of life history for example because of a fundamental change in cognition. If the latter is true, a person who is vulnerable might be a "sleeper" showing no evidence of this state until the right circumstances occur.

Early Loss

The role of predisposing factors in the origin of depression have been investigated on many occasions. Loss in early life, together with social class, have both been identified as key factors. For example, Brown (1961) reported that 41% of 216 depressed patients had lost at least one parent before the age of 15. This compared with 12% in the general population and 19.6% in 267 medical patients. This was confirmed in a study by Beck in which diagnostic groupings and depression inventory ratings were used as a criterion (Beck, 1967). The depression inventory provided a means of comparing severe with moderate depression; 27% of those with more severe depression reported the loss of a parent before the age of 16, as compared with 12% in the nondepressed group. This was statistically significant ($p < .01$). When clinical judgments were used, the difference between severe depression and no depression in terms of the proportions of early bereavement as 36.4% and 15.2%, respectively. For both males and females, paternal loss appeared with greater frequency, and in terms of cases presenting with depression, females were described as "overrepresented." Beck's study also indicated that depression was not the only outcome of apparent loss; a schizophrenic and a neurotic-depressive group did not differ significantly in the incidence of orphanhood. The possibility that early loss does not provide any particular directional preparation for later experiences is in keeping with the views of Gregory (1966), who states that there is no relationship between parental loss and diagnostic groups.

There are two important points that appear to change the risk associated with early loss. Firstly, the loss of a close relative is not as important as the loss of the mother. Secondly, loss of the mother before the age of 11 is likely to be a factor that increases the risk of depression later. Brown and Harris (1978) suggest that the mother is the largest source of appreciation and support, in addition to providing the largest source of control in the child's world. After the age of 11, he may be less dependent on external control. The role played by a dependency factor was supported in a study by Birtchnell (1975), who measured dependency on a scale developed by Navran (1954) and found that women who lost their mothers before the age of 10 were more dependent than those who did not, although loss incurred between the ages of 10 and 19 also introduced a measure of dependency.

The relationship between early loss and subsequent agoraphobia is considered by Bowlby (1973). His notion is that separation and loss move the individual away from an "optimum developmental pathway." The central concept appears to be that of self-reliance defined in terms of a sense of consequence of the individual's own actions. Absence of a mother may provide the nurturant conditions for perceived loss of control. The young individual may find himself facing an environment in which he genuinely has little chance to control events that happen to him. If at this stage he cannot distinguish the reasons, he may develop a cognitive structure that favors the transmission of helplessness.

Circumstantial Factors

A number of important studies have implicated social class as an important factor in mental disorder. We apologize to the reader for what has to be a rather brief discussion of some of the main findings; excellent accounts taking methodological problems into consideration are provided by Dohrenwend (1975); Dohrenwend and Dohrenwend (1974) report that the highest overall rates of psychiatric disorder have been found in the lowest social class in 28 out of 33 studies, with the relationship strongest in studies conducted in urban or mixed urban and rural settings. The relationship is consistent for the main subtypes of schizophrenia and personality disorder.

The explanation provided originally by Jarvis in 1855 (Jarvis, 1971) was the basis for what has become known as the social drift hypothesis: People who are inadequate drift to the lowest level of the class system and to urban settings, which are poor. By contrast, rather similar observations by Faris and Dunham (1939) lead these authors to conclude that social location may be the cause of psychopathology. Many other epidemiological investigations have taken a related view. For example, the much-quoted studies of Hollingshead and Redlich (1958) and recently Brown and Harris (1978) have emphasized that psychopathology has social origins.

Investigations have emphasized the role social factors might play in changing the ingredients in cognition. A study by Jessor et al. (1968) and by Parker and Kleiner (1966) emphasized the importance of discrepancy between goal and achievement produced by impoverished environments. A person cannot find the resources to achieve his goals. This may even include finding the resources to enable external intervention through help-seeking to occur. In the Camberwell study, the authors asserted that the "same social factors that increase the risk of developing psychiatric disorder greatly reduce the chances of reaching psychiatric services" (Brown, Bhrolchain, & Harris, 1975, p. 227). Nearly all the women interviewed in a door-to-door survey in south London who were found to be disturbed had not seen a psychiatrist, and "scarcely half" had seen a medical practitioner. The women were of low social class, with a background of poverty and deprivation.

On first consideration these studies support the notion that sociological background factors create the conditions for mental disorder. However, Dohrenwend (1975) reviews the "Midtown study," in which a significant inverse relationship between respondents' symptoms and socioeconomic status of parents was reported and point out that although this is strong support for the idea that childhood deprivation causes vulnerability, the respondents' own socioeconomic status is more strongly related to symptoms. Moreover, those with psychopathology were more "downwardly

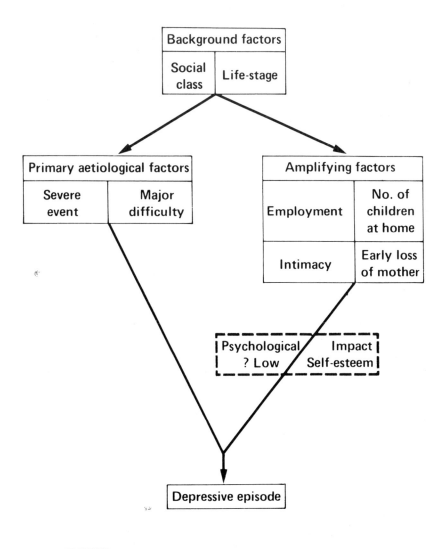

FIG. 9.1. Illustration of possible ways in which background factors predispose the individual to depression. (Redrawn from Brown, Bhrolchain, & Harris, 1975, by permission of the authors and *Sociology*.

213

mobile" relative to parents. In all, a complex "soup" of deprivation, social stress, and social selection would be likely to predict psychopathology.

On the theory that the problem lies in decision making concerning control, both possibilities are likely. As a result of deprivation, a person is weakened in his beliefs that he can exercise control; equally, circumstances present stresses but in ways that confirm the "weak control" hypothesis still further. There are two logical outcomes: One is control by avoidance or withdrawal, the other is helplessness. Both would be expected to increase downward mobility.

The complexity of factors that act to reduce the control a person could expect to exercise through normal channels is illustrated in Fig. 9.1 from Brown, Bhrolchain, and Harris (1975). Background factors such as social class and life stage determine the frequency and severity of primary aetiological factors such as the incidence of events and the background of concurrent difficulty, while at the same time there are factors providing amplifying conditions. Early loss of mother, loss of intimacy, number of children at home, and employment are grouped together as amplifying conditions in this model.

A particular combination of circumstances where there is a problem but lowered capacity for solving it should result in helplessness. Brown and Harris (1978) develop the notion of lowered *self-esteem* as a cognitive state arising from such circumstances. This is, however, a problem that low self-esteem may predate rather than arise from the consequences of the problem. Low self-esteem may have self-confirming results because of, for example, inadequate organization or wrong choice of marriage partner. This raises a very important point: A vulnerable person cannot necessarily be assumed to be in passive receipt of unpleasant events; he may be causing the events by his decision making quite early on in life history. This needs investigating.

RISK FACTORS AND CRISIS

Mediating Links

Behavioral Links

It is possible to specify a number of ways in which environmental experiences may change the risk of mental or physical disorder. Firstly, a person may change the pattern of his behavior for the rest of his life. He may do this abruptly, as when he suddenly decides to move his environment, resign his job, or get married. Some people may be in a role that allows them to make the decision. Others may, because of their dependent relationship, have to accept a change; women in traditional roles or children are in this position.

Secondly, a person may evolve a new pattern of behavior gradually, by changing his attitudes, his friends, or his hobbies. Thus he may change the risks both of incurring stresses and of disordered response. A person who takes up heavy alcohol consumption may visit bars more frequently, meet more friends, risk meeting antigens, increase the risks of divorce and liver damage. Risk may be changed by a major decision that may itself represent attempts to gain control, or it may be a form of helplessness. In turn, this may change the parameters for a subsequent hierarchy of decisions.

Biological Links

A difficulty for a cognitive model of vulnerability is the well-established finding that genetic factors play an important part in specifying the risk of mental illness. Kety has argued that the main concern now is how much of the variance in behavior is attributable to genetic factors; the fundamental issue of nature–nurture is an obsolete controversy (see Kety, 1965; Kety et al., 1968).

Any cognitively based model would be incomplete if it failed to take into account the 40 to 50% genetic vulnerability factor. This form of biological memory seems little explored in terms of what it is that specifies risk. There are a number of possibilities. The first is that there is base "biological tuning" which, in turn, determines the intensity of experiences and the latency in return to resting state. This, in turn, determines intensity of learning and the degree of generalization. In other words, part of concurrent state described in Chapter 5 may be intensity or lability of biological response. Vulnerability may be influenced by compatibility with incoming influences.

In terms of a cognitive model, the genetic factor may determine the outcomes of initial stress scenarios in life, for the reasons outlined above. Vulnerability is a genetically tuned metamemory that comes to represent deprivations and trauma, impoverished social circumstances, undesirable life history experiences, and changes in life. The model must provide a basis for understanding both big bang (single early trauma) and obstacle (gradual encounter with unfortunate conditions) causation.

Vulnerability as an Aspect of Decision Making

A cognitive model that gives primacy to decisions concerning control can provide a useful basis for understanding vulnerability. First, such a model can account for vulnerability in terms of sensitivity to certain stimulus conditions as well as for unrealistic response patterns in everyday situations encountered. Secondly, it can take account of big bang or obstacle developmental processes, because selected aspects of decision making can be gradually refined throughout life history experiences or changed significantly by a major shock during a formative period.

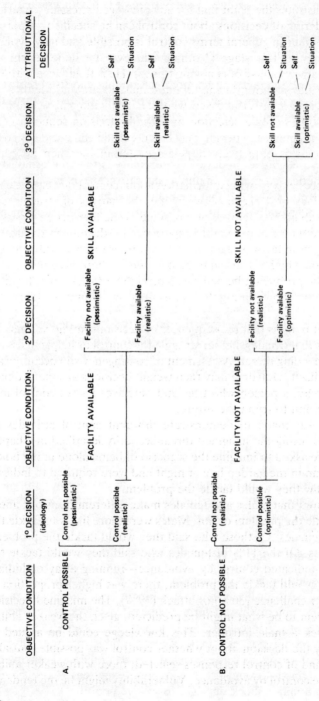

FIG. 9.2.   Selection of some possible sequences of decisions from a matrix of decisions that must logically be involved in determining the outcome of a stressful scenario.

Figure 9.2 illustrates the point that for any envisaged stressful scenario a hierarchical ordering of decisions about control can be specified. A person must decide whether in general terms control is possible and may evoke a personal ideology at this stage (Nothing can ever be done to change things/There is always a way of changing things). He is then faced with the practicalities of the situation facing him and must locate and identify the means of exercising control and see whether it is within his capability. Figure 9.2 illustrates only a selection of possible decision sequences. At each stage in the sequence, a person may be unrealistic and decide to go on when the outcome is objectively hopeless or terminate when he could achieve a result.

Life experiences may provide information about control that can be used to modify the bias in decision between the alternatives of struggle and persist, or give up and be helpless at any stage of the hierarchy. A person who is poor and who has frequently experienced reduced control facility may shift decisions in favor of the view that control is rarely possible in life. Equally, a person who has learned to be pessimistic about his abilities may fail to engage the problem if he believes (correctly or falsely) that he lacks the skill. Again, as shown in Fig. 9.2, pessimistic or optimistic errors may occur.

An important point is that the sequences of decisions in Fig. 9.2 may be the critical ones that decide whether struggle for control or helplessness is a response to impending threat. Assessment of contingency will occur during the experience itself. Outcome may then weight decisions at superordinate levels of hierarchy; a person who tries and perceives loss of control may modify the decision to try in the future.

An attempt was made to demonstrate different control attitudes by symbolic means, using the imagined threat scenario described in Chapter 1. Subjects were asked to imagine the scenario of being alone in the house and seeing a man in the garden late at night and were required to indicate whether and how they would tackle the problem.

Table 9.1 shows that males and females make different decisions about whether to tackle the problem or not. Males were more likely to tackle the problem than females: Of those who said they would tackle the problem, 89% were males. Of the 11% of females who said they would tackle the problem, 91% indicated control by avoidance—running away or hiding. For males who would tackle the problem, there was higher proportion of endorsement for challenge (30%) or attack (39%). The imagined decision making does seem to be what might be predicted, given the weaker ability of girls to attack a male intruder. This knowledge could be argued to dictate not only the decision about whether control was possible, but also influence the kind of control responses selected; those with weaker ability to attack choose control by avoidance. Vulnerability might be the tendency

TABLE 9.1
Imagined Responses to Hypothetical
Scenario of "Stranger in Garden at Night"[a]

a. *Percentage of total*

	F	M	Total
tackle the problem (engage)	11%	89%	34%
do nothing (disengage)	89%	11%	66%

b. *Percentage of those who engaged problem (34%)*

Choice of action	F	M
hide/run	81%	15%
attack	4%	39%
call for help	9%	10%
challenge	4%	30%
other	2%	6%

[a] See Chapter 1.

to make unrealistic (overoptimistic or overpessimistic) decisions in the hierarchy. A proportion of girls did say they would attack; in the case of a male intruder, the outcome could be unpleasant.

Control Ideology

It is important to understand the role played by ideologies of one kind or another in the decision to engage or not to engage a stressful problem. Control ideology may not only be a factor in the decision to engage, it may be responsible for the attribution made. A person who doubts the wisdom of tackling a problem because he is fatalistic should attribute failure to fate as well.

Ever since the classic studies of Battle and his colleagues (e.g., Battle & Rotter, 1963; Rotter, Seeman & Liverant, 1962), there has been evidence that there are population differences concerning control that appear to relate to poverty and underprivilege. For example, Lefcourt and Ludwig reported differences in the score on the Rotter scale between blacks and whites; the former showed significantly higher levels of externality ($p <$

.05). However, in most cases extreme positions in this respect are not reported for normal subjects, even in cases of underprivilege (Gore & Rotter, 1963). In cases where control ideology is not strongly polarized, people might depend on a deeper analysis of the situation confronting them.

There may be reasons for assuming differences in ideology as a function of religious conviction. However, it is not clear how this influences decision making. On first consideration, belief that there is a higher authority should logically lead to passivity, perhaps to praying as a response to a problem. The pattern of behavior in a stress scenario could be much the same as for a person who believes in chance and fate, unless the religion dictates that "God helps those who help themselves" and thus requires that problems be engaged.

Differences in control ideology should determine whether other decisions about control facility and personal capability are made. If a person believes strongly that he can do nothing to change reality, then these other decisions are irrelevant. If stressful experiences with poor outcomes increase the probability of externality, the probability of helplessness as an immediate response increases.

It follows that if control ideology occupies a superordinate position in the hierarchy of decisions, people who are strongly polarized in this respect will differ in fundamental attitudes to a stress scenario. Chapter 7 cited evidence that suggested that information processing attitude distinguished the two extremes: Internalizers constantly seek information, whereas externalizers do not.

One way of considering vulnerability is in terms of modification in control ideology as a result of experience. "Big bang" theory would assume that an early trauma would create increased situations of zero control. Obstacle theory would assume that low control expectancies develop as a function of unpleasant circumstances and deprivations in life. In cases where control ideology is strongly polarized in favor of not engaging the problem, a person may never encounter the information that would tell him he could have succeeded. Therefore, control ideology may have self-confirming properties for "external" cases.

Evidence from performance on questionnaires designed to measure control ideology would suggest that the central tendencies for most populations are not polarized to extremes of internality or externality, and therefore we would expect that many problems encountered do require further decision making for most people (see Lefcourt, 1966, p. 181).

The Principles of the Hierarchical Control Model

Figure 9.3 illustrates the kind of hierarchical decision model we believe is needed to provide a format for understanding decision making in control.

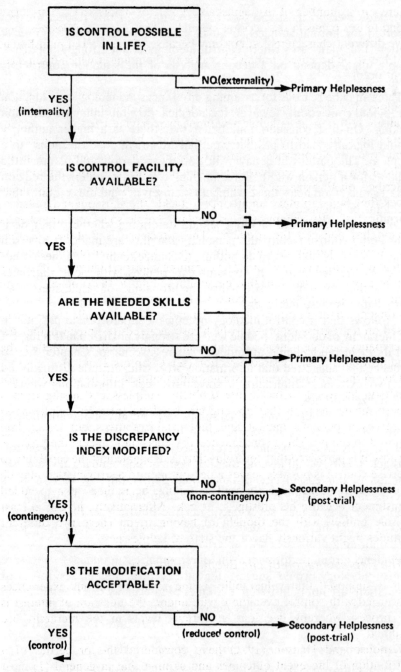

FIG. 9.3. Hierarchy of decisions in determining effort, struggle, and persistence compared with different types of perceived helplessness in a stressful scenario.

There are a number of distinguishable levels of helplessness that correspond to exit points in the decision hierarchy. The state of helplessness may have different characteristics, not only because of the level of punishment that has to be accepted, but also because of the point at which disengagement occurs.

A number of critical questions are involved. The first concerns control ideology: If a person decides that nothing can be done and accepts a totally fatalistic position, he is helpless without ever having tried. If he decides there is no control facility or he lacks capability, he is equally helpless. The term "primary helplessness" is used to distinguish helplessness that arises without any attempt to engage the problem. Seligman's dogs would be so described on this analysis, because after a pretreatment of inescapable shock they failed to make an attempt to tackle the subsequent avoidance-learning task. By comparison, secondary helplessness occurs when a person has engaged the problem. The difference is that he then has information enabling him to examine his successes and failures trial-by-trial and actually decide whether he is gaining control. Figure 9.3 illustrates that as a result of decisions that cause him to engage the problem, he can then make an assessment of control. In some cases he needs to assess contingency data, in others he may depend on a less detailed assessment based on a progress report—in which case he needs to know whether the discrepancy between intention and reality is modified and whether the modification is in the desired direction (see Chapters 2 and 3).

One of the most important distinguishing features will be whether or not a person has tried to tackle the problem. Helplessness arising from a superordinate decision that nothing can be done (primary helplessness) preserves a person's mental and biological resources but leaves him exposed to the punishing consequences. A decision to tackle the problem because it is perceived that control facility is available and the capability to exercise control is possible leaves a person open to a struggle that may be prolonged. If he perceives himself as failing, he is then open to added punishment because his prestige is at risk. Alternatively, he can at least console himself with the thought of having tried. These two different attitudes might variously flavor the state of helplessness.

The Representation of Life Events in Decision

If it is supposed that vulnerability is the result of various experiences concerned with control over the environment, the question of interest is the process whereby decisions at various levels in the hierarchy are modified.

Kanouse and Hanson (1971) have considered the properties of a distribution of life event outcomes and assume that in general (1) most outcomes are good, and (2) extremely bad outcomes are more frequent than extremely good ones. The hypothetical distribution should have a psychologically neutral point half-way between the median and the mid-point (see Parducci, 1963, 1965, 1968), and therefore people will see the majority of outcomes as positive. The authors argue that, for the most part, people will work their way into "good environments" and out of bad ones, and they will not seek *very* good experiences because this will shift the psychologically neutral point for judgments and will render more intermediate experiences "bad." Avoiding negative experiences and seek-ing mildly positive experiences should, therefore, represent the control directives of normal people.

It is possible that a change in early experience arising from trauma or severe deprivation might prevent the optimizing of experiences and therefore increase the proportion of successive unpleasant experiences a person must face. Thus, early decision making may change the properties of a life experience distribution.

A convenient way of understanding the basis for changes in decision is provided by sensitivity measures and criterion changes. In some cases the evidence favoring one kind of decision may be clearly discriminable. In other cases discriminability may be difficult. Equally, a person may change the position of his criterion so that he veers toward one kind of decision rather than another. The proportions of errors made will change accor-dingly. This basic formulation, fundamental to signal detection theory analysis (Green and Swets, 1966), enables us to consider the possibility that for a given set of evidence about control, a disposition is represented on the distributions of likelihoods.

A study by Bekerian (1980) examined the possibility that pretreatment in a helplessness condition might change either d' or β on a signal detection theory analysis of a task involving a same-different judgement. The hypothesis pursued was that helplessness effects might bias perceptual/attentional processes and result in a shift in d', or in interpretive processes resulting in a β criterion shift. Generally, the only significant result was a speeding-up of reaction times following "helpless" pretreatment. How-ever, the helplessness condition was not faster than an untreated control, so the effect was one of relatively increased slowness following helpless pretreatment and may have been because of motivational factors or because of uncertainty. This raises the hypothesis that anxiety associated with loss of control is a factor that may influence performance (e.g., see Roth & Kubal, 1975).

On a signal detection theory analysis, there was no apparent effect on either d' or β of the helplessness pretreatment. Thus, there is effectively no evidence to support the idea that helplessness pretreatment changes the characteristics of sensitivity to, or interpretation of, data on a subsequent task. However, we might expect that situation-specific influences operate and there is a need for research into changes in these measures as a function of life event experiences and performance on tasks relevant to these experiences.

The result might also be explained in terms of the hypothesis proposed by Schwartz (1981). In considering the Alloy and Abramson (1979) results, he points out that correct detection of noncontingency is characteristic of depressives and may be a symptom rather than a cause. The norm for nondepressed people is to resist depression by detecting contingency, even where contingency is absent. Therefore, normals will not produce the criterion shift easily as a result of helplessness treatment; they will continue to create and find control. Depression immunization could be represented by criterion positions in the hierarchy of decisions concerned with control. Thus a normal person will face an unpleasant stress problem by deciding that in general people can exert control (internality), control facility is available, and there is capability to use the control facility. This then leads to engaging the problem and running plans. Equally, normals would be expected to preserve optimism for success in the task by overrepresenting evidence of success. By comparison, depressed subjects will continue to make a more logical assessment of objective contingency, may not increase the effort to find evidence of control (Fisher & Ledwith, 1983), and will not resist the transmission of helplessness.

This raises the question of a more complex definition of vulnerability. In some respects it is as pathological to resist helplessness and continue to struggle with an unsolvable problem as it is to disengage and give up without ever having tried. Different problem scenarios may encourage a different approach. There may be nothing that can prevent the death of a very old terminally ill relative, and to persist with more and more extravagant sacrifices would be unrealistic. On the other hand, a student struggling to write a thesis may make gradual progress that eventually pays off, although in the process the problems seem intractable.

A vulnerable person may be the person whose decision mechanisms are so organized that he is inclined to "get it wrong." He will persist and incur enormous cost in engagement on a problem that most people would not tackle. Or he may never tackle a problem and hence incur the punishment it brings when there were solutions available.

These ideas are developed further in the next chapter. The basic idea developed about vulnerability is that it is a form of risk (extrinsic risk) of inappropriate response that will center on decisions concerned with the perception of control and combine interactively with stressful influences in specific stressful scenario (intrinsic risk) to determine outcome.

10 Decisions, Attributions, and Disorders

ILLOGICAL DECISION PROCESSES IN STRESS

In the previous chapter it was proposed that there is a hierarchical arrangement of decisions concerned with control. The result of these decisions was assumed to determine action patterns and outcome within any particular stressful scenario.

Figure 10.1 illustrates the basis of the concept of vulnerability as a metamemory for stress characteristics and outcome. The figure provides a sample of the kinds of questions a person must ask in order to disambiguate potentially threatening situations. The figure also illustrates that decisions about control form an important subsection. The answer to each question both represents current "extrinsic risk" conveyed as a set of metamemories, and has the capability of changing it. Since sets of decisions are involved, a scan of metamemory should provide an observer with a digital representation of risk, with both positive and negative risk factors present, which may counteract each other in some cases. A person may overrepresent hazards but perceive that he can control them. In this case there would be increased risk of crisis in his life because there are more potential threats, but there is decreased risk of crisis because he sees himself as being able to control them. Level of vulnerability would be assessed by a total scan of the perception of harm and of counterharm resources. A person at high risk for a personal crisis would have high weightings for perceiving threat readily, conceiving of it as probable, and perceiving a low level of ability to cope.

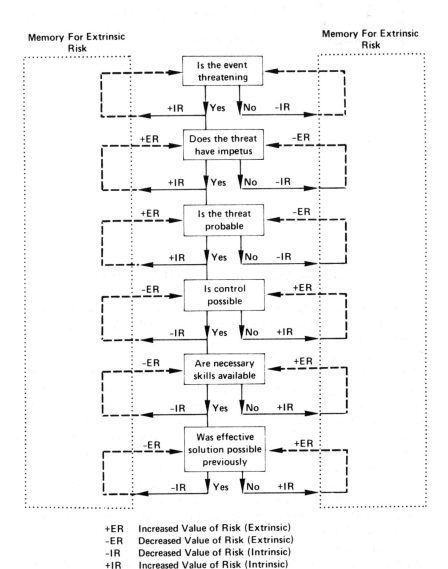

+ER	Increased Value of Risk (Extrinsic)
-ER	Decreased Value of Risk (Extrinsic)
-IR	Decreased Value of Risk (Intrinsic)
+IR	Increased Value of Risk (Intrinsic)

FIG. 10.1.   Schematic illustration of metamemory for risk updated by and contributing to decision and outcome of stress scenarios.

Another aspect of vulnerability identified in the previous chapter is the tendency to be unrealistic. It is as unrealistic to struggle inappropriately with an unsolvable problem as it is to be inappropriately helpless. This aspect of vulnerability may be specifically determined by groups of decisions concerned with control. If a person perceives that control is possible, he engages the problem. If he continues to perceive that there is contingency in the desired direction, he continues to struggle. Error in decisions on various components of the perception of control could drive behavior to the point of crisis.

Inappropriate behavior may be driven by the outcome of decisions concerning control. Figure 10.2 illustrates a hypothetical state of decision making as a profile of independently established criteria on distributions of positive likelihoods and negative likelihoods. A very influential subset of these decisions concerns control. Control decisions are embedded in a logical hierarchy of decisions about threat characteristics as illustrated in Fig. 10.2.

Optimism and pessimism may be variously represented as positions on the distributions. One person may always expect the worst, for example, and always expect that he will have no control. This pessimistic grouping of criteria predicts a very anxious person, who reacts to actual problems with helplessness. Alternatively, an optimistic grouping might be represented by a tendency to think that the threat is unlikely to materialize, but that even if it does, the problem can be tackled—"I'll cross that bridge when I come to it."

Although, as indicated in the hierarchical decision model (Fig. 9.3), it has so far been assumed that there is a logical structure of decision making in stress, it is possible that some decisions are so powerful that outcomes override the logical sequence. First, if a person believes he is a useless failure, then there will be no point in deciding that control facility is available. Secondly, the recognition of threatening events may be dependent on perceptions concerning control. A person who expects low control should locate more potential threats in his world.

Therefore, far from being an independent set of decisions applied independently to properties of different encounters, there may be an organizational matrix of decisions that is rationalized or interpreted at higher levels of intellectual activity. Part of thinking about control may be the attempt to locate and resolve discrepancies. At the same time there will be a development toward abstraction and ideology as a function of experience. It is possible that strong organizational tendencies evolve that are appraised as illogical or inappropriate by higher intellectual processes. A person may seek the help of friends or professional people when strong discrepancies are evident. It is assumed the decisions are normally structured on logical principles.

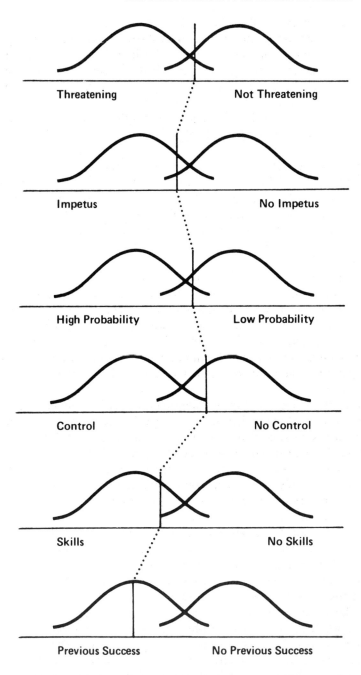

FIG. 10.2.   The representation of risk as a profile of decision criteria for distributions of likelihoods.

Optimism in Normals

Evidence from experimental studies of contingency assessment suggests that normal subjects may best be regarded as immunized against helplessness. As described in Chapter 8, Alloy and Abramson (1979) showed that normals are capable of unrealistic optimism. In a more recent paper Alloy and Abramson (1981) suggest that optimism is self-serving in helping to maintain self-esteem. Langer (1965) advanced a view that suggested that optimism enabled subjects to avoid the negative consequences of perceiving low control. Schwartz (1981) points out that normals may be resistant to depression in that they will not develop the depression-producing expectation in relation to helplessness treatment. In terms of the decision model proposed here, normals may be keeping the "extrinsic" risk for negative outcomes to stress encounters artificially low. It could be argued that the failure to detect noncontingency is an error in normals, but, since the failure is dependent on the presence of rewards, it could equally well be argued that normals are making use of reward in an illogical way because there should be no connection between reward and level of contingency.

Pessimism in Depressed Individuals

In the same group of experiments in which normals are shown to be unrealistic or illogical, there is evidence to suggest that depressed subjects remain extremely logical. If they are more logical than normals, then it follows that they might best be described as "sadder but wiser," as the authors suggest. Perhaps life is a bad deal, and only depressed subjects see it for what it really is; a depressed person recognizes helplessness when he sees it. However, there is evidence of some illogicality in depressed thinking, which may be central to depression itself.

The decisions involved in control assessment should also be evident in attributing the cause of success or failure. For example, if a person believes that there is control available, the demands are simple, and the skill is available, he should logically attribute failure either to a fault in the system (fault in the machine; difficult conditions) or to transient faults in his behavior. This preserves optimism.

It appears that depressed subjects do not necessarily think logically in this respect; there is a tendency toward self-blaming attributions and generalized characterological self-blame. In the study by Brown and Harris (1978) a whole "soup" of factors producing isolation and lack of opportunity was described. The authors themselves observed that the source of the problem also prevented effective solution. Yet a key aspect of the thinking of the women who were depressed was self-blame and lowered self-esteem; the attribution appears illogical.

The reason for this apparent illogicality is important, because although the learned helplessness model provides a useful account of inaction and passive acceptance, which is one aspect of depression, it is clear that characterological self-blame is a recurring feature. It is part of the negative cognitive triad that Beck proposed as the central features of a cognitive model of depression. Beck (1967) investigated the symptomatologies of depressed and nondepressed patients and noted that the tendency for self-blame, self-criticism, indecisiveness, distorted self-image, and negative expectancies was found to be more prevalent with increasing severity of depression. Only 38% of nondepressed psychiatric patients provided evidence of lowered self-esteem, whereas 81% of severely disturbed patients had these beliefs. Beck formalized the attitudes as a tendency to denigrate past, present, and self, and to be pessimistic about the future. This in turn will sensitize a person to the occurrence of failure and increase the chances that stress will be responded to by helplessness and depression.

Bulman (1979) argued that the form of attribution that correlates with depressive symptoms is blame directed at the self rather than at the situation or at behavior. She proposed that characterological blame is associated with helplessness and depression, but behavioral blame is not. Since character is blamed, the transmission of helplessness should be guaranteed. If behavior is blamed, future situations remain potentially controllable; a person could improve his behavior. Bulman reported that depressed college students were more likely than nondepressed students to make a characterological attribution for bad events, but the two groups were not distinguished by behavioral blame.

This hypothesis was confirmed by Peterson, Schwartz, and Seligman (1981), who conducted a longitudinal study and found that for 87 female undergraduates there was a correlation between depressive symptoms and blame directed at their own characters; blame directed at behavior correlated with lack of depressive symptoms. Further, negative events that were attributed to behavior were seen as more controllable, with less stable and less global causes. Interestingly, characterological blame increased with the greater frequency of negative events in the year.

Abramson and Sackheim (1977) locate a conceptual paradox in the notion that depressives might see a situation as uncontrollable and yet blame themselves for it, because learning that a situation is uncontrollable is learning that it could not have been otherwise. This difficulty might be resolved if the cause of the uncontrollability is seen to result from personal inadequacy rather than from transient faults in behavior or irreversible features of the situation. A person may be effectively helpless because of his own perceived lack of skills. This could evolve if he had many experiences in which he received evidence of inadequacy. If the situations are varied, he then could logically begin to see inadequacy as the common denominator. Thus self-blame arises as an inductive generalization from successive observed behavioral faults; the step from assuming behavioral responsibility on successive occasions to making the step of assuming incompetence could be logical. Resistance to this could be failure to accept behavioral blame initially. This is where the evidence we provided in Chapter 7 suggesting that people expect to do badly in stress may be important. A source of attribution that wards off behavioral blame effectively prevents a person from accruing the evidence of successive behavioral incompetence and thus from the generalization of lowered potential for competence in the future.

It is also possible that self-blaming attributions do have an initial usefulness in aiding coping. A study by Bulman and Wortman (1977) examined the attributions of causality made by 29 accident victims against their judged ability to cope. Data was obtained by asking respondents to attribute blame and causality; ratings of coping behavior were obtained from social workers and nurses. Their findings suggested that self-blame was actually functional, a predictor of *good* coping, whereas blaming another or assuming the accident could have been avoided were predictors of poor coping. This result is of great importance in indicating that self-blame may be adaptive as a response to negative encounters. Of particular interest is the fact that the good copers did not feel they could avoid the accident, despite the fact that they indulged in self-blame. Responses to the question "Why me?" were found to fall into 6 categories: "predetermination," "probability," "chance," "God had a reason," "deservedness," and "reevaluation of the events as positive." Regression analysis on coping data did not suggest that any one of these was a predictor of coping. One interesting predictor turned out to be the nature of the activity at the time of the accident; those who were engaged in leisure activities were more likely to show better signs of coping.

The opposite view is advanced by Walster (1966), who argued that to assign blame to others is adaptive in reassuring a person that similar disasters can be avoided. If causality is assigned to unpredictable, uncontrollable circumstances, control over the future is reduced. Thus, according to the Walster hypothesis, blame directed at the self should be unadaptive. Blame directed at others encourages optimism; Walster shows that there is a greater tendency to attribute blame to others as a function of the severity of the accident.

Attributional styles in response to artificially induced failures were reported by Funkenstein, King, and Drolette (1957) in the Harvard studies; given exactly the same circumstances, "anger-out" students blamed the situation, "anger-in" students blamed themselves. The two different response modes were accurately predicted by close friends and associates of the subjects and were reported as having some relation to social origin in that lower-income individuals were more likely to be blamers of the situation.

Thus, not only should those who face insurmountable difficulties be expected to attribute blame correctly to circumstances, but those of lower-class origins should tend in any case toward external blame. Lowered self-esteem and self-denigration should not be logical consequences of loss of control when the environment is hostile and provides no opportunity for solution and should be less likely in those regularly exposed to these conditions.

In addition, it might be reasonable to suppose that since women in traditional roles have rather less chance to exercise effective control than their male counterparts, they would correctly deduce this in attributing blame for perceived control loss.

Men are still at a survival disadvantage and are still more vulnerable to chronic disease, although women have been argued to make more use of health care resources, to take more prescriptions than men (see Nathanson, 1977; Weissmann & Klerman, 1977), and to be more prone to depression (Weissman & Klerman, 1977; Pearlin, 1975). It is tempting to consider the possibility that changes in control facility might determine the difference: In traditional roles men struggle for control and are more likely to react with illness; women are presented with change, perceive the lack of facility for control, and react with lethargy, boredom, and depression.

This hypothesis has been neatly investigated by some Boston researchers concerned with the changing roles of women in society. As increasing numbers of women work, we may be provided with vital information about the difference in reaction. Stewart and Salt (1981) compared the relationship between life stress, depression, and physical illness in 122 normal adult women divided into groups according to occupation and marital status. Results showed that work stresses are associated with illness, not depression, and the relationship is strongest among work-centered women. By comparison, family stresses appeared to relate to depression rather than illness and were strongest among housewives. The authors point out that two groups may be distinguished by form of life stresses. Firstly, there is the group (traditionally men) who are faced with a constant demand for instrumentality; secondly, there is the group (likely to be women) who encounter the futility of instrumentality. The difference disappears when the women are divided into those who are work-centered and those who are home-centered.

Helplessness, because of lack of "instrumentality" in life, should not lead to depression, because a source of situational attribution is provided. Both the women in traditional roles in the Stewart and Salt study and the Camberwell women in the Brown and Harris study were in this position. In terms of the hierarchical decision model, the decision that there is little control should arise from the perception of lack of control facility. This should have provided the basis for the attribution "because I am poor," or "because of my role in the household." This is a logical deduction of the form $(A \rightarrow B)$ depends on X; X is not present, therefore (not $A \rightarrow B$). It would be logical to resist self-blaming attributions. Depressed people do not seem to be logical in this respect.

It is possible that the attribution of loss of control is sensitive to a number of other factors we have not taken into account. There is an impressive literature in social psychology concerning the attribution of causality (see Heider, 1958; Festinger, 1954). A question central to the development of attribution theory is whether an individual who fails in a particular test blames himself or the test.

Two sources of data for attribution judgments are generally identified. The first involves covariation between an observed effect and possible cause. If a person sees himself to fail consistently, then he may come to believe that the cause is in himself rather than in the task. The second involves the configuration of factors present, which provides plausible causes of the effect. If an individual finds that he fails at a task but learns that everyone else did too, he may attribute the cause of the failure to the task.

An important article by Weiner et al. (1971) proposed that when reacting to failure, individuals use four causal elements of ascription to interpret and predict outcome; these are ability, task difficulty, effort, and luck. The former two elements are supposedly stable, and the latter two are supposedly unstable. It is assumed that attribution of change in control as being due to luck rather than ability will lead to instability in future prediction. The "gambler's fallacy" may operate, so that a person expects a loss after a gain and vice versa.

Experiments conducted by Weiner and Frieze (reported by Weiner et al., 1971, 1972), investigated how an individual might make use of contextual information, perhaps from a number of sources, in making his judgments. Subjects were given information on a hypothetical person who achieved a percentage of success at a task and a percentage of success for previous tasks. In addition, subjects were told the percentage of other individuals successful at the task, but they were given *no* information about the task. The discrepancy between outcome and prior performance increased the frequency at attributions made to luck and effort. Conversely when past behavior correlated with current outcome, ability or task difficulty were more likely to be the outcome of attribution. The percentage of prior success and the perceived successes of others contributed to the probability that ability would provide the source of attribution. However, outcome on a particular task was important; greater attributions to ability and effort are made following a success, and a greater proportion of inferences about task difficulty were made following a failure.

A number of anomalies arising from the application of the learned helpless model to human laboratory and psychosocial experience have suggested that an attributional reformulation is more appropriate (Abramson et al., 1978). Not only did experimental studies show that passivity was not always shown in experience of uncontrollable events, but on some occasions facilitated performance was reported. The reformulated learned helplessness model assumes that experience with uncontrollable events with noncontingency are not sufficient conditions for helplessness and depression. Causal attributions which are internal, stable, and global in character are prerequisites and lead to lowered self-esteem.

As argued previously, factors involved in the detection of the reasons for noncontingency may provide a basis for the attributions made if the evidence is correctly utilized. Figure 10.3 illustrates an ordering of questions that both affect control estimation *and* provide the evidence for an attribution. For example, a negative answer to the question "is control facility available" should provide the basis for attributing failure "I failed because there was no means for control" (situational blame). However, some control estimation questions load heavily on the individual's appraisal of his own capabilities. Lowered self-esteem should thus jointly influence decisions on the degree of control *and* the basis for the attribution. (I am helpless because I cannot cope).

Low self-esteem could be assumed to be of primary causal significance, whether it arises by assessment of personal failure or by comparison with the perceived success of others. One plausible hypothesis is that reported experience of stressful experiences with negative outcomes could predispose toward self-blame and lead to lowered self-esteem. A person perceives that he fails in A, B, C, etc., and by inductive logic assumes that he is a failure. However, Fisher (1983e) has argued that failing in stressful conditions should *protect against lowered self esteem*. Since people expect to perform less well in stressful conditions (Table 7.3), the same evidence provides a basis for *situational* rather than *self* blame. However, depressed subjects judging the performance of a (hypothetical) typist in stress were found to be less likely to make compensatory allowances than nondepressed subjects (Table 6.5). If depressed subjects operate a criterion in judgments that do not allow for the effects of circumstances, than the protective elements of expectancies about poor performance in stress will be lost and depressed people could be described as "sadder but harder."

A person will frequently encounter cases where A–B is weakened by error trials and detection and tolerance of error will be important. If a person expects to make more errors under stress, then roughly the same logical argument outlined above applies. A person should make a behavioral

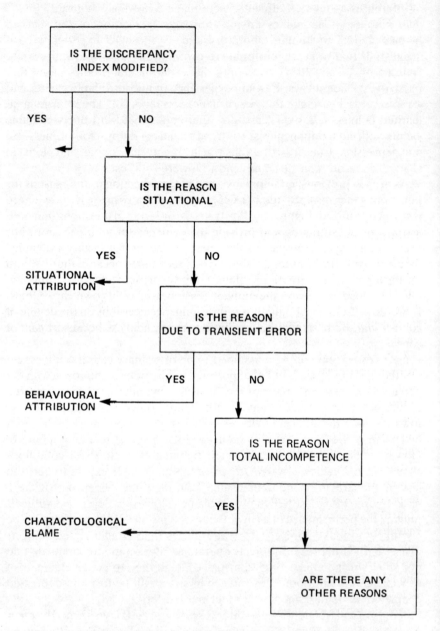

FIG. 10.3.   Representation of a number of possible attributions that derive
from perceived loss of control.

attribution when he detects the error, but a situational attribution protects him if normal conditions (N) are absent: $A \rightarrow B$ if N; not B; not A (error detection); not N. The proportion of errors that may be tolerated and protected by a situational attribution needs investigating, both for depressed and for normal subjects.

Errors that arise from memory and attention failure will not necessarily be detected. Therefore the person may note "not B" but not detect the reason. However, he may still use a situational attribution and assume that he is not behaviorally responsible: "The task does not respond in the same way in noise."

WORK STRESS AND DECISION PROCESSES

Different Levels and Functions of Control

Further information about factors in decision making is provided by investigations into stress at work. Available evidence suggests that some job characteristics are associated with depression and others with anxiety. However, a no-control work situation may not necessarily result in increased depression, and a number of conditions present at the time may change or alleviate the effects of work stress.

Control structure may be quite different for the white-collar/professional worker, as compared with the blue-collar worker. In the former case, there is an opportunity, often exercised by skill and initiative, to influence company policy and work structure; there is less concern with the details of control on the features of daily tasks, because control is not constrained. In the latter case, the worker may have very little control over major variables such as these and may even have zero control over factors affecting the actual task. His only "control" may be whether to accept work or not; if he is poor and relatively uneducated, "control facility" is not available in this respect; he has no options. In this case, accepting a daily task with no control may be seen as part of the plan for daily existence. Lack of control may not result in depression because it has been selected and is seen to be true for everyone.

This may help to explain results reported by Broadbent and Gath (1981) and Broadbent (1982), which showed that no-control paced assembly work is more likely to be associated with high demand and anxiety than with depression. This was found to be true for car workers, but also for other groups such as electricity workers. Comparisons showed that paced workers had greater anxiety levels than unpaced workers, but depression was not a factor.

By comparison, a study by Parkes (1980) on the differences between wards and on their effect on the mental health of student nurses suggests that control and involvement might be direct determinants of satisfaction and mental state. The comparison was between surgical and medical wards in two hospitals. Both ward types were associated with high work pressure, but the surgical wards offered greater staff support, autonomy, and task orientation, and the nurse played a greater instrumental role. The students showed higher levels of anxiety and depression as measured by questionnaires on the medical wards. There were also lower reported levels of satisfaction.

Parkes considers a number of explanations. One is that the degree of control or instrumentality is reduced in medical wards. In this case, depression is a factor likely to be associated with control loss. This perhaps suggests that a distinction needs to be made about levels of control; a worker faced with a paced assembly task does not expect control to be present and is therefore incurring "primary helplessness," but not depression. His work stress symptoms are decided by the nature of the punishment exclusively; on paced assembly work he is overstimulated and anxious. By contrast, a nurse may need to have control over the welfare of a patient in order to gain the satisfaction required as a member of the caring professions. The role played by loss of control in the context of total life plans may be quite different.

The Ameliorating Role of Independent Variables

Social Support

An aspect of decision making that is also emphasized by findings from the above studies concerns the moderating effect of social support. Parkes' observations lead to the proposal that surgical wards might produce a better working environment because of social support factors. Equally, in the study of depression by Brown and Harris (1978), an important observed difference between middle-class mothers and children at home and working-class mothers in the same predicament was the tendency of the former to have a confiding relationship with another person. This appeared to be a factor acting against the risk of depression.

In his studies in car factories, Broadbent (1982) noted a significant difference between two factories in terms of the incidence of reported depression. When the factories were compared on all the questions asked about jobs, there were key questions on which the factories showed significant difference. A main difference was that in the factory with more depression, ability to communicate was reduced by the presence of ear defenders to protect against high noise levels. Equally, Broadbent noted that with a group of electricity workers, inability to talk to others correlated with depression but not with anxiety. Depression was associated with time spent alone.

The question of interest is the locus of influence of social support on decision making. One hypothesis, that it provides incentive and encourages "illusion of control" or optimism when some control is possible, seems more appropriate for nurses than car workers and perhaps less appropriate for the Brown and Harris women who were effectively helpless. It is perhaps more likely that social support has another role in influencing decision making and helping to ward off depression. If the analysis presented earlier is accepted, a person may be helpless but not necessarily depressed if he blames the situation and does not incur lowered self-esteem. This is in keeping with the Bulman hypothesis that characterological self-blame is a fundamental factor. Social support would reduce the risk of illogical self-blaming attributions by providing information suggesting that others feel the same way about the task. Therefore the pessimistic attributions are warded off when they are not logical.

A third hypothesis worth considering is that social support provides distraction and reduces the time for a person to become mentally preoccupied with his unhappiness. If, as has been argued in these chapters, the tendency to be depressed is the outcome of successive failure experiences conveyed as a metamemory in decision making about control, then reduced time to rehearse the unpleasant source of information present during daily work could be effective.

Equally, the effect of social support may be to direct attention away from the self, again by distraction. Koch (1956) proposed that there are two exclusive motivational states, one of which concerns general ineffectiveness, self-depreciation, and guilt. Distraction may provide a means of reducing the time a person is mentally preoccupied in this way. An interesting point made by Duval and Wickland (1972) was that self-awareness may increase the tendency to assume responsibility for outcomes. An experiment in which subjects were positioned in front of a mirror supposedly to direct attention to the self and asked to rate responsibility for positive and negative outcomes associated with hypothetical events showed that subjects facing a mirror assumed greater responsibility than did controls. A comparable experiment (Duval & Wickland, 1973) showed that the presence of a mirror affected the degree of control reported by subjects on a task involving tracking of a finger position on a rotating turntable. It might follow that distraction, by reducing the time available for preoccupations of this kind, could reduce the likelihood of perceived helplessness as well as perceived responsibility.

External Leisure Activities

Broadbent also emphasized the importance of interest in leisure activity as a means of ameliorating the effects of stress at work. In electricity workers, Broadbent reports a three-way interaction between stress, satisfaction with work, and satisfaction with leisure, but only for depression. He suggests that it acts as a buffer or protective wall; stress principally results in depression among those unhappy with their leisure and unhappy with their job. No such interactions were reported for anxiety.

A straightforward distraction hypothesis is perhaps less valid, because leisure activities take place after work. However, there is the possibility of indirect distraction; leisure provides a topic to think about during work and provides a source of social support.

An equally attractive idea is that a person is fortified against depression because he has an alternative area where he can establish control. As was described earlier in the book, Dolgun (1965) claimed to ward off the effects of deprivation and interrogation stresses in Stalin's prisons by establishing control of walking activities in his own cell. An irrelevant source of control might be argued to provide a contradictory input to the decision system. A normal person might resist depression and increase optimism by selecting or even generating evidence of success. This would be an extension of the helplessness-immune hypothesis.

Equally, success at leisure activities may reduce the risk of self-blaming attributions. A person cannot generalize and incur lowered self-esteem while continuing to experience conditions where this is clearly not the case. This should create logical inconsistencies.

Rewards

Broadbent's studies with industrial groups have also provided some useful information about the value of monetary reward in creating an apparent change in mental states accompanying less than comfortable working conditions. In particular among car workers, monetary rewards for paced, "high-demand" work is associated with reduction in anxiety levels. Broadbent notes that the protective factor lies in motives. These findings, however, were based not on physiological indices but on self-rating responses; it remains conceivable that a person is more tolerant of the effects of high demand tasks if there are rewards. He may incur high arousal but feel less inclined to interpret it in terms of feelings of anxiety.

Monetary reward was one of the factors inducing a move towards overoptimism in the Alloy and Abramson subjects; reward for wins produced the illusion of control. On the hypothesis that normal people will resist pessimism by structuring their world so as to emphasize positive features such as success, it might follow that assessment of unpleasant working conditions will change if rewards are high enough. Monetary rewards may also introduce the possibility of future control over life events, including work.

PATTERNS OF OUTCOME IN STRESS SCENARIOS

In predicting the influence of stress on mental disorder or physical illness, there are two decision elements. Firstly, there is the decision of whether the problem is engaged, and there is a struggle for control. Secondly, there is the question of what method is selected if the decision favors engagement.

The selection of action/no action, the degree of persistence, and the character of the action itself may dictate not only whether or not a person is seen by others to be mentally ill, but whether he perceives himself as disturbed and whether he becomes physically unwell.

An important point to remember is that an unexpected life event may occur when a person is not prepared. He comes under pressure immediately and may have to make a series of quite critical decisions just when psychologically he is ill-equipped to do so.

Three basic options have already been identified: engage the problem (struggle for control); disengage (helplessness); operate "control by avoidance." These three possibilities may be implemented inappropriately or appropriately, and this in itself may determine whether others see the behavior as odd or normal. The outcome may create effects that persist beyond the scenario; or the individual may be locked in a prolonged scenario. Additionally, associated hormone-related changes may alter the risk of illness.

It has been traditional to assume that there are two independently functioning neuroendocrine systems. The first route, associated with the research of Cannon (1932, 1936), is via the sympathetic–adrenal-medullary system, resulting in a balance of adrenaline and noradrenaline. The second route is much associated with the research of Selye (1956) and is via the pituitary-adrenal system, which involves the adrenal cortex in the secretion of corticoid hormones such as cortisol.

With some notable exceptions (Mason, 1968; Mason, Brady, et al., 1968; Mason, Mangan, et al., 1968; Frankenhaeuser & Johansson, 1982), there has been a tendency only to report the levels of one hormone system. Yet a balance of both may accompany some conditions.

Equally, there has been a tendency to assume that the two hormone systems have different independent effects, which change the risks associated with different kinds of illness. High catecholamine levels increase the risk of illnesses such as cardiovascular disease because hyperarousal is associated with changes in the release of sugars and fats, as well as with increased function in the cardiovascular system and changes in gastrointestinal function. These functional changes, if prolonged, may eventually lead to structural damage leading to atheroma, changes in blood viscosity, and angina and hence may increase the risk of a heart attack (somatization). High ACTH and corticoid response levels have been argued to lower disease resistance. ACTH is associated with suppression of the immune response (Amkraut & Solomon, 1975), which raises the risk of disease from antigens. Frequency of response may be critical; the waiting-time effect (Feller, 1966) would predict that if antigens arrive at random in time, the antigens will be more likely to catch the long intervals. Rassmussen (1957) investigated the stress of avoidance learning in mice using as stresses electric shock, constraint, or loud noise (120 dB). The result of daily 6-hour sessions was hypertrophy of the adrenals, leukopenia, hypertrophy of spleen, hypertrophy of thymus. There was increased susceptibility to herpes simplex, poliomyelitis, and Coxsackie B and polyoma virus infections. There was delay in the rejection of skin grafts, but no changes in resistance to influenza and related respiratory viruses. Results were generally interpreted in terms of raised corticosteroids; catecholamine responses were not reported.

However, the hypothesis that raised catecholamine levels increase the risk of diseases due to structural change, whereas raised corticosteroids increase the risk of diseases arising from antigens, may well turn out to be an oversimplification. Elevated catecholamine levels may also affect the bodily immune response because of the changes produced in the spleen, and also because of the effect of lymphocyte activity (Wang, Sheppard, & Foker, 1978).

Many of these complex issues have yet to be resolved. They are important because there is now evidence to suggest that situations that require effort and involve demand are likely to be characterized by raised catecholamine levels, whereas these situations, which create some distress, are likely to have raised catecholamine levels and raised corticosteroid levels (Frankenhaeuser & Johansson, 1982). The outcome of decision making may thus set a pattern of activity with direct influence on certain categories of disorder. These issues are now discussed further under the headings of the different control strategies identified in Chapter 8.

"The Struggle for Control"

This paradigm will characterize situations where a person engages a problem as a result of his earlier decision making. He may do so appropriately or inappropriately, depending on objective conditions; to persevere and never give up may be a pathological response when a situation is objectively hopeless.

It is assumed that struggle for control will require effort and be experienced as "high demand." A person may have to maintain this over a period of time if he is initially unsuccessful or the problem recurs. Therefore there may be an important duration factor, which increases the chances for somatization to take place, resulting in structural damage.

In a laboratory experiment quoted by Frankenhaeuser and Johansson (1982), subjects performed a choice reaction task where there was a high degree of personal control. Subjects first established preferred work pace and then were given an opportunity to make modifications during the task. Self-reports showed that the task was seen to induce "effort" but no "distress"; the work conditions were thus perceived as pleasant. Hormone balance appeared to reflect these perceptions; adrenaline levels were increased, but cortisol decreased relative to a low-control situation.

Frankenhaeuser compared this result directly with an industrial situation involving control-room operators in which telephone, radio, and computer-based coordination of a steel plant was involved (Johansson & Sanden, 1982). The operators faced high demand, had high motivation and job satisfaction, and their physiological pattern was accompanied by raised adrenaline levels and decreased cortisol.

An additional comparison was made by Frankenhaeuser with a situation involving high work demand. A subgroup of white-collar professionals, who spent more than 50% and as much as 90% of their time at a computer terminal, was compared with a group consisting of typists and secretaries who spent less than 10% of their time on the terminal. The former had raised adrenaline levels during work relative to the latter, and the difference was more apparent later at home. Frankenhaeuser makes the point that the computer terminal might become a "mental assembly line" for those whose job it is to feed in data.

An obvious problem with comparisons between groups of workers is that of self-selection for the job. Just as the ulcerated monkeys in Brady's (1958) experiments could have been those who best learned avoidance tasks, so those highly capable and attracted to computer work might be those who spend most time engaged in it.

Professional groups with high demand and high control levels might be thought of as engaged in stress scenarios involving some struggle for control. Raised demand levels might be reflected in anxiety. Increased failure may raise anxiety levels further (e.g., see Coulter, 1970) and may begin to lead to distress. People confronting a serious life event will be in a comparable situation.

There is little information concerning the beginnings of distress, perceived failure, and disengagement from the struggle. Klinger (1975) denotes "current concern" as a continuing state of sensitivity to a problem that has an onset (commitment) and an offset (consummation or disengagement). A progression of initial commitment leading to disengagement, with accompanying mood changes, is envisaged. Generalizing, the person engaged in the struggle for control could be expected to be principally characterized by high demand, high anxiety, high mental preoccupation, and raised catecholamine or cholesterol. This pattern may be expected to change toward distress patterns if control fails. The duration of the experience may be a key factor adding to the risk of structural disease result from functional disorder.

Loss of Control

Loss of control (secondary helplessness) is argued in the previous chapter to be different from never having engaged the problem (primary helplessness).

The essential difference is that in the latter case a person has not shown himself to fail and may remain protected by the fact that he can always suppose that had he tried he might have succeeded. In addition, as mentioned at the beginning of this chapter, a person may accept a no-control task as part of a wider plan and may opt to accept it. Not having control might be regarded as a necessary but not a sufficient condition for perceived helplessness in human beings.

Loss of control, for whatever reason, leaves a person exposed to conditions that he might ordinarily seek to avoid. Thus the flavor of the mood and even the hormone balance might be determined by the severity of the unpleasantness. Seligman's dogs experienced high shock and reacted passively. Broadbent's paced-assembly-line workers experienced high work demand and reacted with anxiety.

Frankenhaeuser also showed that high demand and low distress were associated with high control, whereas low control evoked both high demand and high distress. The low control task was a vigilance task involving 1-hour duration of work at light intensity detection. Self reports and hormone levels suggested effort (raised adrenaline) and distress (raised cortisol). When the subject was given control over work pace, increased effort was associated with raised adrenaline, cortisol levels decreased relative to base, and there was absence of distress (e.g. Frankenhaeuser, Lundberg, & Foresman, 1980; Lundberg & Foresman, 1979; Lundberg & Frankenhaeuser, 1980).

A study by Gatchel and Proctor (1976) involved the measurement to physiological correlates of learned helplessness; they reported that lack of escape from loud tones resulted in greater feelings of helplessness in human beings. However, this was accompanied by lowered arousal levels, as indexed by skin conductance, and by a decrease in task involvement, relative to those who could escape tones by depressing a microswitch. This might be taken to suggest that for human beings, being able to control by avoidance is in some respects more stressful than being helpless.

In an industrial setting, as part of the study by Johansson and Sanden (1982), a group of process controllers who regularly worked in monotonous conditions were investigated. The low-control monotonous task was found to give rise to feelings of boredom and slight uneasiness. There were slightly increased levels of adrenaline and a small increase in cortisol.

These studies indicate that loss of control effects may vary from mild distress, with a relatively small change in levels of corticoid and medullary hormones, to rather greater distress, with high levels. There will be a number of determining factors: (1) the nature of the "punishment," (2) whether the person ever engages the problem, (3) whether failure is important to his prestige. If distress is an outcome, the risk of illness through the process of somatization (catecholamines) and immunological incompetence (corticoid response) is increased.

Helplessness may only lead to distress when conditions are unpleasant. If it arises from involvement, failure and loss of prestige may be the punishment. Helplessness may be a necessary but not a sufficient condition for depression. The existence of depression depends on characterological self-blame as an added factor. This may occur only in some scenarios where there is loss of control. A prerequisite for characterological self-blame is perceived failure; therefore it is perhaps more likely to arise at the point of secondary helplessness (tried but failed).

In animal studies there is now considerable evidence to suggest that tumor development is exacerbated or inhibited by stressful conditions. In a recent review of research in this area, Sklar and Anisman (1981) point to the conclusion that acute exposure to uncontrollable physical stress following viral innoculation or tumor cell transplantation enhances tumor growth. When control is possible, tumor growth is less likely to be affected. By contrast, in the case of chronic uncontrollable physical stresses, tumor development is likely to be inhibited. Finally, in the case of social stresses tumor growth is more likely to be exacerbated, at least for mature animals. The issues are beyond the scope of this book but raise a number of questions about the possible conditions experienced by patients who develop tumors. The review of the aetiology and development of cancers by Cox and Mackay (1982) points to the possible importance of the loss of a key relative (likely to be a parent) early in life, the inability to handle emotion or express hostile feelings, and the lack of adequate coping resources. The first and last items listed may be seen as closely associated with loss of control.

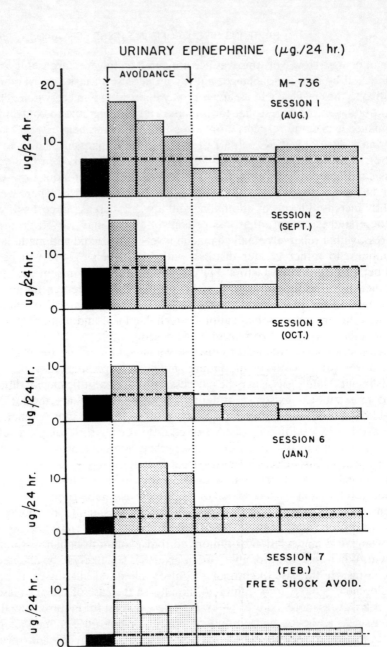

URINARY EPINEPHRINE (μg./24 hr.)

M−736

SESSION I
(AUG.)

SESSION 2
(SEPT.)

SESSION 3
(OCT.)

SESSION 6
(JAN.)

SESSION 7
(FEB.)
FREE SHOCK AVOID.

AVOIDANCE

DAYS

FIG. 10.4 Urinary epinephrine response to free shock-avoidance in monkeys after six regular 72-hr. avoidance experiences. (Reprinted by permission of the publisher from Mason, J. W., Tolson, W. W., Brady, J. Tolliver, G., & Gilmore, L. "Urinary epinephrine and norepinephrine responses to 72-hr. avoidance sessions in the monkey," *Psychosomatic Medicine, 30*, p. 657.

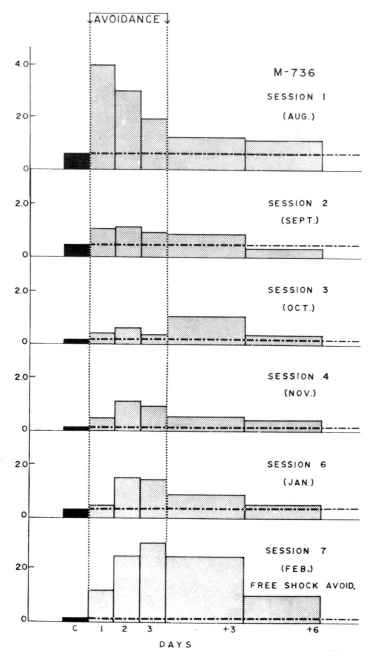

FIG. 10.5. Urinary 17-OHCS (milligrams per day) to free-shock avoidance
ʼin monkeys after six regular 72-hr. avoidance experiences. (Reprinted by
permission of the publisher from Mason, J. W., Tolson, W. W., Brady, J.
Tolliver, G., & Gilmore, L. "Urinary epinephrine and norepinephrine
responses to 72-hr. avoidance sessions in the monkey," *Psychosomatic
Medicine, 30,* p. 657.

Control by Avoidance

As has been emphasized previously, control by avoidance might be maximally stressful because the threat is severe enough that avoidance is required but a person does not really know whether or not he has been successful. He therefore operates a form of control under conditions of maximum uncertainty about outcome. Figures 10.4 and 10.5 from Mason (Mason, 1968; Mason, Tolson, et al., 1968; Mason, Brady, et al., 1968) show that for animals on the same avoidance task, *both* catecholamine and corticoid responses are high. From conclusions drawn by Frankenhaeuser concerning these hormones in human beings it could be inferred that the animals were distressed and faced with high demand. Both figures illustrate that over a spaced-out series of sessions, the magnitudes of both hormone responses do show some small decrease, but levels remain elevated relative to base levels.

Control by avoidance is applicable to cases of phobic fear and possibly to states such as schizophrenia as well as to states of withdrawal. Elaborate means may be necessary to avoid social situations, especially those involving family members. Processes such as denial may also be ways of exerting control by avoidance.

The hypothesized mental state would be distress and effort, with high catecholamine and corticoid levels during avoidance periods. A person afraid of dogs will respond in this way during periods when the presence of a dog is remotely likely. Equally, a person who responds to the presence of a key relative or threatening social encounter by elaborate means, including schizophrenic speech and behavior, may continue to experience high demand and high distress. In all cases, risk of damage by somatization or illness by immunological incompetence should be raised as a function of the frequency and duration of avoidance sessions.

Final Summary

It is too difficult to undertake a complete summary of the various issues and ideas discussed in this book within the confines of this space. It would perhaps be more acceptable to end with one or two speculations that, it is hoped, will at least stimulate research hypotheses. A point that must have been obvious in this final chapter is that in work-stress situations, the control conditions are partly set in advance; a person's only real control decision is whether to take the job and accept the conditions of work. In life-stress conditions this is less likely to be the case; a person has more freedom for deciding on courses of action. His decision making may be very influential in determining any outcomes in terms of both mental health and illness.

In conditions where people make free decisions about life events, the points of differences between normals and depressives might be rather easier to identify. The evidence we have covered suggests that the helplessness-resistance approach of normals has many forms. These include seeking cause for optimism, putting extra effort into meeting a challenge, and attempting control by irrelevant means. The behavior of depression-resistant people might be argued to involve not only resisting depression but failing to lower self-esteem by accepting responsibility for failure. Acccepting behavioral responsibility will provide the cognitive basis for an inductive generalization of characterological blame if there is sufficient exposure to negative events.

A possibility is that depression-resistant people have a major overall decision bias that almost has the status of an ideology. If we were to build a model of depression-resistant decision making, there are two conflicting elements that would be built in. The first is what is traditionally regarded as "locus of control" decisions: "I can always do something to change a situation I dislike." The second may appear contradictory in some cases: "I am never totally responsible for my own failures." These apparent contradictions may never be put to the test as long as a person continues to find evidence of success. This driving motive may be part of the thinking of depression-resistant people.

References

Abramson L. Y., & Sackheim, H.A. A paradox in depression uncontrollability and self-blame. *Psychological Bulletin*, 1977, *84*,(5), 838–851.

Abramson, L. Y., Seligman, M., & Teasdale, J. D. Learned helplessness in humans: Critique and reformulation. *Journal of Abnormal Psychology*, 1978, *87*, 49–74.

Alloy, L. B., & Abramson, L. Y. Judgements of contingency in depressed or non-depressed students: sadder but wiser? *Journal of Experimental Psychology (General)*, 1979, *108*(4), 441–485.

Alloy, L. B., & Abramson, L. Y. Learned helplessness, depression and the illusion of control. *Journal of Personality and Social Psychology* (1981).

Alloy, L. B., Abramson, L. Y., & Viscusi, D. Induced mood and judged control. *Journal of Personality and Social Psychology* (1981).

Alloy, L. B., & Seligman, M. E. P. On the cognitive component of learned helplessness and depression. In J. Garber, & M. E. P. Seligman (Eds.), *Human helplessness: Theory and application*. New York: Academic Press, 1979.

Allport, A., Antonis, B., & Reynolds, P. On the division of attention: a disproof of the single channel hypothesis. *Quarterly Journal of Experimental Psychology*, 1972, *124*, 225–235.

Alluisi, E. A. & Chiles, W. D. Sustained performance, work-rest scheduling, and diurnal rhythms in man. *Acta Psychologica*, 1967, *27*, 436–442.

Amkraut, A., & Solomon, G. F. From the symbolic stimulus to the parthophysiologic response immune mechanisms. *International Journal of Psychiatry in Medicine*, 1975, *5*, 541–563.

Amsel, A. Frustrative non-reward in partial reinforcement and discrimination learning. *Psychological Review*, 1962, *69*, 306–328.

Atkinson, J. W. Motivational determinants of risk taking behaviour. *Psychological Review*, 1957, *64*, 359–372.

Atkinson, J. W., & Feather, N. (Eds.). *A theory of achievement motivation*. New York: Wiley, 1966.

Averill, J. Personal control of aversive stimulation and its relationship to stress. *Psychological Bulletin*, 1973, *80*(4), 286–303.

Averill, J. R. Autonomic response patterns during sadness and mirth. *Psychophysiology*, 1969, *5*, 399–414.

Ax, A. F. The physiological differentiation between fear and anger in humans. *Psychological Medicine*, 1953, *15*, 433–442.

Bacon, S. J. Arousal and the range of cue utilisation. *Journal of Experimental Psychology*, 1974, *102*, 81–87.

Baddeley, A. D. How does acoustic similarity influence short term memory. *Quarterly Journal of Experimental Psychology*, 1968, *20*, 249–264.

Bahrick, H. P., & Shelley, C. Time sharing as an index of automatization. *Journal of Experimental Psychology*, 1958, *56* (3), 288–293.

Baker, C. H. Further toward a theory of vigilance, Chapter 11 in D. Buckner & J. McGrath (Eds.), *Vigilance: A syposium*. New York: McGraw-Hill, 1963, pp. 127–154.

Balke, B., & Wells, J. G. Ceiling altitude tolerance following physical training and acclimatization. *Journal of Aviation Medicine*, 1958, *29*, 40–47.

Ball, T. S., & Vogler, R. E. Uncertain pain and the pain of uncertainty. *Perceptual Motor Skills*, 1971, *33*, 1195–1203.

Bartlett, F. C. *Remembering*. Cambridge: Cambridge University Press, 1932.

Battig, W. R., & Montague, W. E. Category norms for verbal items in 56 categories: A replication and extension of the Connecticut category norms. *Journal of Experimental Psychology Monograph*, 1969, *80*, 3, Pt.2, 1–46.

Battle, E., & Rotter, J. B. Childrens' feelings of personal control as related to social class and ethnic groups. *Journal of Personality*, 1963, *31*, 482–490.

Beck, A. T. *Depression: Clinical, experimental and theoretical aspects*. New York: Harper & Row, 1967.

Beck, A. T. The core problem in depression: The cognitive triad. *Science and Psychoanalysis*, 1970, *17*, 47–55.

Beck, A. T., Ward, C. H., Mendelson, M., Mock, J., & Erbaugh, J. An inventory for measuring depression. *Archives of General Psychiatry*, 1967, *4*, 561–571.

Beck, J. C., & Worthen, K. Precipitating stress crisis theory and hospitalisation in schizophrenia and depression. *Archives of General Psychiatry*, 1972, *26*, 123–129.

Becker, J. *Depression: Theory and research*. New York: Wiley, 1974.

Beebe-Center, J. G. *The psychology of pleasantness and unpleasantness*. New York: Russell and Russell, 1932 (reprinted 1965).

Bekerian, D. A. The effects of helplessness manipulations on perceptual responding: a signal detection theory analysis. *Quarterly Journal of Experimental Psychology*, 1980, *32*, 571–584.

Berkowitz, L. Aggressive cues in aggressive behaviour and hostility cartharsis. *Psychological Review*, 1964, *71*, 104–122.

Berlyne, D. *Conflict, arousal and curiosity*. New York: McGraw-Hill, 1960.

Berlyne, D. E., Borsa, D. M., Craw, M. A., Gelman, R. S., & Mandell, E. E. Effects of stimulus complexity and induced arousal on paired-associate learning. *Journal of Verbal Learning and Verbal Behaviour*, 1965, *4*, 291–299.

Berlyne, D. E., Borsa, D. M., Hamacher, J. H., & Koenig, I. D. Paired-associate learning and the timing of arousal. *Journal of Experimental Psychology*, 1966, *72*, 16.

Bettelheim, B. Individual mass behaviour in extreme situations. *Journal of Abnormal and Social Psychology*, 1943, 38, 417–452.

Bettelheim, B. *The informed heart*. New York: Free Press of Glencoe, 1960.

Bexton, W. H., Heron, W., & Scott, T. H. Effects of decreased variation in the sensory environment. *Canadian Journal of Psychology*, 1954, *8*, 70–76.

Bills, A. Blocking: A new principle in mental fatigue. *American Journal of Psychology*, 1931, *43*, 230–245.

Birnbaum, R. *Autonomic reaction to threat and confrontation conditions of psychological stress*. Doctoral dissertation, University of California, 1964.

Birtchnell, J. The personality characteristics of early bereaved psychiatric patients. *Social Psychiatry*, 1975, *10*, 97–103.

Blake, M. Temperament and time of day. In W. P. Colquhoun (Ed.), *Biological rhythms and human performance*. London: Academic Press, 1971.

Boggs, D. H., & Simon, R. J. Differential effects of noise on tasks of varying complexity. *Journal of Applied Psychology*, 1968, *52*(2), 148–153.

Bonvallet, M., & Allen, M. B. Prolonged spontaneous and evoked reticular activation following discrete bulbar lesions. *Electroencephalography Clinical Neurophysiology*, 1963, *15*, 968–988.

Bower, G. H., Gilligan, S. G., & Monteiro, K. P. Selectivity of learning caused by affective states. *Journal of Experimental Psychology, General*, 1981, *110*(4), 451–473.

Bowers, K. Pain, anxiety and perceived control. *Journal of Clinical and Consulting Psychology*, 1968, *32*, 596–602.

Bowlby, J. *Attachment and loss. Volume 2: Separation anxiety and anger*. London: Hogarth Press, 1973.

Brady, J. V. Ulcers in "executive monkeys." *Scientific American*, 1958, *199*, 95–100.

Brady, J. V., Porter, R. W., Conrad, D. G., & Mason, J. W. Avoidance behaviour and the development of gastroduodenal ulcers. *Journal of the Experimental Analysis of Behaviour*, 1958(b), *1*, 69–72.

Broadbent, D. E. The twenty dials and twenty lights tests under noise conditions. *Applied Psychological Unit Report*, 1951, No. 160.

Broadbent, D. E. Noise, paced performance and vigilance tasks. *British Journal of Psychology*, 1953, *44*, 295–303.

Broadbent, D. E. Some effects of noise on visual performance. *Quarterly Journal of Experimental Psychology*, 1954, *6*, 1–5.

Broadbent, D. E. *Perception and communication*. New York: Pergamon Press, 1958.

Broadbent, D. E. Differences and interactions between stresses. *Quarterly Journal of Experimental Psychology*, 1963(a), *15*, 205–211.

Broadbent, D. E. Possibilities and difficulties with the concept of arousal. In D. E. Buckner, & J. J. McGrath (Eds.), *Vigilance: A symposium*. New York: McGraw-Hill, 1963(b).

Broadbent, D. E. A reformulation of the Yerkes–Dodson law. *British Journal of Mathematical and Statistical Psychology*, 1965, *18*, 145–157.

Broadbent, D. E. Word frequency and response bias. *Psychological Review*, 1967, *74*, 1–15.

Broadbent, D. E. *Decision and stress*. London: Academic Press, 1971.

Broadbent, D. E. Noise and the detail of experiments: A reply to Poulton. *Applied Ergonomics*, 1976, *7*, 231–235.

Broadbent, D. E. Precautions in experiments in noise. *British Journal of Experimental Psychology*, 1977, *68*, 427–429.

Broadbent, D. E. The current state of noise research: A reply to Poulton. *Psychological Bulletin*, 1978, *85*, 1052–1067.

Broadbent, D. E. *Some relations between clinical and occupational psychology*. Paper delivered at the 20th International Congress of Applied Psychology, Edinburgh, July 25–31, 1982.

Broadbent, D. E., & Gregory, M. Effects of noise and signal rate upon vigilance organised by means of decision theory. *Human Factors*, 1965, *7*, 155–162.

Broadbent, D. E., & Gath, D. Ill-health on the line: Sorting out myth from fact. *Employment Gazette*, 1981 (March), 157–160.

Broadbent, D. E., Cooper, P. F., Fitzgerald, P., & Parkes, K. R. The Cognitive Failures Questionnaire (CFQ) and its correlates. *British Journal of Clinical Psychology*, 1981, *21*, 1–16.

Broadhurst, P. L. The biometrical analysis of behavioural inheritance. *Science Programme*, Oxford, 1960, *55*, 123–129.

Broen, W. E., & Storms, L. H. A reaction potential ceiling and response decrements in complex situations. *Psychological Review*, 1961, *68*, 405–415.

Bronstein, P. M., & Hirsch, S. M. Ontogeny of defensive reactions in Norway rats. *Journal of Comparative and Physiological Psychology*, 1976, *90*, 620–629.

Brown, F. Depression and childhood bereavement. *Journal of Mental Science*, 1961, *107*, 754–777.

Brown, G. W., & Birley, J. L. T. Crises and life changes and the onset of schizophrenia. *Journal of Health and Social Behaviour*, 1968, *9*, 203–214.

Brown, G. W., & Birley, J. L. T. Social precipitants of severe psychiatric disorders. In E. H. Hare & J. K. Wing (Eds.), *Psychiatric epidemiology; Proceedings of the International Symposium* (Aberdeen, June/July, 1969). New York: Oxford University Press, 1970.

Brown, G. W., Bhrolchain, M., & Harris, T. Social class and psychiatric disturbance among severely handicapped women in an urban population. *Sociology*, 1975, *9*, 225–254.

Brown, G. W., & Harris, T. H. *Social origins of depression: A study of psychiatric disorders in women*. Great Britain: Tavistock, 1978.

Brown, I. The measurement of perceptual load and reserve capacity. *Transactions of the Association of Industrial Medical Officers*, 1964, *14*, 44–49.

Brown, J. S., & Forbes, I. R. Emotions conceptualised as intervening variables: With suggestions towards a theory of frustration. *Psychological Bulletin*, 1951, *48*, 45–495.

Brown, I. D. Measurement of perceptual load and reserve capacity. *The Transactions of the Associated Medical Officers*, 1964, *14*, 44–49.

Bulman, R. J. (Janoff-Bulman). Characterological versus behavioural self blame: Inquiries into depression and rape. *Journal of Personality and Social Psychology*, 1979, *37*, 1798–1809.

Bulman, R. J., & Wortman, C. B. Attributions of blame and coping in the real world. Severe accident victims react to their lot. *Journal of Personality and Social Psychology*, 1977, *35*, 351–363.

Burch, N. R., & Greiner, T. H. Drugs and human fatigue: GSR parameters. *The British Journal of Psychology*, 1958, *45*, 3–10.

Bursill, A. E. The restriction of peripheral vision during exposure to hot and humid conditions. *Quarterly Journal of Experimental Psychology*, 1958, *10*, 113–129, 1798–1809.

Callaway, E., & Dembo, D. Narrowed attention: A psychological phenomenon that accompanies a certain physiological change. *Archives of Neurology and Psychiatry*, 1958, *79*, 74–90.

Callaway, E., & Stone, G. Re-evaluating the focus of attention. In L. Uhr & J. G. Miller (Eds.), *Drugs and behavior*. New York: Wiley, 1960.

Cameron, N. A., & Margaret, A. *Behavior pathology*. New York: Houghton, Mifflin, 1951.

Campbell, D., Sanderson, R. E., & Laverty, S. G. Characteristics of a conditioned response in human subjects during extinction trials following a single traumatic conditioning trial. *Journal of Abnormal and Social Psychology*, 1964, *68*, 627–639.

Canfield, A. A., Comrey, A. L., Wilson, R. C., & Zimmerman, W. S. The effect of increased positive radial acceleration upon discrimination reaction time. *Journal of Experimental Psychology*, 1950, *40*, 733–737.

Cannon, W. B. *The wisdom of the body.* New York: Norton, 1932.

Cannon, W. B. *Bodily changes in pain, hunger, fear and rage.* New York: Appleton-Century-Crofts, 1936.

Caplan, G. *Principles of preventative psychiatry.* London: Tavistock Publications, 1964.

Caplan, I., & Lindsay, J. K. An experimental investigation of the effects of high temperatures on the efficiency of workers in deep mines. *Bulletin of the Institute of Mineralogy and Metallurgy,* 1946, (480).

Carlton, P. L. Cholinergic mechanisms in the control of behavior by the brain. *Psychological Review,* 1963, *70,* 19–39.

Carruthers, M. *The western way of death.* London: Davis-Poynter, 1974.

Chambers, R. M. Operator performance in acceleration environments. In N. M. Burns, R. M. Chambers, & E. Hendler (Eds.), *Unusual environments and human behaviour.* London: Free Press of Glencoe, 1963.

Chase, R. A., Harvey, S., Standfast, S., Rapin, I., & Sutton, S. Studies on sensory feedback: Effect of delayed auditory feedback on speech and key tapping. *Quarterly Journal of Experimental Psychology,* 1961, *13,* 141–152.

Christenson, W. W., & Hinkle, L. E. Differences in illness and prognostic signs in two groups of young men. *Journal of the American Medical Association,* 1961, *177,* 247–253.

Clark, R. E., & Jones, C. E. Manual performance during cold exposure as a function of practice level and thermal conditions of training. *Journal of Applied Psychology,* 1962, *46,* 276–280.

Clark, W. C. Sensory-decision theory analysis of the placebo effect on the criterion for pain and thermal sensitivity. *Journal of Abnormal Psychology,* 1969, *74,* 363–371.

Clayton, S., Halikas, J. A., & Maurice, W. L. The depression of widowhood. *British Journal of Psychiatry,* 1972, *120,* 71–78.

Cofer, C. N., & Appley, M. H. *Motivation: Theory and research.* New York: John Wiley and Sons, 1964.

Cohen, S., & Lezak, A. Noise and inattentiveness to social cues. *Environment and Behaviour,* 1977, *9*(4), 559–571.

Collett, C. *Category organisation dominance effects on a sentence verification task.* Unpublished thesis toward Master of Arts degree, University of Dundee.

Colquhoun, W. P. The effect of unwanted signals on performance in a vigilance task. *Ergonomics,* 1961(4), 41–42.

Colquhoun, W. P. Circadian variations in mental efficiency. In W. P. Colquhoun (Ed.), *Biological rhythms and human performance,* London: Academic Press, 1971.

Colquhoun, W. P., & Goldman, R. F. The effect of raised body temperature on vigilance performance. *Ergonomics,* 1968, *11,* 408.

Conrad, R. Speed and load stress in a sensori-motor skill. *British Journal of Industrial Medicine,* 1951, *8,* 1–7.

Conrad, R. Missed signals in a sensory motor skill. *Journal of Experimental Psychology,* 1954(a), *48,* 1–9.

Conrad, R. Speed stress. In W. F. Floyd & A. T. Welford (Eds.), *Symposium on human factors in equipment design.* London: H. K. Lewis, 1954(b).

Corcoran, D. Noise and loss of sleep. *Quarterly Journal of Experimental Psychology,* 1962, *14*(3), 178–182.

Corcoran, D. W. J. *Individual differences in performance after loss of sleep.* Ph.D. Thesis, University of Cambridge.

Coulter, X. The effect of performance relevance and feedback upon resistance to anticipatory stress. U.S. Army Aeromedical Research Laboratory, Naval Aerospace Medical Research Laboratory, *USAARL Report* 1970, No. 6190.

Courts, F. A. Relationship between muscular tension and performance. *Psychological Bulletin*, 1942, *39*, 347–367.

Cox, T., & Mackay, C. Psychosocial factors and psychophysiological mechanisms in the aetiology and development of cancers. *Society of Science and Medicine*, 1982, *16*, 381–396.

Craik, F. I., & Blankstein, K. R. Psychophysiology and human memory. In P. H. Venables & M. J. Christie (Eds.), *Research in psychophysiology*. London: John Wiley, 1975.

Crown, S., & Crisp, A. H. A short clinical diagnostic self-rating scale for psychoneurotic patients. *British Journal of Psychiatry*, 1966, *112*, 917–923.

Cruze-Coke, W. W., Etcheverry, R., & Nagel, R. Influences of migration on the blood pressure of Easter Islanders. *Lancet*, 1964(March), *28*, 697–699.

Daee, S., & Wilding, J. M. Effects of high intensity white noise on short term memory for position in a list and sequence. *British Journal of Psychology*, 1977, *68*, 335–349.

Davis, D. R. Pilot error. *Air Ministry Publication A.P 3139A*, London: H.M.S.O., 1948.

Davis, D. R. Depression as an adaptation to crisis. *British Journal of Medical Psychology*, 1970, *43*, 109–116.

Davis, D. R., & Jones, D. M. The effects of high intensity white noise and incentive upon attention in short term memory. *British Journal of Psychology*, 1975, *66*, 61–68.

Deese, J., & Ormond, E. Studies of detectability during continuous visual search. *USAF WADC Technical Report*, 1953, No. TR-53-8.

Denenberg, V. H. Critical periods, stimulus input and emotional reactivity: A theory of infantile stimulation. *Psychological Review*, 1964, *71*, 335–351.

Dittes, J. E. Impulsive closure as a reaction to failure-induced threat. *Journal of Abnormal and Social Psychology*, 1961, *63*(3), 562–569.

Dohrenwend, B. P. Sociocultural and social-psychological factors in the genesis of mental disorders. *Journal of Health and Social Behaviour*, 1975, *16*, 365–392.

Dohrenwend, B. P., & Dohrenwend, B. S. Social class and stressful events. In E. H. Hare & J. K. Wing (Eds.), *Psychiatric epidemiology: Proceedings of the international symposium* (Aberdeen University, June/July 1969). New York: Oxford University Press, 1970.

Dohrenwend, B. P., & Dohrenwend, B. S. Social and cultural influences on psychopathology. *Annual Review of Psychology*, 1974, *5*, 417–452.

Dohrenwend, B. S. Life events as stressors: A methodological inquiry. *Journal of Health and Social Behaviour*, 1973, *14* (June), 167–175.

Dolgun, A. *Alexander Dolgun's story: An American in the Gulag*. New York: Knopf, 1965.

Dollard, J., & Miller, N. E. *Personality and psychotherapy*. New York: McGraw-Hill, 1950.

Doris, J., & Sarason, S. B. Test anxiety and blame assignment in a failure situation. *Journal of Abnormal and Social Psychology*, 1955, *50*, 335–338.

Dornic, S. *Some studies on the retention of order information*. Reports from the Psychological Laboratories, University of Stockholm, 1974.

Duval, S., & Wickland, R. A. Effects of objective self-awareness on attribution of causality. *Journal of Experimental Psychology*, 1973, *9*, 17–31.

Duval, S., & Wickland, R. A. A theory of objective self awareness. New York: Academic Press, 1972.

Easterbrook, J. A. The effect of emotion on cue utilisation and the organisation of behaviour. *Psychological Review*, 1959, *66*, 187–201.

Ebbinghaus, H. Memory: A contribution to experimental psychology. Republished in translation. New York: Dover Publications, 1885.

Egeth, H., & Smith, E. E. On the nature of errors in choice reaction time. *Psychonomic Science*, 1967, *8*, 345–346.

Ellis, A. W. Slips of the pen. *Visible Language*, 1979, *13*, 265–282.

Ells, J. G. Analysis of temporal and attentional aspects of movement control. *Journal of Experimental Psychology*, 1973, *99*, 10–21.

Epstein, S. Toward a unified theory of anxiety. In B. A. Maher (Ed.), *Progress in experimental personality research. Volume 4.* New York: Academic Press, 1967.

Epstein, S., & Clarke, S. Heart rate and skin conductance during experimentally induced anxiety: The effects of anticipated intensity of noxious stimulation and experience. *Journal of Experimental Psychology*, 1970, *84*, 105–112.

Eysenck, M. W. Extraversion, arousal and retrieval from semantic memory. *Journal of Personality*, 1974, *42*, 319–331.

Eysenck, M. W. Effects of noise activation level and response dominance on retrieval from semantic memory. *Journal of Experimental Psychology*, 1975, *104*, 143,148.

Faris, R. E. L., & Dunham, H. W. *Mental disorders in urban areas: An ecological study of schizophrenia and other psychoses.* Chicago: Chicago University Press, 1939.

Farley, F. Memory storage in free learning as a function of arousal; and time with homogenous and heterogenous lists. *Winconsin University Center in Cognitive Learning Technical Reports*, 1969, 87.

Feather, N. T. The relationship of persistence at a task to expectation of success and achievement-related motives. *Journal of Abnormal and Social Psychology*, 1961, *63*, 552–561.

Feller, W. *An introduction to probability theory and its applications. Volume 2.* New York: John Wiley, 1966.

Fenz, W. D. Arousal and performance of novice parachutists to multiple sources of conflict and stress. *Studia Psychologica*, 1964.

Fenz, W. D. Strategies for coping with stress. In I. G. Sarason and C. D. Spielberger (Eds.), *Stress and anxiety: Volume 2.* Washington: Hemisphere Publishing Corporation, 1975.

Fenz, W. D., & Epstein, S. Measurement of approach-avoidance conflict along a stimulus dimension by a thematic apperception test. *Journal of Personality*, 1962, *30*, 613–632.

Fenz, W. D., & Epstein, S. Changes in gradients of skin conductance, heart rate and respiration, as a function of experience. *Psychosomatic Medicine*, 1967, *29*, 33–51.

Fenz, W. D., Kluck, B. L., & Bankart, C. P. The effect of threat and uncertainty on the mastery of stress. *Journal of Experimental Psychology*, 1969, *79*, 473–479.

Festinger, L. A theory of social comparison processes. *Human Relations*, 1954, *7*, 117–140.

Finkleman, J. M., & Glass, D. C. Re-appraisal of the relationship between noise and human performance by means of a subsidiary task measure. *Journal of Applied Psychology*, 1970, *54*(3), 211–213.

Fiorca, V., Higgins, E. A., Iampietro, P. F., Lategola, M. T., & Davis, A. W. Physiological responses of man during sleep deprivation. *Journal of Applied Physiology*, 1968, *24*, 167–176.

Fischer, S. L., & Turner, R. M. Standardisation of the fear survey schedule. *Journal of Behaviour Research and Therapy*, 1978, *9*, 129–133.

Fisher, S. A distraction effect of noise bursts. *Perception*, 1972, *1*, 223–236.

Fisher, S. A possible artifact in serial response behaviour. *Acta Psychologica*, 1973, *37*, 249–254.

Fisher, S. The microstructure of dual task interaction: 1. The patterning of main task responses within secondary task intervals. *Perception*, 1975(a), *4*, 267–290.

Fisher, S. The microstructure of dual task interaction: 2. The effect of task instructions and a model of attention-switching. *Perception*, 1975(b), *4*, 459–474.

Fisher, S. The microstructure of dual task interaction: 3. Incompatibility and attention switching. *Perception*, 1977, *6*, 467–77.

Fisher, S. The microstructure of dual task interaction: 4. Sleep deprivation and the control of attention. *Perception*, 1980, *9*, 327–337.

Fisher, S. Pessimistic noise effects: The perception of reaction times in noise. *Canadian Journal of Psychology*, 37(2), 258–271.

Fisher, S. Memory and search in loud noise. *Canadian Journal of Psychology*, *37*(3), 439–449.

Fisher, S. *The microstructure of attentional deployment on a dual task in loud noise*. 1983(c), submitted for publication.

Fisher, S. *The detection of lapses in anxious and busy people: The double lapse hypothesis*. 1983(d), submitted for publication.

Fisher, S. *The judgements of depressed and nondepressed students concerning performance in stress: Sadder but harder?* 1983(e), submitted for publication.

Fisher, S. *Homesickness in University students: A preliminary report*. 1983(f), submitted for publication.

Fisher, S. *Cognitive processes in the recognition of threat*. 1983(g), submitted for publication.

Fisher, S., & Ledwith, M. *The perception of control in loud noise*. 1983, submitted for publication.

Fitts, P. M. The information capacity of the human motor system in controlling the amplitude of movement. *Journal of Experimental Psychology*, 1954, *47*, 381–391.

Fitts, P. M. Cognitive aspects of information processing: III Set for speed versus accuracy. *Journal of Experimental Psychology*, 1966.

Flavell, J. H., Draguns, J., Feinberg, L. D., & Budin, W. A microgenetic approach to word association. *Journal of Abnormal and Social Psychology*, 1958, *57*, 1–8.

Folkard, S. Time of day and level of processing. *Memory and Cognition*, 1979, *7*(4), 247–252.

Folkard, S. Circadian rhythms and human memory. In F. M. Brown & R. C. Graeber (Eds.), *Rhythmic aspects of behavior*. Hillsdale, New Jersey: Lawrence Erlbaum Associates, 1980.

Folkhard, S., & Greeman, A. L., Salience, induced muscle tension and the ability to ignore irrelevant information. *Quarterly Journal of Experimental Psychology*, 1974, *26*, 360–367.

Forster, P. M., & Grierson, A. T. Noise and attentional selectivity: A reproducible phenomenon? *British Journal of Psychology*, 1978, *69*, 489–498.

Foster, J. H. Blood pressure of foreigners in China. *Archives of International Medicine*, 1927, *40*, 38–45.

Fowler, C. J. H., & Wilding, J. M. Differential effects of noise and incentives on learning. *British Journal of Psychology*, 1979, *70*, 149–153.

Frankenhaeuser, M. Behaviour and Circulating Catecholamines. *Brain Research*, 1971, *31*, 241–262.

Frankenhaeuser, M., & Gardell, B. Underload and overload in working life: Outline of a multidisciplinary approach. *Journal of Human Stress*, 1976, *2*, 35–46.

Frankenhaeuser, M., & Johansson, J. *Stress at work: Psychobiological and psychosocial aspects*. Paper presented at the 20th International Congress of Applied Psychology, Edinburgh. July 25–31, 1982.

Frankenhaeuser, M., & Lundberg, U. The influence of cognitive set on performance and arousal under different task loads. *Motivation and Emotion*, 1977, *1*, 139–149.

Frankenhaeuser, M., Lundberg, U., & Foresman, L. Dissociation between sympathetic-adrenal and pituitary adrenal response to an achievement situation characterised by high controllability. *Biological Psychology*, 1980, *10*, 79–91.

Frankenhaeuser, M., & Patkai, P. Interindividual differences in catecholamine excretion during stress. *Scandinavian Journal of Psychology*, 1965, *6*, 117–123.

Frankenhaeuser, M., & Rissler, A. Effects of punishment on catecholamine release and the efficiency of performance. *Psychopharmacologia*, 1970, *17*, 378–390.

Freedman, J., & Loftus, E. F. Retrieval of words from long term memory. *Journal of Verbal Learning and Behaviour*, 1971, *10*, 107–115.

Freud, S. *A General Introduction to Psychoanalysis*. New York: Garden City Books, 1943.

Fried, M. Grieving for a Lost Home. In L. J. Duhl (Ed.), *The Environment of the Metropolis*. New York: Basic Books, 1962.

Friedman, M., Rosenman, R., & Carroll, V. Changes in the serum cholesterol and blood clotting time in men subjected to cyclic variation of occupational stress. *Circulation*, 1958, *17*, 825–861.

Fry, P. S., & Ogston, D. G. Emotion as a function of the labeling of interruption produced arousal. *Psychonomic Science*, 1971, *24*, 53–154.

Funkenstein, D. H., King, S. H., & Drolette, M. E. *The mastery of stress*. Cambridge: Harvard University Press, 1957.

Furneaux, W. D. The psychologist and the University. *University Quarterly*, 1962, *17*, 33–47.

Garcia, J., & Koelling, R. A. Relation of cue to consequence in avoidance learning. *Psychonomic Science*, 1966, *4*, 123–124.

Garner, W. R. *Uncertainty and structure as psychological concepts*. New York: John Wiley, 1962.

Gatchel, R., & Proctor, J. D. Physiological correlates of learned helplessness in man. *Journal of Abnormal and Social Psychology*, 1976, *85*, 27–34.

Gates, A. L. Diurnal variation in memory and association. *University of California Publications in Psychology*, 1916, *1*, 323–344.

Geer, J. H., & Maisel, E. Evaluating the effects of the prediction-control confound. *Journal of Personality and Social Psychology*, 1972, *23*, 314–319.

Glass, D. C., & Singer, J. E. *Urban stress: Experiments on noise and social stressors*. New York: Academic Press, 1972.

Glass, D. C., Singer, J. E., & Friedman, L. N. Psychic cost of adaptation to an environmental stressor. *Journal of Personality and Social Psychology*, 1969, *12*, 200–210.

Glass, D. C., Rheim, B., & Singer, J. E. Behavioural consequences of adaptation to controllable and uncontrollable noise. *Journal of Experimental Social Psychology*, 1971, *7*, 244–257.

Gopher, D., & North, R. A. Manipulating the conditions of training in time sharing performance. *Human Factors*, 1977, *19*, 583–593.

Gore, P. S., & Rotter, J. B. A personality correlate of social action. *Journal of Personality*, 1963, *31*, 58–64.

Gray, J. *The psychology of fear and stress*. World University Library, London: Weidenfeld and Nicolson, 1971.

Green, D., & Swets, J. *Signal detection theory and psychophysics*. New York: John Wiley, 1966.

Greenwald, A. G. Sensory feedback mechanisms in performance control: With special reference to the ideomotor mechanism. *Psychological Review*, 1970, *77*, 73–99.

Gregg, V. Word frequency recognition and recall. In J. Brown (Ed.), *Recall and recognition*. London: John Wiley, 1976.

Gregory, I. W. Retrospective data concerning childhood loss of a parent, II. Category of parental loss of a parent by decade, birth, diagnosis and MMPI. *Archives of General Psychiatry*, 1966, *15*, 362–367.

Griffin, J. H. *Black like me?* Boston: Houghton Mifflin, 1962.

Grinker, R. R., & Spiegel, J. P. *Men under stress*. New York: McGraw-Hill, 1945.

Haggard, E. A. Experimental studies in affective processes: I. Some effects of cognitive structure and active participation on certain autonomic reactions during and following experimentally induced stress. *Journal of Experimental Psychology*, 1943, *33*, 257–284.

Hale, D. Speed/error trade-off in serial choice reaction time tasks. *Paper to the Experimental Psychology Society*, Nottingham, July, 1968.

Hale, D. J. Speed error trade-off in a three-choice serial reaction task. *Journal of Experimental Psychology*, 1969, *81*(3), 428–435.

Hall, C. S. The genetics of behavior. In S.S. Stevens (Ed.), *Handbook of experimental psychology*, New York: John Wiley, 1951.

Haltmeyer, G. C., Denenberg, V. H., & Zarrow, M. X. Modification of plasma corticosterone response as a function of infantile stimulation and electric shock parameters. *Physiology and Behaviour*, 1967, *2*, 61–63.

Hamilton, P. *Selective attention in multisource monitoring tasks*. Ph.D. Thesis, University of Dundee, Scotland, 1967.

Hamilton, P., Hockey, G. R. J., & Quinn, G. Information, selection, arousal and memory. *British Journal of Psychology*, 1972, *63*, 181–190.

Hamilton, P., Hockey, G. R. J., & Rejman, M. The place of the concept of activation in human information processing theory: An integrative approach, Sixth International Symposium on Attention and Performance, Stockholm. In S. Dornic (Ed.), *Attention and performance, Vol.VI*. New York: Academic Press, 1977.

Hamilton, V. *Socialisation anxiety and information processing: A capacity model of anxiety-induced performance deficits*. Paper presented at a conference on Dimensions of Anxiety and Stress, Athens, Greece, September, 1974. Scientific Advisory Committee of NATO and Roche Laboratories.

Harrison, G. A., Palmer, C. D., Jenner, D. A., & Reynolds, V. Associations between rates of urinary catecholamine excretion and aspects of life style among adult women in some Oxfordshire villages. *Human Biology*, 1981, 53(4), 617–633.

Hartley, L. R. Effect of prior noise or prior performance on serial reaction. *Journal of Experimental Psychology*, 1973(a), *101*, 255–261.

Hartley, L. R. Performance during continuous and intermittent noise and wearing ear protection. *Journal of Experimental Psychology*, 1973(b), *102*, 515–516.

Hartley, L. R. Noise does not impair by masking: A reply to Poulton's "composite model for human performance in continuous noise." *Psychological Bulletin*, 1981a, *88* (1), 86–89.

Hartley, L. R. Noise attentional selectivity, serial reactions and the need for experimental power. *British Journal of Psychology*, 1981b, *72*, 101–107.

Hartley, L. R., & Adams, R. G. Effects of noise on the stroop test. *Journal of Experimental Psychology*, 1974, *102*(1), 62–66.

Hartley, L. R., & Carpenter, A. A comparison of performance with headphone and free-field noise. *Journal of Experimental Psychology*, 1974, *103*, 377–380.

Haveman, J. E., & Farley, F. H. Arousal and retention in paired associate, serial and free learning. *Wisconsin University Center for Cognitive Learning Technical Reports*, 1969, 91.

Hebb, D. O. *Organization of Behavior*, New York: John Wiley, 1949.

Heider, F. *The psychology of interpersonal relations*. New York: John Wiley, 1958.

Held, R. Exposure history as a factor in maintaining stability of perception and co-ordination. *The Journal of Nervous and Mental Disease*, 1961, *132*(1), 938, 26–32.

Henderson, D. K. & Gillespie, R. D. *Textbook of psychiatry*. London: Oxford University Press, 1962. Revised by I. Batchelor, 1969.

Hermon, L. M., & Kantowitz, B. H. The psychological refractory period effect: Only half the double stimulation story. *Psychological Bulletin*, 1970, *73*, 74–88.

Hick, W. E. On the rate of gain of information. *Quarterly Journal of Experimental Psychology*, 1952, *4*, 11–26.

Hiroto, D. S. Locus of control and learned helplessness. *Journal of Experimental Psychology*, 1974, *102*, 187–193.

Hiroto, D. S., & Seligman, M. E. P. Generality of learned helplessness in man. *Journal of Personality and Social Psychology*, 1975, *14*, 263–270.

Hirschman, R. Cross modal effects of anticipatory bogus heartrate feedback in a negative emotional context. *Journal of Personality and Social Psychology*, 1975, *31*, 13–19.

Hockey, G. R. J. Effects of loud noise on attentional selectivity. *Quarterly Journal of Experimental Psychology*, 1970(a), *22*, 28–36.

Hockey, G. R. J. Signal probability and spatial location as possible bases for increased selectivity in noise. *Quarterly Journal of Experimental Psychology*, 1970(b), *22*, 37–42.

Hockey, G. R. J., & Hamilton, P. Arousal and information selection in short term memory. *Nature, London*, 1970, *226*, 866–867.

Hockey, G. R. J. Changes in the information-selection patterns in multisource monitoring as a function of induced arousal shifts. *Journal of Experimental Psychology*, 1973, *101*, 35–42.

Hollingshead, A. B., & Redlich, F. C. *Social class and mental illness*. New York: John Wiley, 1958.

Hollister, L. E. Drug induced psychoses and schizophrenic reactions: A critical comparison. *Annals of the New York Academy of Science*, 1962, *96*, 80–88.

Holmes, D. S., & Houston, B. K. Effectiveness of situation redefinition and affective isolation in coping with stress. *Journal of Personality and Social Psychology*, 1974, *29*, 212–218.

Holmes, T. H. Multidiscipline studies of tuberculosis. In P. J. Sporer (Ed.), *Personality, stress and tuberculosis*. New York: International Universities Press, 1956.

Holmes, T. H. Life situations, emotions and disease. *Psychosomatics*, 1978, *19*, 747–754.

Holmes, T. H., & Rahe, R. H. The social readjustment rating scale. *Journal of Psychosomatic Research*, 1967, *11*, 213–218.

Horney, K. *Neurotic personality of our times*. New York: Norton, 1937.

Houston, B. K. Control over stress, locus of control and response to stress. *Journal of Personality and Social Psychology*, 1972, *21*, 249–255.

Howell, W. C., & Burnett, S. A. Uncertainty measurement: A cognitive taxonomy. *Organizational Behavior and Human Performance*, 1978, *22*, 45–68.

Hudgens, R. W. Personal catastrophe and depression: A consideration of the subject with respect to medically ill adolescents and a requiem for retrospective life-event studies. In B. S. Dohrenwend & B. P. Dohrenwend (Eds.), *Stressful life events: Their nature and effects*. New York: John Wiley, 1974.

Hudgens, R. W., Morrison, J. R., & Barchha, R. G. Life events and the onset of primary affective disorders. *Archives of General Psychiatry*, 1967, *16*, 134–145.

Hull, C. L. *Principles of behavior*. New York: Appleton-Century-Crofts, 1943.

Hunt, J. Mc.V. Intrinsic motivation and its role in psychological development. In D. Levine (Ed.), *Nebraska Symposium on Motivation, Vol 13*. Lincoln: University of Nebraska Press, 1965.

Hyman, R. Stimulus information as a determinant of reaction time. *Journal of Experimental Psychology*, 1953, *45*, 188–196.

James, W. What is an emotion? *Mind*, 1884, *9*, 188–205.

James, W. *Principles of psychology, Volumes 1 and 2*. New York: Holt, 1890.

Janis, I. L. *Psychological stress*. New York: John Wiley, 1958 (2nd edition 1974).

Janis, I. L. Psychological effects of warnings, In G. W. Baker & D. W. Chapman (Eds.), *Man and society in disaster*. New York: Basic Books, 1962.

Jarvis, E. *Insanity and idiocy in Massachusetts: Report of the Commission of Lunacy 1855*. Cambridge: Harvard University Press, 1971.

Jastrow, J. The lapses of consciousness. *The Popular Science Monthly*, 1905 (October), *67*, 481–502.

Jenkins, H. M. Performance on a visual monitoring task as a function of the rate at which signals occur. *Massachusetts Institute of Technology Laboratory Technical Report*, 1953, *47*.

Jenkins, H. M., & Ward, W. C. Judgements of contingency between response and outcome. *Psychological Monographs*, 1965, *79*, 594.

Jenner, D. A., Reynolds, V., & Harrison, G. A. Catecholamine excretion rates and occupation. *Ergonomics*, 1980, *23*, 237–246.

Jennings, J. R., Wood, C. C., & Lawrence, E. E. Effect of graded doses of alcohol on speed-accuracy trade-off in choice reaction time. *Perception and Psychophysics*, 1976, *19*, 85–91.

Jerison, H. J. Differential effects of noise and fatigue on a complex counting task. *USAF WADC Technical Report*, 1956, TR55–359.

Jerison, H. J. Performance on a simple vigilance task in noise and quiet. *Journal of Acoustical Society of America*, 1957, *29*, 1163–1165.

Jerison, H. J. Experiments on vigilance IV. Duration of vigil and decrement function. *USAF WADC Technical Report*, 1958, No.TR–58–369.

Jerison, H. J., & Wallis, R. A. Experiments in vigilance: Performance on a simple vigilance task in noise and quiet. *USAF WADC Technological Report*, 1957, No.TR–57–317, & No. 57–206.

Jersild, A. T. Studies of Childrens' Fears, In R. G. Barker, J. S. Kounin, & H. F. Wright (Eds.), *Child behavior and development*. New York: McGraw-Hill, 1943.

Jenson, A. R., & Rohwer, W. D. The stroop colour word test: A review. *Acta Psychologica*, 1966, *25*, 36–93.

Jessor, R., Graves, T. D., Hanson, R. C., & Jessor, S. L. *Society, personality and deviant behaviour: A study of a tri-ethnic community*. New York: Holt, Rinehart and Winston, 1968.

Johansson, G., & Sanden, P. Mental load and job satisfaction of control room operators. *Rapparter*, 1982, Department of Psychology, University of Stockholm, No 40.

Jones, E. E., & Davis, K. E. From acts to dispositions: The attribution process in perception. In Berkowitz (Ed.), *Advances in experimental social psychology*, New York: Academic Press, 1965.

Julian, W., & Katz, S. B. Internal versus external control and the value of reinforcement. *Journal of Personality and Social Psychology*, 1968, *76*, 43–48.

Jung, C. G. *Analytical psychology,* New York: Moffat Yard, 1916.

Jung, C. G. *Psychological types*, New York: Harcourt, 1933.

Kahneman, D. Remarks on attention control. *Acta Psychologica, 33*; also in A. F. Sanders (Ed.), *Attention and performance I,* Amsterdam: North-Holland, 1969, 118–131.

Kahneman, D. *Attention and effort*. Englewood Cliffs, New Jersey: Prentice-Hall, 1978.

Kahneman, D., & Tversky, A. Subjective probability: A judgement of representativeness. *Cognitive Psychology*, 1972, *3*, 430–454.

Kahneman, D., & Tversky, A. 1973, On the psychology of prediction. *Psychological Review*, 1973, *80*, 237–251.

Kanouse, D. E., & Hanson, L. R. Negativity in evaluations. In E. Jones, D. Kanouse, H. Kelley, R. Nisbett, S. Valins, & B. Weiner (Eds.), *Attribution: Perceiving the causes of behavior*. Chapter 3. Morristown, N.J.: General Learning Press, 1971.

Kantowitz, B. H., & Knight, J. L. Testing, tapping, timesharing. *Journal of Experimental Psychology*, 1974, *103*, 331–336.

Kantowitz, B. H., & Knight, J. L. Testing, tapping, timesharing, II: Auditory secondary task. *Acta Psychologica*, 1976, *40*, 343–362.

Kay, H., & Weiss, A. D. Relationship between simple and serial reaction time. *Nature*, 1961, *191*, 790–791.

Kerr, B. Processing demands during mental operations. *Memory and Cognition*, 1973, *1*, 401–412.

Kelly, H. H. The processes of causal attribution. *American Psychologist*, 1973 (February), 107–128.

Kety, S. Biochemical theory of schizophrenia. *International Journal of Psychiatry*, 1965, *1*, 409–430.

Kety, S., Rosenthal, D., Wender, P. H., & Schulsinger, F. The types and prevalence of mental illness in the biological and adoptive families of adopted schizophrenics. In D.

Rosenthal & S. S. Kety (Eds.), *The transmission of schizophrenia*, London: Pergamon Press, 1968.

Kleinsmith, L. J., & Kaplan, S. Paired associate learning as a function of arousal and interpolated rest interval. *Journal of Experimental Psychology*, 1963, *65*, 190–193.

Kleitman, N. *Sleep and wakefulness*. Chicago: University of Chicago Press, 1939. Revised 1963.

Klinger, E. Consequences of commitment to and disengagement from incentives. *Psychological Review*, 1975, *82*(1), 1–7.

Kluver, H., & Bucy, P. C. Preliminary analysis of functions of the temporal lobes in monkeys. *Archives of Neurology and Psychiatry*, 1939, *42*, 979–1000.

Kobasa, S. C. Stressful life events and health: An inquiry into hardness. *Journal of Personality and Social Psychology*, 1979, *37*, 1–11.

Koch, S. Behavior as intrinsically regulated: Work notes towards a pre-theory of phenomena called motivational. In M. R. Jones (Ed.), *Nebraska Symposium on Motivation: Vol 4.* Lincoln: University of Nebraska Press, 1956.

Kogan, N., & Wallach, M. A. Risk taking as a function of the situation the person and the group. In *New directions in psychology III.* New York: Holt, Rinehart and Winston, 1967.

Korchin, S. Anxiety and cognition. In C. Sheerer (Ed.), *Cognition: Theory, research and promise*, New York: Harper & Row, 1964.

Korchin, S. J., & Levine, S. Anxiety and verbal learning. *Journal of Abnormal Social Psychology*, 1957, *54*, 234–240.

Kowalewski, A. *Arthur Schopenhauer und seine Weltanschauung*. Berlin: Halle, 1908.

Kryter, K. D. The effects of noise on man. *Journal of Speech and Hearing Disorders*, Monograph Supplement, 1950, 1.

Kryter, K. D. *The effects of noise on man*. New York: Academic Press, 1970.

Kubzansky, P. E., & Leiderman, P. H. Sensory Deprivation: An overview. In A. D. Biderman & H. Zimmer (Ed.), The manipulation of human behavior. *Proceedings of Sensory Deprivation Symposium* at Harvard University. Cambridge: Harvard University Press, 1958.

Kukla, A. Cognitive determinants of achieving behaviour. *Journal of Personality and Social Psychology*, 1972, *21*, 166–174.

Lacey, J. I. Somatic response patterning: Some revisions of activation theory. In M. H. Appley & R. Trumbell (Eds.), *Psychological stress: Issues in research.* New York: Appleton-Century-Crofts, 1967.

Lacey, J., Bateman, D., & Van Lehn, R. Autonomic response specificity: An experimental study. *Psychosomatic Medicine*, 1953, *15*, 1.

Laming, D. R. J. *Information theory of choice reaction times*. London, New York: Academic Press, 1968.

Landis, C., & Hunt, W. A. *The startle pattern*. New York: Farrer and Rhinehart, 1939.

Lane, D. M. Attention allocation and the relationship between primary and secondary task difficulty: A reply to Kantowitz and Knight. *Acta Psychologica*, 1977, *41*, 493–495.

Lane, D. Developmental changes in attention-deployment skills. *Journal of Experimental Child Psychology*, 1979, *28*, 16–29.

Langer, E. J. The illusion of control. *Journal of Personality and Social Psychology*, 1975, *32*, 311–328.

Langer, E. J., & Roth, J. Heads I win, tails it's chance: The illusion of control as a function of the sequence of outcomes in a purely chance task. *Journal of Personality and Social Psychology*, 1975, *32*, 951–955.

Langer, T. S. A twenty-two item screening score of psychiatric symptoms indicating impairment. *Journal of Health and Human Behaviour*, 1962, *3*, 269–276.

Lazarus, R. *Psychological stress and the coping process*. New York: McGraw-Hill, 1966.

262 REFERENCES

Lazarus, R. *Patterns of adjustment*. Tokyo: McGraw-Hill-Kogakush, 1968.

Lefcourt, H. M. *Locus of control*. Hillsdale, N.J.: Lawrence Erlbaum Associates, 1966.

Lefcourt, H. M., & Ludwig, G. W. The American Negro: A problem in expectancies. *Journal of Personality and Social Psychology*, 1965, *1*, 377–380.

Lefcourt, H. M., & Wine, J. Internal versus external control of reinforcement and the deployment of attention in experimental situations. *Canadian Journal of Science*, 1969, *1*, 167–181.

Leff, M. J., Roatch, J. F., & Bunney, W. E. Environmental factors preceding the onset of severe depression. *Psychiatry*, 1970, *33*, 293–311.

Levi, L. The urinary output of adrenaline and noradrenaline during pleasant and unpleasant emotional states. *Psychosomatic Medicine*, 1965, *27*, 80–85.

Levine, S. Sex differences in the brain. *Scientific American*, 1966, *214*(4), 84–90.

Levine, S., Haltmeyer, G., Karas, G., & Denenberg, V. Physiological and behavioural effects of infantile stimulation. *Physiology and Behaviour*, 1967, *2*, 55–59.

Levine, S., & Mullins, R. F. Hormonal influences on brain organisation in infant rats. *Science*, 1966, *152*, 1585–1592.

Levitt, E. *The psychology of anxiety*. London: Staples Press, 1968.

Lewin, K. *A dynamic theory of personality*. New York: McGraw-Hill, 1935.

Link, S. W. The relative judgement theory analysis of response deadline experiments. In N. Castellan & F. Restle, *Cognitive theory*. Volume 3, Chapter 5. Hillsdale, New Jersey: Lawrence Erlbaum Associates, 1978.

Lloyd, G. G., & Lishman, W. A. Effect of depression on the speed of recall of pleasant and unpleasant experiences. *Psychological Medicine*, 1975, *5*, 173–180.

Lockhart, J. M. Extreme body cooling and psychomotor performance. *Ergonomics*, 1968, *11*, 249–269.

Loeb, A., Beck, A., & Diggory, J. Differential effects of success and failure on depressed and nondepressed patients. *The Journal of Nervous and Mental Disease*, 1971, *152*(2), 106–113.

Lorenz, K. The comparative method in studying innate behaviour patterns. *Symposium of Experimental Biology*, 1950, *4*, 221–268.

Luby, E., & Gottlieb, J. Model psychoses. In J. Howells (Ed.), *Modern perspectives in world psychiatry*, Chapter II. Edinburgh: Oliver and Boyd, 1966.

Luce, G. G. *Body time: The natural rhythms of the body*. St.Albans, Herts.: Paladin, 1973.

Luce, S. W. Detection and recognition. In R. D. Luce, R. R. Bush, & E. Galanter (Eds.), *Handbook of mathematical psychology*, Vol. I. New York: John Wiley, 1963.

Lundberg, U. Psychophysiological aspects of performance and adjustment to stress. In H. W. Krohne & L. Laux (Eds.), *Achievement in stress and anxiety*. Washington: Hemisphere Publishing Corporation, 1979.

Lundberg, U., & Foresman, L. Andrenal-medullary and adrenal-cortical responses to understimulation and overstimulation. *Biological Psychology*, 1979, *9*, 79–89.

Lundberg, U., & Frankenhaeuser, M. Pituitary-adrenal and sympathetico-adrenal correlates of distress and effort. *Journal of Psychosomatic Research*, 1980, *24*, 125–130.

Lundin, R. W. *Principles of psychopathology*. Columbus, Ohio: Merrill International Psychology Series, 1965.

Mace, C. A. Incentives: some experimental studies. *Industrial Health Research Report*, 1935, *72*.

Mackworth, N. H. Researches on the measurement of human performance. *Medical Research Council Special Report Series*, No. 268, 1950.

Maddison, D. The relevance of conjugal bereavement for psychiatry. *British Journal of Medical Psychology*, 1968, *41*, 223–333.

Malmo, R. B., & Shagass, C. Physiologic study of symptom mechanisms in psychiatric patients under stress. *Psychosomatic Medicine*, 1949, *11*, 25–29.

Maltzman, I., & Wolff, C. Preference for immediate versus delayed noxious stimulation and the concomitant GSR. *Journal of Experimental Psychology*, 1970, *83*, 76–79.

Mandler, G. The interruption of behavior. In D. Levine (Ed.), *Nebraska symposium on motivation*. Lincoln: University of Nebraska Press, 1964.

Mandler, G. The conditions for emotional behavior. In D. C. Glass (Ed.), *Neurophysiology and Emotion*. New York: Rockefeller Press and Russell Sage Foundation, 1967.

Mandler, G. *Mind and emotion*. New York: John Wiley, 1975.

Mandler, G., & Sarason, S. B. A study of anxiety and learning. *Journal of Abnormal and Social Psychology*, 1952, *47*, 166–173.

Mandler, G., & Watson, D. L. Anxiety and the interruption of behavior. In C. D. Spielberger (Ed.), *Anxiety and behavior*. New York: Academic Press, 1966.

Marks, I., & Lader, M. Anxiety states (anxiety neurosis): A review. *Journal of Nervous and Mental Disease*, 1973, *156*, 3–18.

Marks, R. A review of empirical findings. In S. L. Syme & L. G. Reeder (Eds.), Social stress and cardiovascular disease. *Milbank Memorial Fund Quarterly*, 1967, *45*.

Marques, T., & Howell, W. *Intuitive frequency judgements as a function of prior expectations, observed evidence and individual processing strategies*. Prepublication offprint, 1979.

Mason, J. W. A review of psychoendocrine research on the pituitary-adrenal cortical system. *Psychosomatic Medicine*, 1968, *30*, 576–607.

Mason, J. W., Brady, J. V., & Tolliver, G. A. Plasma and urinary 17-hydrocorticosteroid responses to 72 Hr. avoidance sessions in the monkey. *Psychosomatic Medicine*, 1968, *30*, 608–630.

Mason, J. W., Mangan, G. F., Brady, J. W., Conrad, D., & Rioch, D. McK. Concurrent plasma epinephrine and 17-hydroxycorticosteroid levels during conditioned emotional disturbance. *Psychosomatic Medicine*, 1961, *23*, 344–353.

Mason, J. W., Tolson, W. W., Brady, J., Tolliver, G., & Gilmore, L. Urinary epinephrine and norepinephrine responses to 72 Hr. avoidance sessions in the monkey. *Psychosomatic Medicine*, 1968, *30*, 640–665.

Masserman, J. H. *Behavior and neurosis*. Chicago, Illinois: University of Chicago Press, 1943.

Masuda, M., & Holmes, T. H. The social readjustment scale: A cross-cultural study of Japanese and Americans. *Journal of Psychosomatic Research*, 1967, *11*, 227–237.

Matarazzo, J. D., Ulett, G. A., & Saslow, G. Human maze performance as a function of increasing levels of anxiety. *Journal of General Psychology*, 1955, *53*, 79–95.

Matarazzo, R., & Matarazzo, J. D. Anxiety learning and pursuitmeter performance. *Journal of Consulting Psychology*, 1956, *20*(1), 70.

Mayer-Gross, W., Slater, E., & Roth, M. *Clinical psychiatry*. London: Cassell and Company, 1960.

Medalie, J. H., & Kahn, H. A. Myocardial infarction over a five-year period. I. Prevalence, incidence and mortality experience. *Journal of Chronic Diseases*, 1973, *26*, 63–84.

Meichenbaum, D. *Cognitive behaviour modification*. New York: Plenum, 1979.

Mellstrom, M., Cicala, G. A., & Zuckerman, M. General versus specific trait anxiety measures in the prediction of fear of snakes, heights and darkness. *Journal of Consulting and Clinical Psychology*, 1976, *44*, 83–91.

Melzak, R., & Casey, K. L. Sensory motivational and central control determinants of pain: A new conceptual model. In D. Kenshalo (Ed.), *The skin senses*. Springfield, Illinois: C. C. Thomas, 1968.

Melzak, R., & Wall, P. D. Pain mechanisms: A new theory. *Science*, 1965, *150*, 971–979.

Mendelson, J., Kurbzansky, P., Leiderman, P. H., Wexler, D., DuToit, C., & Solomon, P. Catechol Amine excretion and behaviour during sensory deprivation. *Archives of General Psychiatry*, 1960, *2*, 147–155.

Millar, K. Word recognition in loud noise. *Acta Psychologica*, 1979, *43*, 225–237.

Millar, K. Noise and the rehearsal masking hypothesis. *British Journal of Psychology*. 1979, *70*, 565–577.

Millar, K. *Loud noise and the retrieval of information*. Dissertation for the degree of Doctor of Philosophy, University of Dundee, 1980.

Miller, J. G. Adusting to overloads of information. In D. Rioch and E. Weinstein (Eds.), Disorders of communication, *Proceedings of the Association*, Chapter 7. New York: Hafner Publishing Company, 1962.

Miller, N. E. Experimental studies in conflict. In J. McV. Hunt (Ed.), *Personality and behaviour disorders*, New York: Ronald Press, 1944.

Miller, G., Galanter, E., & Pribram, K. *Plans and the structure of behavior*. New York: Holt, Rhinehart and Winston Inc., 1960.

Miller, S. M. Controllability and human stress: Method evidence and theory. *Behaviour Research and Therapy*, 1979, *17*, 287–304.

Mills, I. H. Biological factors in international relations. *The year book of world affairs, Volume 27*. The London Institute of World Affairs: Stevens and Sons Ltd. 1973.

Morris, R., & Morris, D. *Men and snakes*. London: Hutchison, 1965.

Morton, J. A preliminary functional model for language behaviour. *International Audiology*, 1964, *3*, 216–225.

Morton, J. Interaction of information in word recognition. *Psychological Review*, 1969, *76* (2), 165–178.

Morton, J. Structuring experience- Some discussion points. In R. A. Kennedy & A. Wilkes, (Eds.), *Studies in long term memory*. London: John Wiley, 1974.

Mouton, R. Effects of success and failure on level of aspiration as related to achievement motives. *Journal of Personality and Social Psychology*, 1965, *1*, 399–406.

Mowrer, O. H. Preparatory set (expectancy): Some methods of measurement. *Psychological Monographs*, 1940, *52* (2), whole no. 233.

Mowrer, O. H., & Viek, P. An experimental analogue of fear from a sense of helplessness. *Journal of Abnormal and Social Psychology*, 1948, *43*, 193–200.

Murphy, C. W., Kurlents, E., Cleghorn, R. A., & Hebb, D. O. Absence of increased corticoid excretion with the stress of perceptual deprivation. *Canadian Journal of Biochemical Physiology*, 1955, *33*, 1062–63.

Murray, D. J. The effect of white noise upon the recall of vocalised lists. *Canadian Journal of Psychology*, 1965, *19*, 333–345.

Murray, E. J., Schein, E. H., Erikson, K. T., Hill, W. F., & Cohen, M. The effects of sleep deprivation on social behaviour. *Journal of Social Psychology*, 1959, *49*, 229–236.

McClelland, D. C. *The achieving society*. New York: Van Nostrand, 1961.

McClelland, D. C., Atkinson, J. W., Clark, R. W., & Lowell, E. L. *The achievement motive*. New York: Appleton-Century-Crofts, 1953.

McGill, W. J. Stochastic latency mechanisms. In R. D. Luce, R. R. Bush, & E. Galanter, (Eds.), *Handbook of mathematical psychology*. Vol. 1. New York: John Wiley, 1963.

McGrath, J. J. Irrelevant stimulation and vigilance performance. In D. Buckner & J. McGrath, (Eds.), *Vigilance: A symposium*. New York: McGraw-Hill, 1963.

McGrath, J. E. *Social and psychological factors in stress*. New York: Holt, Rinehart & Winston, 1970.

Näätänen, R. The inverted-U relationship between activation and performance: a critical review. In S. Kornblum, (Ed.), *Attention and performance, IV*. New York: Academic Press, 1973.

Nathanson, A. Sex, illness and medical care: A review of data, theory and method. *Social Science and Medicine*, 1977, *11*, 13–25.

Navon, D., & Gopher, D. On the economy of the human information processing system. *Psychological Review*, 1979, *86*, 214–225.

Navran, L. A rationally derived MMPI scale to measure dependence. *Journal of Consulting Psychology*, 1954, *18*, 192–194.

Nickerson, R. S. Psychological refractory phase, and the functional significance of signals. *Journal of Experimental Psychology*, 1965, *73*, 303–312.

Nisbett, R. E., & Schacter, S. Cognitive manipulation of pain. *Journal of Experimental and Social Psychology*, 1966, *2*, 227–236.

Nokwicki, S., & Strickland, B. R. A locus of control scale for children. *Journal of Consulting and Clinical Psychology*, 1973, *40*, 148–154.

Norman, D. A., & Wickelgren, W. A. Strength theory of decision rules, and latency on the retrieval from short term memory. *Journal of Mathematical Psychology*, 1969, *6*, 192–208.

Ohman, A. Fear relevance. Autonomic conditioning and phobias. In P. O. Sjoden & S. Bets, (Eds.), *Trends in behavior therapy*. New York: Academic Press, 1979.

Olds, J., & Olds, M. Drives, rewards and the brain. In *New directions in psychology II*. New York: Holt, Rhinehart and Winston, 1965.

Pachella, R. The interpretation of reaction time in information processing research. In B. Kantowitz (Ed.), *Human information processing: Tutorials in performance and cognition*. Hillsdale, New Jersey: Lawrence Erlbaum Associates, 1974.

Pachella, R. G. *Memory scanning under speed stress*. Paper presented at Meeting of Midwestern Psychological Association, Cleveland, Ohio. May, 1972.

Pachella, R., Smith, J., & Stanovich, K. Qualitative error analysis and speeded classification. In N. J. Castellan and F. Restle (Eds.), *Cognitive theory. Volume 3*. Hillsdale, New Jersey: Lawrence Erlbaum Associates, 1978.

Parducci, A. Range-frequency compromise in judgement. *Psychological Monographs*, 1963, *77*, 2.

Parducci, A. Category judgement: A range frequency model. *Psychological Review*, 1965, *72*, 407–418.

Parducci, A. The relativism of absolute judgements. *Scientific American*, 1968, *219*, 84–90.

Parker, S., & Kleiner, R. J. *Mental illness in the urban negro community*, New York: Free Press, 1966.

Parkes, C. M. Bereavement and mental illness. *British Journal of Medical Psychology*, 1965, *38*, 1–26.

Parkes, C. M. *Bereavement*. New York: International Universities Press, 1978.

Parkes, K. R. Occupational stress among student nurses: 1. A comparison of medical and surgical wards. *Nursing Times*, 1980(a), *76*, 25, 113–116.

Parkes, K. R. Occupational stress among student nurses: 2. A comparison of male and female wards. *Nursing Times*, 1980(b), *6*, 117–120.

Pascal, G. R. The effect of relaxation upon recall. *American Journal of Psychology*, 1949, *62*, 33–47.

Pavlov, I. P. *Lectures on conditioned reflexes*. New York: International Publishers, 1928.

Paykal, E. S., Myers, J. K., Dienalt, M. N., Klerman, G. L., Lindenthal, J. J., & Pepper, M. P. Life events and depression. *Archives of General Psychiatry*, 1969, *21*, 753–760.

Pearlin, L. J. Sex roles and depression. In N. Datan and L. H. Ginsberg (Eds.), *Life-span developmental psychology: Normative life crises*. New York: Academic Press, 1975.

Pepler, R. D. Warmth and performance: An investigation in the tropics. *Ergonomics*, 1958, *2*, 63–88.

Pepler, R. D. Warmth and lack of sleep: Accuracy or activity reduced. *Journal of Comparative Physiological Psychology*, 1957, *52*, 446–450.

Pervin, L. A. The need to predict and control under conditions of threat. *Journal of Personality*, 1963, *31*, 570–587.

Peterson, C., Schwartz, S. M., & Seligman, M. E. P. Self-blame and depressive symptoms. *Journal of Personality and Social Psychology*, 1981, *41* (2), 253–259.

Phares, E. J. Differential utilisation of information as a function of internal-external control. *Journal of Personality*, 1968, *36*, 649–662.

Posner, M. I. Information reduction in the analysis of sequential tasks. *Psychological Review*, 1964, *71* (6), 491–504.

Posner, M. M., & Boies, S. J. Components of attention. *Psychological Review*, 1971, *78*, 391–408.

Posner, M. I., Klein, R., Summers, J., & Buggie, S. On the selection of signals. *Memory and cognition*, 1973, *1*, 2–12.

Posner, M. I., & Rossman, E. Effect of size and location of information transforms upon short-term retention. *Journal of Experimental Psychology*, 1965, *70*, 496–505.

Poulton, E. C. Measuring the order of difficulty of visual motor tasks. *Ergonomics*, 1958, *1*, 234–239.

Poulton, E. C. *Environment and human efficiency*. Springfield, Illinois: Charles C Thomas, 1970.

Poulton, E. C. Arousing environmental stresses can improve performance whatever people say. *Aviation Space and Environmental Medicine*, 1976(a), *47*, 1193–1204.

Poulton, E. C. Continuous noise interferes with work by masking auditory feedback and inner speech. *Applied Ergonomics*, 1976(b), *7*, 79–84.

Poulton, E. C. Continuous intense noise masks auditory feedback and inner speech. *Psychological Bulletin*, 1977(a), *84*, 977–1001.

Poulton, E. C. Arousing stresses increase vigilance. In R. R. Mackie (Ed.), *Vigilance: Theory, operational performance and physiological correlates*. New York: Plenum Press, 1977(b).

Poulton, E.C. A note on the masking of acoustic clicks. *Applied Ergonomics*, 1978(a), *9*, 103.

Poulton, E. C. A new look at the effects of noise: A rejoinder. *Psychological Bulletin*, 1978(b), *85*, 1068–1079.

Poulton, E. C. Composite model for human performance in continuous noise. *Psychological Review*, 1979, *86* (4), 361–375.

Poulton, E. C. Not so! Rejoinder to Hartley on masking by continuous noise. *Psychological Review*, 1981(a), *88* (1), 90–92.

Poulton, E. C. Masking beneficial arousal and adaptation level: A reply to Hartley. *British Journal of Psychology*, 1981(b), *72*, 109–116.

Poulton, E. C., & Edwards, R. S. Asymmetric transfer in within subject experiments on stress interactions. *Ergonomics*, 1979, *22* (8), 945–961.

Powers, W. T. *Behavior: The control of perception*. Chicago: Aldine Publishing Company, 1973.

Price, J. The dominance hierarchy and the evolution of mental illness. *Lancet*, 1967, *2*, 243–246.

Rabbitt, P. M. A. Errors and error correction in choice response tasks. *Journal of Experimental Psychology*, 1966(a), *71* (2), 264–272.

Rabbitt, P. M. A. Error correction time without external error signals. *Nature, London*, 1966(b), *212*, 438.

Rabbitt, P. M. A. Three kinds of error-signalling responses in a serial choice task. *The Quarterly Journal of Experimental Psychology*, Part 2, 1968, *20*, 179–188.

Rabbitt, P. M., & Vyas, S. M. An elementary preliminary taxonomy for some errors in laboratory choice RT tasks. In A. F. Sanders (Ed.), *Attention and performance III*. Amsterdam: North Holland Publishing Company, 1970.

Rabbitt, P., & Vyas, S. Processing a display even after you make a response to it. How perceptual errors can be corrected. *Quarterly Journal of Experimental Psychology*, 1981, *33A*, 223–239.

Rahe, R. H. Life change as a predictor of illness. *Proceedings of the Royal Society of Medicine*, 1968, *61*, 44–46.

Rapaport, D. Emotions and memory. *The Menninger Clinic monograph series, No 2*, New York: Science Editions, Inc, 1961.

Rasmussen, A. F. Emotions and immunity. *Annals of the New York Academy of Science*, 1957, *254*, 458–461.

Read, P. P. *Alive*. Philadelphia: Lippincott, 1974.

Reason, J. Absent minds. *New Society*, 1976, *4*, 244–245.

Reason, J. Skill and error in everyday life. In M. Howe (Ed.), *Adult learning*. London: John Wiley, 1977.

Reason, J. Absent-mindedness and cognitive control. In J. Harris & J. P. Morris (Eds.), *Everyday memory, actions and absent-mindedness*. Copy to author in advance of publication, 1982.

Reid, D., & Ware, E. F. Multidimensionality of internal versus external control. Addition of a third dimension and non-distruction of self versus others. *Canadian Journal of Behavioural Science*, 1974, *6*, 131–142.

Reynolds, D. Effects of double stimulation: Tempory inhibition of response. *Psychological Bulletin*, 1964, *62*, 338–347.

Reynolds, D. Time and event uncertainty in unisensory reaction time. *Journal of Experimental Psychology*, 1966, *71*, 286–293.

Reynolds, V., Jenner, D. A., Palmer, C. D., & Harrison, G. A. Catecholamine excretion rates in relation to life styles in the male population of Otmoor, Oxfordshire. *Annals of Human Biology*, 1981, *8*, 197–209.

Rioch, D. McK. Problems of preventative psychiatry at war. In P. H. Hock & J. Zubin (Eds.), *Psychopathology of childhood*. New York: Grune and Stratton, 1955.

Roth, S., & Kubal, L. Effects of non-contingent reinforcement on tasks of differing importance: Facilitation of learned helplessness. *Journal of Personality and Social Psychology*, 1975, *32*, 680–691.

Rotter, J. B. *Social learning and clinical psychology*. Englewood Cliffs, New Jersey: Prentice-Hall, 1954.

Rotter, J. B. Generalised expectancies for internal versus external control of reinforcement. *Psychological Monographs*, 1966, *80*, 609.

Rotter, J. B., & Mubry, R. C. Internal versus external control of reinforcements and decision time. *Journal of Personality & Social Psychology*, 1965, 598–604.

Rotter, J. B., Seeman, M., & Liverant, S. Internal versus external control of reinforcement: A major variable in behaviour therapy. In N. F. Washburne (Ed.), *Decision, values and groups, Vol 2*. Oxford: Pergamon Press, 1962.

Ruff, G. E., Levy, E. Z., & Thaler, V. H. Factors influencing the reaction to reduced sensory input. In P. Solomon (Ed.), *Sensory deprivation*. Symposium held at Harvard Medical School, 1958. Cambridge: Harvard University Press, 1961.

Russell, P. A. Fear-evoking stimuli. In W. Sluckin (Ed.), *Fear in animals and man*, Chapter 4. New York: Van Nostrand and Reinhold Company, 1979.

Rutenfranz, J., Aschoff, J., & Mann, H. The effects of cumulative sleep deficit, duration of preceding sleep period and body temperature on multiple choice reaction time. In W. P. Colquhoun (Ed.), *Aspects of human efficiency: Diurnal rhythm and loss of sleep*. London: English Universities Press, 1972.

Salame, P., & Wittersheim, G. Selective noise disturbance of the information input in short term memory. *Quarterly Journal of Experimental Psychology*, 1978, *30*, 693–704.

Sarason, I. G. Experimental approaches to test anxiety: Attention and the uses of information. In C. D. Spielberger (Ed.), *Anxiety: Current trends in theory and research, Volume 2*. New York: Appleton-Century-Crofts, 1972.

Sarason, I. G. Test anxiety and cognitive modelling. *Journal of Personality and Social Psychology*, 1973, *28*, 58–61.

Sarason, I. G. Anxiety and self-preoccupation. In I. G. Sarason & C. D. Spielberger (Eds.), *Stress and anxiety, Volume 2*. Washington: Hemisphere Publishing Company, 1975.

Schacter, S., & Singer, J. Cognitive, social and physiological determinants of an emotional state. *Psychological Review*, 1962, *69*, 378–399.

Schless, A. P., Schwartz, L., Goetz, C., & Mendels, J. How depressives view the significance of life events. *British Journal of Psychiatry*, 1974, *125*, 406–410.

Schouten, J. F., & Beckker, J. A. Reaction time and accuracy. *Acta Psychologica*, 1967, *27*, 143–153.

Schulberg, H., & Sheldon, A. The probability of crisis and strategies to preventative intervention. *Archives of General Psychiatry*, 1968, *18*, 553–558.

Schwartz, B. Does helplessness cause depression, or do only depressed people become helpless? Comment on Alloy and Abramson. *Journal of Experimental Psychology*, 1981, *110*, 429–435.

Schwartz, S. Arousal and recall: Effects of noise on two retrieval strategies. *Journal of Experimental Psychology*, 1974, *102* (5), 896–898.

Seeman, M., & Evans, J. W. Alienation and learning in a hospital setting. *American Sociological Review*, 1962, *27*, 772–783.

Seligman, M. E. P. Phobias and preparedness. *Behaviour Therapy*, 1971, *2*, 307–321.

Seligman, M. E. P. *Helplessness: On depression development and death*. San Francisco: Freeman, 1975.

Selye, H. *The stress of life*. London, New York: Longmans Green and Co., 1956.

Selye, H. *Stress without distress*. Philadelphia and New York: Lippincott, 1974.

Shannon, C. E., & Weaver, W. *The mathematical theory of communication*. Urbana: University of Illinois Press, 1948.

Shannon, I. L., & Isbell, G. M. Stress in dental patients: Effect of local anesthetic procedures. *Technical Report No. SAM-IDR-63-29*, 1963, USAF School of Aerospace Medicine, Brooks Airforce Base, Texas, U.S.

Sheatsley, P. B., & Feldman, J. The assassination of President Kennedy: Public reaction. *Public Opinion Quarterly*, 1964, *28*, 189–215.

Sher, M. A. Pupillary dilation before and after interruption of unfamiliar sequences. *Journal of Personality and Social Psychology*, 1971, *20*, 281–286.

Siegman, A. W. The effect of manifest anxiety on a concept formation task, a non-directed learning task and on timed and untimed intelligence tests. *Journal of Consulting Psychology*, 1956, *20*, 176–178.

de Silva, P., Rachman, S., & Seligman, M. E. P. Prepared phobias and obsessions: Therapeutic outcome. *Behaviour Research and Therapy*, 1977, *15*, 65–77.

Silverman, R. E. Anxiety and the mode of response. *Journal of Abnormal and Social Psychology*, 1954, *49*, 538–542.

Singleton, W. J. T. Deterioration of performance on a short term perceptual motor task. In W. F. Floyd, & A. T. Welford (Eds.), *Symposium on fatigue*. London: H. K. Lewis, 1953, 163–172.

Sklar, L. S., & Anisman, H. Stress and cancer. *Psychological Bulletin*, 1981, *89* (3), 369–406.

Sloboda, W., & Smith, E. E. Distruption effects in human short-term memory: Some negative findings. *Perceptual Motor Skills*, 1968, *27*, 575–582.

Smelser, N. J. *Theory of collective behaviour*. New York: The Free Press of Glencoe, 1963.

Sokolov, E. N. Neural models and the orienting reflex. In M. A. Brazier (Ed.), *The central nervous system and behaviour*. New York: Josiah Macy Jr. Foundation, 1960.

Sokolov, E. N. *Perception and the conditioned reflex*, (Tr: S. W. Waydenfeld). Oxford: Pergamon, 1963.

Solomon, R. L., & Corbit, J. D. Motivation: Temporal dynamics of affect. *Psychological Review*, 1974, *81*, 119–145.

Solomon, R. L., & Wynne, L. C. Traumatic avoidance learning. *Psychological Monographs*, 1953, *67* (4), (No. 354).

Speisman, J. C., Lazarus, R. S., Mordkoff, A. M., & Davison, L. A. The experimental reduction of stress based on ego defense theory. *Journal of Abnormal and Social Psychology*, 1964, *68*, 367–380.

Spence, K. W. *Behaviour theory and condition.* London: Oxford University Press, 1956.

Stagner, R. The redintegration of pleasant and unpleasant experiences. *American Journal of Psychology*, 1931, *43*, 463–468.

Staub, E., & Kellett, D. S. Increasing pain tolerance by information about aversive stimuli. *Journal of Personality and Social Psychology*, 1972, *1*, 198–203.

Steinberg, H. Effects of drugs on performance and incentives. In B. R. Lawrence (Ed.), *Quantitative methods in human pharmacology and therapeutics.* London: Pergamon Press, 1959.

Stern, R. M., Botto, R. W., & Herrick, C. D. Behavioural and physiological effects of false heart rate feedback: A replication and extension. *Psychophysiology*, 1972, *9*, 21–29.

Sternbach, R. A. *Pain: A psychophysiological analysis.* New York: Academic Press, 1968.

Sternberg, S. Memory scanning: Mental processes revealed by reaction time experiments. *American Scientist*, 1969, *57*, 421–457.

Sternberg, S. Memory scanning: New findings and current controversies. *Quarterly Journal of Experimental Psychology*, 1975, *27*, 1–32.

Stevens, S. S. Stability of human performance under intense noise. *Journal of Sound and Vibration*, 1972, *21*, 35–56.

Stewart, A., & Salt, P. Life stress, life styles, depression and illness in adult women. *Journal of Personality and Social Psychology*, 1981, *40* (6), 1063–1069.

Stroop, J. R. Studies of interference in serial verbal reaction. *Journal of Experimental Psychology*, 1935, *18*, 643–662.

Swensson, R. G. The elusive trade-off: Speed versus accuracy in visual discrimination tasks. *Perception and Psychophysics*, 1972, *12*, 16–32.

Symington, T., Currie, A. R., Curran, R. C., & Davidson, J. N. The reaction of the adrenal cortex in conditions of stress. *Ciba Foundation colloquia on endocrinology, Vol. VIII.* Boston: Brown and Co, 1955.

Szpiler, F. A., & Epstein, S. Availability of an avoidance response as related to autonomic arousal. *Journal of Abnormal Psychology*, 1976, *85*, 73–82.

Tanner, W. P., & Swets, J. A. A decision making theory of visual detection. *Psychological Review*, 1954, *61*, 401–409.

Teichner, W. The attentional bandwidth hypothesis: Interaction of behavioural and physiological stress reactions. *Psychological Review*, 1968, 75 (4), 271.

Thayer, R. E. Measurement of activation through self-report. *Psychological Reports*, 1967, *20*, 663–678.

Thayer, R. E. Activation states as assessed by verbal report and four psychophysiological variables. *Psychophysiology*, 1970, *7*, 86–94.

Theios, J. Reaction time measurements in the study of memory processes: Theory, and data. In G. Bower (Ed.), *The psychology of learning and motivation: Advances in research and theory, Vol. 7.* New York: Academic Press, 1973.

Theorell, T., & Rahe, R. H. Life changes in relation to the onset of myocardial infarction. In T. Theorell, *Psychosocial factors in relation to the onset of myocardial infarction: A pilot study.* Stockholm: Seraphimar Hospital, 1970.

Thompson, S. C. Will it hurt less if I can control it? A complex answer to a simple question. *Psychological Bulletin*, 1981, *90* (1), 89–101.

Tinbergen, N. *The study of instinct.* London: Oxford University Press, 1951.

Tompkins, S. Affect as the primary motivational system. In M. B. Arnold (Ed.), *Feelings and emotions.* New York: Academic Press, 1970.

Townsend, J. T. Theoretical analysis of an alphabet matrix. *Perception and Psychophysics,* 1971, *9,* 40–50.

Trumbo, M., & Milone, F. Primary task performance as a function of encoding retention and recall in a secondary task. *Journal of Experimental Psychology,* 1971, *91,* 272–279.

Tung, C. L. Relative hypertension of foreigners in China. *Archives of International Medicine,* 1927, *40,* 153–158.

Tversky, A., & Kahneman, D. Judgment under uncertainty: Heuristics and biases. *Science,* 1974, *185,* 1124–1131.

Uehling, B., & Sprinkle, R. Recall of a serial list as a function of arousal and retention interval. *Journal of Experimental Psychology,* 1968, *78,* 103–106.

Usdansky, G., & Chapman, J. Schizophrenic-like responses in normal subjects under time pressure. *Journal of Abnormal and Social Psychology,* 1960, *1,* 143–146.

Valins, S. Cognitive effects of false heart rate feedback. *Journal of Personality and Social Psychology,* 1966, *4,* 400–408.

Valins, S., & Ray, A. Effects of cognitive desensitisation on avoidance behaviour. *Journal of Personality and Social Psychology,* 1967, *7,* 345–350.

Van Bergen, A. *Task interruption.* Amsterdam: North Holland Publishing Company, 1968.

Velton, E. C. A laboratory task for the induction of mood states. *Behaviour Research and Therapy,* 1968, *6,* 473–482.

Venables, P. H. Input dysfunction in schizophrenia. In B. A. Maher (Ed.), *Progress in experimental personality research Vol. 1.* New York: Academic Press, 1964.

Van Holst, E. Relations between the central nervous system and the peripheral organs. *British Journal of Animal Behaviour,* 1954, *2,* 89–94.

Wachtel, P. L. Conceptions of broad and narrow attention. *Psychological Bulletin,* 1967, *6,* 417–429.

Wade, J. E. Psychomotor performance under conditions of weightlessness. *Report No. MRL IDR 62–73.* Dayton, Ohio: Wright Patterson Air Force Base Aerospace Medicine Research Laboratories, 1962.

Wald, A. *Sequential analysis.* New York: John Wiley, 1947.

Walker, E. L. Action decrement and its relation to learning. *Psychological Review,* 1958, *65,* 129–142.

Walley, R. E., & Weiden, T. D. Lateral inhibition and cognitive masking. A neuropsychological theory of attention. *Psychological Review,* 1973, *80,* 284–302.

Walsh, J.T., & Cordeau, J. P. Responsiveness in the visual system during various phases of sleep and waking. *Experimental Neurology,* 1965, *11,* 80–107.

Walster, E. Assignment of responsibility for an accident. *Journal of Personality and Social Psychology,* 1966, *3,* 73–79.

Wang, T., Sheppard, J. R., & Foker, J. E. Rise and fall of cyclic AMP required for onset of lymphocyte DNA synthesis. *Science,* 1978, *201,* 155–157.

Ward, W. C., & Jenkins, H. M. The display of information and the judgements of contingency. *Canadian Journal of Psychology,* 1965, *19,* 231–241.

Warren, L. R., & Harris, L. J. Arousal and memory phasic measures of arousal in a free recall task. *Acta Psychologica,* 1975, *39,* 303–310.

Warren, N., & Clarke, B. Blocking in mental and motor tasks during a 65-hour vigil. *Journal of Experimental Psychology,* 1937, *21,* 97–105.

Wartman, C. B. Some determinants of perceived control. *Journal of Personality and Social Psychology,* 1975, *31,* 282–294.

Waters, R. H. The principle of least effort in learning. *Journal of General Psychology,* 1937, *16,* 3–20.

Weiner, B., Heckhausen, H., Meyer, W. V., & Cook, R. E. Causal ascriptions and achievement motivation. *Journal of Personality and Social Psychology*, 1972, *21*, 239–248.

Weiner, B., Frieze, I., Kukla, A., Reed, L., Rest, S., & Rosenbaum, R. M. Perceiving the causes of success and failure. In E. E. Jones, D. E. Kanouse, H. H. Kelley, R. E. Nisbett, S. Vallins, & B. Weiner, *Attribution: Perceiving the causes of behavior*. New York: General Learning Press, 1971.

Weinstein, N. Effect of noise on intellectual performance. *Journal of Applied Psychology*, 1974, *59* (5), 548–554.

Weiss, J. M. Effects of coping responses on stress. *Journal of Comparative and Physiological Psychology*, 1968, *65*, 251–260.

Weiss, J. M. Somatic effects of predictable and unpredictable shock. *Psychosomatic Medicine*, 1970, *32*, 397–408.

Weiss, J. M. Effects of coping behaviour in different warning signal conditions on stress pathology in rats. *Journal of Comparative and Physiological Psychology*, 1971(a), *17*, 1–13.

Weiss, J. M. Effects of coping behaviour with and without a feedback signal on stress pathology in rats. *Journal of Comparative and Physiological Psychology*, 1971(b), *77*, 22–30.

Weiss, J. M. Effects of punishing the coping response (conflict), on stress pathology in rats. *Journal of Comparative and Physiological Psychology*, 1971, *77*, 14–21.

Weissman, M. M., & Klerman, G. L. Sex differences and the epidemiology of depression. *Archives of General Psychiatry*, 1977, *34*, 98–111.

Welford, A. T. The psychological refractory period and the timing of high speed performance. *British Journal of Psychology*, 1952, *43*, 2–9.

Welford, A. T. Stress and achievement. *Australian Journal of Psychology*, 1965, *17*, 1–11.

Welford, A. T. Stress and performance. *Ergonomics*, 1973, *16* (5), 567–580.

Welford, A. T., Norris, A. H., & Shock, N. W. Movement time and age: A preliminary report. *Ergonomics*, 1963, *6*, 310.

Wherry, R. J., & Curran, P. M. A study of some determinants of psychological stress. *US Naval School of Aviation Medicine Report*, July, 1965.

White, R. W. Motivation reconsidered: The concept of competence. *Psychological Review*, 1959, *66*, 297–333.

Wilding, J. M., & Mohindra, N. Effects of subvocal suppression, articulating aloud and noise on sequence recall. *British Journal of Psychology*, 1980, *71*, 247–261.

Wilkinson, R. T. Interaction of sleep with knowledge of results, repeated testing and individual differences. *Journal of Experimental Psychology*, 1961, *62*, 263–271.

Wilkinson, R. T. Interaction of noise with knowledge of results and sleep deprivation. *Journal of Experimental Psychology*, 1963, *66*, 332–337.

Wilkinson, R. T. Effects of up to 60 hours sleep deprivation on different types of work. *Ergonomics*, 1964, *7*, 175–186.

Wilkinson, R. T. Sleep deprivation. In O. G. Edholm & A. L. Bacharach (Eds.), *The physiology of survival*. London and New York: Academic Press, 1965.

Wilkinson, R. T. Some factors influencing the effects of environmental stressors on performance. *Psychological Bulletin*, 1969, *72*, 260–272.

Wilkinson, R. T. *Noise, incentive and prolonged work: Effects on short term memory*. Paper presented to the Annual Meeting of the American Psychological Association. Chicago. 1975.

Wine, J. Test anxiety and the direction of attention. *Psychological Bulletin*, 1971, *76*, 92–104.

Wolff, J. G. Language acquisitions, data compression and generalisation. *Language and Communication*, 1982, *2* (1), 57–89.

Wolpe, S., & Lang, P. J. *Fear survey schedule*. San Diego: Educational and Industrial Testing Service, 1969.

Wood, C. G., & Hokanson, J. E. Effects of induced muscular tension on performance and the inverted "U" function. *Journal of Personality and Social Psychology*, 1965, *1*, 506–510.

Woodhead, M. Effect of a brief loud noise on decision making. *Journal of the Acoustical Society of America*, 1959, *31* (10), 1329–1331.

Woodrow, H. Time perception. In S. S. Stevens (Ed.), *Handbook of experimental psychology*. New York: John Wiley, 1951.

Wortman, C. B. Some determinants of perceived control. *Journal of Personality and Social Psychology*, 1975, *31*, 282–294.

Yellott, J. I. Correction for fast guessing and the speed accuracy trade-off in choice reaction time. *Journal of Mathematical Psychology*, 1971, *8*, 159–199.

Yerkes, R. M., & Dodson, J. D. The relation of strength of stimulus to rapidity of habit formation. *Journal of Comparative Neurological Psychology*, 1908, *18*, 459–482.

Zeigarnik, B. Das Behalten erledigter und unerledigter Handlungen. *Psychologische Forschung*, 1927, *9*, 1–85.

Zipf, G. K. *Human behavior and the principle of least effort. An introduction to human ecology*. New York: Hafner Publishing Company, 1949 (revised 1965).

Author Index

A

Abramson, L. Y., 26, 27, 187, 188, 190, 191, 223, 228, 229, 233, 238
Adams, R. G., 162
Allens, M. B., 102
Alloy, L. B., 26, 27, 51, 187, 188, 190, 191, 223, 228, 238
Allport, A., 4, 76
Alluisi, E. A., 108
Amkraut, A., 105, 240
Amsel, A., 45
Anisman, H., 243
Appley, M. H., 3
Aschoff, J., 108
Atkinson, J. W., 35
Averill, J., 21, 22, 96
Ax, A. F., 70, 96

B

Bacon, S. J., 162
Baddeley, A. D., 169
Bahrick, H. P., 76, 156
Baker, C. H., 87
Balke, B., 116
Ball, T. S., 22
Bankart, C. P., 43
Barchha, R. G., 207, 208

Bartlett, F. C., 109, 110
Battig, W. R., 16
Battle, E., 218
Beck, A. T., 9, 27, 151, 181, 182, 191, 195, 204, 206, 211, 229
Beck, J. C., 207, 208, 209
Becker, J., 204
Beebe-Center, J. G., 206
Bekerian, D. A., 222
Bekker, J. A., 122
Berkowitz, L., 45
Berlyne, D., 38, 39, 106, 168
Bettelheim, B., 13
Bexton, W. H., 85
Bhrolchain, M., 212, 213, 214
Bills, A., 130
Birley, J. L. T., 207, 208
Birnbaum, R., 11
Birtchnell, J., 211
Blake, M., 107, 108
Blankstein, K. R., 168
Boggs, D. H., 78, 79, 80
Boies, S. J., 4, 78
Bonvallet, M., 108
Botto, R. W., 197
Bower, G. H., 110
Bowers, K., 27

273

Subject Index